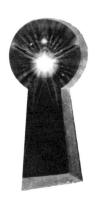

ANSWER TO CANCER

A guide to living cancer-free

ANSWER TO CANCER

A guide to living cancer-free

Dr. Douglas R. Levine

Printed by Worzalla Publishing, U.S.A.
Book orders: Please go to *www.drdouglevine.com*

Unless otherwise specified, the images contained in this book have been created and provided by *www.chillibreeze.com*

Book cover design, interior book design, and editing provided by Harvard Girl Word Services at *www.harvardgirledits.com*

Dedication

I dedicate this book to all those who have allowed the pain of cancer to thrust them to live above the hand that life has dealt them and to all those who find the courage to transform yesterday's struggles into today's devotion.

Acknowledgments

Thank you to the medical community that saved my life and the complementary community that has kept me alive and well. Special thanks to my mother, who said to me, "This is a temporary setback in your life," as I lay in my hospital bed, sick and lifeless. I never forgot it, Mom...thank you.

Answer to Cancer: A guide to living cancer-free

TABLE OF CONTENTS

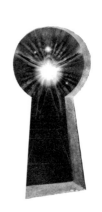

1. Answer to Cancer...
The Story Behind the Story

Answer to cancer

As I sat down to write the introduction for this book, I drew a blank. Sitting with laptop in front of me, I asked myself what I could possibly have to say to all those who have been touched by cancer. I thought long and hard, until suddenly it came to me. I would simply speak from my heart and, in doing so, dedicate my book to each and every one of the people I care about so much, respect, and want to reach with every fiber of my being—in other words, every individual whose life has been directly or indirectly affected by cancer. Because this book is for all of you—for all of us: for the fighters, the survivors, and the families…every single one. I know if you are reading this, you are likely included on this list, as I am, and are someone who has personally or peripherally been forever changed by this disease.

I have to say right up front that I'd like to think I didn't need an experience like cancer to change me, and quite possibly you'd like to think you didn't either. But it happened and change I did. And although I can't pinpoint exactly where, when, or how this change occurred, looking back I can admit that the shift has been for the better. For cancer teaches what can't be taught: to appreciate and to understand, to empathize and to prioritize, to learn and to be humble. It brings with its suffering a humility and dignity that cannot be denied.

It makes us human—and more.

It is my belief that we each have within us an innate determination to live, that unwavering tenacity to keep going, to get through it—whatever *it* is. This determination underscores a powerful will to live that can go unrecognized for years, as it is only when threatened with the possibility of death that out of necessity we instinctively rise to the occasion. In this case, in this book, the threat we're discussing is the one brought about by cancer, a disease of unparalleled proportions, one that often shrouds us in unparalleled fear. For some reason, however, even when we are in the very midst of our deepest fear, we find a way to move past it in order to defeat the disease. How? By resolutely setting about the task and expecting—yes, expecting—to emerge victorious, and by seeking help from those who have the tools to help us, while we work on finding that inner strength to go on. Somehow, we just seem to do what we have to do.

Instinctively we know that conquering cancer will only be possible by combining our own efforts with the efforts of the people who are willing to help us on our journey. These guides are the doctors "outside," the ones with the diplomas on the wall. The "doctor outside" is my way of describing the physician who is not only courageous in his or her work to cure all kinds of diseases throughout the world, including cancer, but who treats those of us in need. The other equally important guide in our life, however, is someone I call the "doctor inside." This guide has been with us since birth and is like our own personal physician, available to guide us and support us along the way to ensure our battle with cancer will be over for good. This "physician" is an individualized, intrinsic system that functions to keep us well, even as we know with the certainty born of experience, that we will never be quite the same again and that we must continue to strive to rekindle our hope and rebuild the people we once were.

When you are a patient receiving treatment for cancer, you find yourself in the midst of a dilemma that you have never encountered before. While you may be a thriving, strong, or opinionated person in the other parts of your life, in this one area you must accept—and submit to, often without objection—all the advanced medicine available to rid your body of disease. This may be the first time you find yourself faced with having to relinquish control of your life, accepting help from others in a way you may never have accepted it before. You must learn to acknowledge that sometimes you don't understand the specifics or that you're not the authority in areas of disease treatment. Your role, therefore, becomes predominantly passive as you allow others to make the best decisions for you and for your illness.

Eventually though, when you have completed your treatment, the passive role you have accepted must come to an end as well. That's where this book begins, because *Answer to Cancer* enters at the very moment you accept responsibility for your new life, the new life you have been given and which you are now ready to live. For this book is not about the end, but about the beginning of everything to come. It's a rebirth, so to speak, of the part of us that is inborn, but which many of us are unaware exists—the part that has supported us through our tough times and still exists and awaits our continued connection. The word "doctor" comes from the Latin *docere*, "to teach." It is that teacher, that "other doctor," *the doctor inside us*, whom we address in the following pages.

This book represents the more than 30 years of my life in which I have grown to appreciate the multifaceted doctor inside and the role this intrinsic healer plays in my continuing growth and renewal. If I were asked to define this quality, I think the words "innate intelligence" describe it the best. It is the innate intelligence that expresses itself through us on a daily basis: the innate intelligence that is manifested through our lungs that breathe and our heart that beats with no conscious effort from us whatsoever, and the undeniable, ever-present, invisible, and powerful force that needs our support so it can, in return, support us. The doctor within each of us needs us to take an *active* role in our health and wellbeing, because an active role is necessary to ensure that the disease we ousted remains gone forever.

If you have dealt with cancer in some form or another, gotten a clean bill of health, and then been pronounced "cured," you might well ask yourself why you have to take such an active role now. Isn't it over now? Can't your life go back to "normal" now? Can't you forget about it now?

Well, you can. Every one of us has the power of choice. For me, it was not a question of forgetting, however. Instead, I found myself asking, *How can I remember in a way that will inspire me to continue to live the longest and healthiest life possible?*

In my case, the answer was about self-preservation. Over time, my determined self-preservation grew slowly and distinctly into self-awareness, and this self-awareness helped ensure that after suffering such a devastating life-threatening disease I would be prepared to do everything in my power to make sure it wouldn't come back. I imagine many of my readers feel the same way—that you, or someone you care about, got cancer once (or more than once) and that you darn well want to make sure you, or they, don't get it again. Taking an active role in the ongoing process of staying healthy to ensure we're doing everything we possibly can to stay healthy seems to be the next logical step to lowering our risk every day of our lives.

Reading the following statistics may encourage you to take on this more purposeful role.

Currently, there are over 1 million new cases of cancer diagnosed each year in the United States. By the year 2030 this number is expected to double. Currently the National Cancer Institute (NCI) predicts that one in every two men and women will have cancer in their lifetimes. In an article written by Dr. Ernest Rosenbaum, et al. for the National and International Cancer Supportive Care Programs (at *www.cancersupportivecare.com*), research cited states that 50% of cancer survivors show lingering effects from their treatment, over 25% develop recurrence or new cancers, and that an estimated 75% can expect to have some kind of health concern associated with their treatment. If these facts aren't discouraging enough, cancer patients also die of *non-cancer* causes at a higher rate than the general population.

Needless to say, being clinically cured of cancer doesn't mean that when your treatment ends you're finished. Rather, your journey—the one of becoming and staying healthy—is just beginning.

It is my goal in this book to provide an adjunct source to any science-based tools you may already be putting to good use along your path. I hope to help you not only lower your risk of getting cancer, but to prevent it altogether. If I'm lucky, I will inspire you, through these words, to travel the road to better health. To that end, the guidelines outlined in this book address health—not illness. The research-based concepts support living—not dying. This book is about being given an opportunity at a second chance, the same kind of second chance I created for myself many years ago.

This book will pose the questions: *How would you do things differently this time around?* and *How might you change your approach if you knew more than you did before?*—and discuss many possible options. That's why this book is for you if you want to do more than "hope for the best" or maintain the status quo. My intention is to set the groundwork so that you have many more—and many different—tools at your disposal that you can use to establish a very different experience from this moment forward. And while there are no guarantees in life, I strongly believe that trying something new is better than trying nothing at all. This belief comes from my own experience, which taught me that if you keep thinking the same old way, you will keep doing the same old thing—and ultimately get the same old result. Here is an opportunity to think a new way, do something different, and achieve a different result. And that result just might be living, and staying cancer-free.

Cancer-free is the standard with which I live and is, I believe, the only way to be. In fact, taking a second chance may be our only chance to fulfill that goal and the goal of a healthy life. As the actor Harrison Ford once said, "We all have big changes in our lives that are more or less a second chance."

Let this second chance be our fighting chance to win the war against cancer.

The story behind the story

> *"Nothing is predestined. The obstacles of your past can become*
> *gateways to new beginnings."*
>
> - Ralph Blum, writer and cultural anthropologist

Did you ever read something that suddenly really hit home, I mean REALLY hit home? Well, Ralph Blum's quote did for me. Who would have thought that a simple statement like this could have such a deep meaning for me in my everyday life? But the obstacles of my past really *did* become gateways to a new beginning. I could never have imagined that my loss of health, my destitution, and my near loss of life would lead to my greatest triumphs; that my biggest loss would actually become my greatest gain. I feel blessed and thankful for the gifts that this experience has bestowed on my life. It may sound strange, but it's the truth, because it is my life-altering experience with cancer that has made me who and what I am today.

Looking back, of course, I did not wish to set any kind of example. I was simply a 19-year-old college student studying my courses, playing sports, partying, eating fast food, and doing what every young person does as a matter of course. As a typical, normal teenager, I had the world in front of me and was busy trying to figure out who I was and how I fit into the spectrum of careers available to me. Now, more than 30 years later, I realize that I was unwittingly given an opportunity to set an example for those around me. I see how, with no real conscious effort whatsoever, I have since touched the lives of many people who share the same or similar experiences as I had then. By describing what it was like to surface out of the overwhelming turmoil that at one time drained the very life out of me and how it felt to calm the unrest that gnawed at me on a daily basis, I have found another way of reaching out. I read somewhere once that a kite rises against the wind rather than with it; I finally started to understand the meaning of those words as I gradually began not to fear the winds of adversity, but to embrace them.

A quote by Napoleon Hill, personal-success author, explains it so simply: "Every adversity, every failure, every heartache carries with it the seed of an equal or greater benefit." What follows is the cause and effect of the adversity and heartache I faced, and the sweeping, ultimately positive change it had on me.

My story begins in 1976, while I was living at college, when out of nowhere I woke up sweating in the middle of the night. My hair, forehead, and body were drenched from sweating so profusely that I had been startled out of a deep sleep. Unable to sleep in a perspiration-soaked T-shirt, I got up, changed it for a dry one, and tried to go back to sleep. It didn't take long before these incidences of sweating were happening every night to the degree that I found myself changing my wringing-wet T-shirt three to four times a night and sleeping on a towel to avoid saturating the mattress.

As the sweat-infused, sleep-interrupted nights continued, I began to get really scared. To prevent the inevitable from occurring, I tried to stay up as late as I could. There I was, a teenage college student, young, enthusiastic and fearless...yet scared to sleep and scared to give voice to my fears. The episodes of unrelenting night sweats went on for weeks, filling me with anxiety and exhaustion. I felt utterly forlorn. My fears soon verged on the paranoid as I became more and more confused from sleep deprivation. I couldn't figure out what was happening to me.

During this time, I started experiencing a sharp, constant, left-sided rib pain. My ribs felt bruised and tender to touch. As the days passed, both the rib pain and the sweating continued to get worse.

I finally took myself to the campus clinic doctor who, after a brief examination, concluded that I had something called "broken rib virus." In his opinion this virus was causing both the night sweats and rib pain. After the examination I was given medication and told to rest. The sweating and pain did not abate, however, and were soon followed by weight loss. Not just an ounce or two, but more like twenty pounds in two weeks.

Weak, tired, and listless, I was dominated by a life of confusion and terror. I began suffering from debilitating migraine headaches that started in the early morning and stayed with me all day long. During the same period, I discovered a golf ball-sized lump over my left clavicle, the long bone that attaches the sternum, or the chest bone, to the front of the shoulder. After the appearance of this hard, well-defined growth, the people around me began to share a variety of unsolicited medical opinions, all of which concluded that I was suffering from nothing more than a harmless cyst. Ultimately, however, when an unexplained high fever and uncontrolled vomiting compounded my other symptoms, I took a bus home. I was admitted to the hospital the next day.

Lying on the examination table, all focus and concern seemed to be on the mysterious cyst that was growing bigger by the day. It was as if the growth had a mind of its own, increasing at a rate that my 19-year-old body couldn't handle. A biopsy in the hospital confirmed what the doctors now suspected: the lump was a cancerous growth. I was diagnosed with Stage 1 Hodgkin's disease, a type of lymphoma and a malignant form of cancer. After being told the news, I shook my head in total disbelief. I lay in my hospital bed staring at the ceiling in utter and persistent denial. Wasn't this the kind of thing that was supposed to happen to somebody else? You know, the neighbor's kid or someone in the news, or some unknown student on campus. Certainly not me!

As time passed, reality finally set in. I was faced with making decisions regarding options that I knew little about. From a medical point of view, my first priority was to treat the problem by getting rid of the invading cancer. That meant having the growth above my clavicle surgically removed. Sure enough, when the growth was completely removed I immediately started to feel a little better. The headaches, the night sweats, and the vomiting all subsided. It was as if a demon had been exorcised from my body and I felt I was on the road to recovery. But what I didn't realize was that this was just the beginning. I found out that the surgery I'd had above the clavicular area wasn't enough. I needed another surgery, this one in my abdominal area. I had to undergo a splenectomy—total surgical removal of the spleen. This kind of surgery by itself is a relatively safe procedure, especially by today's standards. The spleen, it turns out, is a major organ of the lymphatic system, which plays an important role in the immune system by regulating blood flow to the liver and filtering foreign substances and worn-out blood cells from the blood. Splenectomies are performed for a variety of reasons, such as primary cancer of the spleen, a blood disorder called Hereditary Spherocytosis (HS), rupture (such as after a trauma like a car accident), thalassemia (a painfully enlarged spleen), and to assess the progress of a disease. In my particular case, removing the spleen at that time was a necessary precaution to make sure the cancer had not spread.

You can see that the spleen is a very important organ in protecting against infection in general. That's why it's amazing that a person can continue to live a normal, healthy life without one. Still, it's not a procedure to be undertaken lightly, and even now is only performed in those cases where the benefits outweigh the risks. This undoubtedly was the case for me, way back in my 19th year of life.

To this day, I am thankful for the medical care that I received from my doctors, nurses, therapists, and support staff. They all saved my life. Without their outstanding care at that time, I doubt very much I would be here today, writing this book. To be honest though, it was also a very difficult time in my life. My career options were put on hold. I had to drop out of school and move back home, which meant losing most of my friends. I found that people behaved awkwardly around me and seemed to walk on eggshells after they found out I had cancer. Some were at a loss about how to relate to me and my situation. I felt their uneasiness, and soon my own confidence began to shake. I began to feel disconnected and disassociated from the world, afraid of the feelings of those around me as well as of my own. I was alienated from all I had known to be real for the first two decades of my life.

Frankly, I was miserable. I was tempted to curl up into a ball, hide, and never come out. But I had no choice. Despite my ongoing feelings of alienation, I had to go on. I realized I had to become my own foundation of courage, strength, and self-reliance. It was a slow and painful process, but I eventually discovered that with acceptance, determination, and faith I had the power to transform a difficult situation and make it better.

After one month in the hospital recovering from my surgeries, I embarked on my next steps: radiation and chemotherapy treatments on an outpatient basis for the next six months. In 1976, radiation followed by chemotherapy was the primary treatment for early Hodgkin's disease. Radiation therapy uses high-energy ionizing radiation to destroy cancer cells. It is delivered by way of an external radiation beam, and it works in a similar fashion as an x-ray, radioactive implantation, and short-lived radioactive chemicals. Today, with improvements in chemotherapy, radiation therapy can be modified or eliminated completely.

Before my treatment program began, my chest and abdomen areas were sketched with ink markers to denote the areas to be radiated. I looked like a red and black Etch A Sketch, with squiggles, rectangles, squares, and L-shaped lines. My chest area was first with a few weeks of radiation, then the abdominal area in subsequent weeks, with a week's rest in between. I still have the permanent ballpoint-sized tattoo marks on my chest and back that denote where the chest radiation stopped and the abdominal radiation began. As I was undergoing radiation treatment as an outpatient, I felt the effects all the way home. Having no car, I commuted back and forth to the hospital by bus and subway. Knowing what to expect a few minutes after each radiation treatment, I carried a bag similar to the ones provided on airplane flights for air sickness. Retching violently a few minutes after my treatment, as well as in the bus and subway on the way home, was an everyday affair. I carried sickness bags in my back pocket the way someone else might carry a handkerchief for the sniffles.

I was prepared to do whatever I had to do to get through this second phase of treatment. Hair loss ensued, a phenomenon with which I had to learn to cope. Not only was I grappling with the cancer, I was now coping with the multiple side effects as well. One day, at the end of one of my radiation treatments, I began vomiting uncontrollably on the ride home. As soon as I arrived at the house, I borrowed a car from a friend. Then, with one hand on the steering wheel and the other clutching my abdomen, I drove myself back to the hospital, where I was again admitted.

At that time my mother was working full time as a medical secretary at Columbia Presbyterian Hospital. She was alone in supporting and raising me and my sister after my father had left. My parents had divorced when I was 12, so she was my only support system, and if anyone deserves high honors it's my mother. While I was in treatment she was at my side daily, an amazing pillar of strength, always telling me my illness was a "temporary setback." She smuggled tuna sandwiches into my room to make sure I was adequately fed because the hospital food was so bad, and her constant reassurance became my strength on the road to recovery. My mother's efforts never waned, but because we didn't own a car and my mother had no driver's license, there were many times I was still pretty much on my own.

At the hospital, after numerous tests, I was diagnosed with an intestinal obstruction, which had occurred from the radiation treatment I had received. I was hospitalized for another week and fed intravenously until the obstruction finally unblocked itself. Once this condition had cleared, I reluctantly finished the remainder of my radiation therapy.

The next and last stage of my treatment was chemotherapy. Chemotherapy is the use of drugs to shrink tumors and kill cancer cells. These drugs are administered by way of oral medication, single-shot injection, or intravenous (IV) drip. Unlike radiation and surgery, which are localized treatments, chemotherapy is systemic, where the medicine circulates throughout the whole body. Chemotherapy also has many side effects, though these reactions differ from person to person. Age, the type of medicine, extent of the cancer, and intensity of the chemotherapy are just a few of the factors that create variables in potential side effects. The most common generalized side effects of chemotherapy are fatigue, loss of appetite, total or partial baldness, skin eruptions, ulcerations, and digestive problems. On the emotional end, it is not uncommon to suffer from anxiety, fear, despair, loneliness, and depression. Despite my attempt to believe that I was winning my own personal war on cancer, I was about as low as

I could go on both fronts, mentally and physically. I was all of the above: depressed, confused, lonely, and afraid.

My body was so tired and battered by this time that I could only endure two out of the six months of the prescribed chemotherapy. I was exhausted, despondent, and weak, living in a 6′5″-inch body, weighing only 160 pounds.

Not a day passed that I didn't feel the cancer would return. With every ache and pain came the immediate conviction that the disease had indeed come back. Every sniffle or sneeze was the cancer recurring. Sweating during exercise or from a fever was a painful reminder of my T-shirt-soaked nights in college—and a warning light of things to come. My mind became the master of catastrophe. My thinking became so fear-based that I just knew getting sick again was only a matter of time. I began to ask myself why, if I were clinically cured from the disease, was I so afraid of getting it again? Wasn't I "all better"?

I eventually realized that the reason I felt so completely horrible and life looked so bleak was because my surgically spent, radiated, and all-too-chemotherapied body still felt vulnerable, weak, tired, and listless—despite the fact that I had been told I was "clinically cured." When I pushed open the glass doors of the hospital toward the street for what was supposed to be the "last time," I still felt ill. But this time it was a different type of ill. I felt almost as vulnerable being *cured* of cancer as I did *having* cancer. I asked myself how that could be. I began recounting all the treatment I had received in the past year to determine what was missing. I had been told I was free of cancer, yet it didn't seem to add up. I still didn't understand why I was feeling such a void. I continued to rack my brain, while at the same time feeling this sense of loss, the sense of not having what it was that I needed, even though I didn't know what that was.

It didn't take too long before it became glaringly apparent exactly what was lacking. It dawned on me that I had never been given any kind of advice about what I should do next—in the "meantime," between checkups—or, more importantly, what I could do for myself to *stay* cancer-free. No one had approached me to say, "Here, Doug, here is what you need to do not to get this disease again." When you go to the dentist and have a cavity filled, you come out with an arsenal of toothbrushes, floss, and toothpaste to help you stay cavity-free. When it comes to cancer, it's "See you for your next checkup," and you leave empty-handed. At least that's the way it was in those days. So, the question that came to mind and repeated itself over and over again as I walked toward the bus stop to go home that day was, "Now what do I do?"

Not having an answer to that question and not knowing where to look, it occurred to me that a good place to start would be to talk with other cancer survivors who had recently ended their treatment. Perhaps I would be able to find out what, if anything, they were doing now that their treatment programs were over. I was unaware of any "survivor groups" or of ways to meet other survivors, but through word of mouth I managed to locate two other students on campus who had also recently recovered from cancer. They agreed to meet with me, and standing outside a classroom, they both admitted that other than routine, scheduled checkups, no one had ever told them what to do either. It seemed that the three of us were all in a giant fend-for-yourself boat, set out to sea with no clear direction and no tools for navigation. Discouraged, I knew I'd been left to my own devices. And basically, at that point, that meant I had nothing more than a big fat zero.

As the weeks passed, my thoughts whirled and my dissatisfaction grew. I needed to *do* something, even though I was still at a loss about how or what. My own quiet self-reliance, the self-reliance I had always had prior to my battle with cancer, was beginning to surface once again. If there were no one to help me at this critical juncture, I would simply have to help myself. But not only did I need and want to help myself, it became clear that I also wanted to help as many other people as I could, people who were also looking for the same kind of answers. The problem was that any "answers" were scattered, at best, even if I'd known where to look. No single resource guide, handbook, or outline existed to address the issues of preventing the recurrence of cancer. Additionally, little information was available to inform people of what they could do to reduce their risk of getting the disease in the first place. Can you begin to understand why I needed to write this book as both a reminder to myself and to help others with similar questions?

From my experience, I can tell you that almost every cancer survivor is aware that this gap exists. It can be defined as the "end of treatment and the beginning of living again" gap, or the "Now what do I do?" gap, but it's the question that resonates in every cancer survivor's mind and heart. It's the divide that now becomes that single moment in time where new conscious choices start laying the groundwork for how you need to start living. In essence, it is the moment of a new beginning, a rebirth, of the cancer-free you.

For me, it was during this gap that I became aware of how tired I was of "living illness," as I called it. It was during this gap that I consciously began "living healthy" instead. I began to explore any and all health information I could get my hands on. From books on how the body worked to articles on vegetarianism—you name it, I read it. The problem was that though I was continuing to learn new information, the publications I read were also incredibly confusing. One article said one thing and then another article contradicted the one I had just read. For the most part, I was finding the published health information to be sketchy and clouded at best. I started to feel bewildered on top of already feeling inadequate relative to my quest for knowledge. All I knew was that I was sick of being sick—and confused—and that I had to start somewhere.

Despite the informational chaos, I was determined to stay with it. What I began to notice about myself in the process was that aside from the muddled presentation, the more I learned the more I continued to grow. I found myself gravitating to less-than-well-known health practices. Like a match to dry wood, I started to become engrossed with everything and anything having to do with alternative and complementary health practices, and became fascinated by these healing arts that worked *with* the body. It soon became apparent during the process that I was becoming inspired and more hopeful, and that I was starting to wake up and move out of the rut of my illness.

I was beginning to move in the direction of being the prime facilitator of my own health.

As it says in the Bible, "As a man thinketh, so shall he be" (Proverbs 23:7). In my quest for answers I pushed myself to continue thinking and focusing on health, *not illness*. Having been told I was "cured" by my doctors, I was standing at a crossroad in my life: Would I continue to follow a road that almost figuratively and literally led me to a dead end, or would I take a new road, a road never before traveled? From my reading and research I was getting the feeling that my cancer—and maybe all cancers—could be prevented from recurring. So, with an inquisitive mind and blind faith, I continued my studies to validate my theory. Certainly, getting older is a fact of life, and admittedly, the aging process has its challenges by increasing our odds of getting diseases, including cancer. However, the choices we make on a day-to-day basis as we naturally age are in our hands. I have come to understand that most chronic diseases can be attributed—to a marked extent—to lifestyle. Self-inflicted stress, negativity, diet, drug dependence, smoking, and lack of exercise are all examples of elements that play significant roles in the development of chronic, debilitating, and life-threatening diseases. Deciding to be responsible and acting as the ones responsible for our health is something that needs to come from within us. We have to take responsibility for ourselves, and do the best we can with the things we can and do control.

I continued my exploration of alternative and complementary medicine practices. The field is surprisingly vast, encompassing some of the more traditional therapies, such as chiropractic, acupuncture, naturopathy, Ayurveda, and Oriental medicine, modalities that express themselves through body movement, such as yoga and tai chi, and meditative techniques for calming the mind. And when it comes to our dietary daily requirements, nature provides herbs, fruits, and vegetables to sustain the body's complex systems. I was becoming convinced that the best approach to health had to include both an emphasis on the principles of prevention and a willingness to meet the body's needs every single day and that together these elements would form a solid foundation for healthy living.

I began a regimen of proper rest, exercise, and stress reduction. While my old self wanted to go back to my prior poor eating habits and indulge in a Big Mac in front of the TV, my new self was disciplined to stay on the road to health. I was unknowingly living the proverb, "When the student is ready, the teacher appears." Nutrient-absent fast food was replaced with whole foods. Skipping meals was replaced with structured eating at regular intervals. Quick fixes were replaced with well-thought-out balanced meals. Plenty of water and fruit snacks became the norm. It didn't take long before the way I was eating was becoming a way of life. I was becoming conscious about the decisions I was making, about what I chose to eat, and why I needed to eat it. It was as if my life depended on it.

And it did.

H. Jackson Brown, Jr., bestselling author, once wrote, "In the confrontation between the stream and the rock, the stream always wins, not through strength, but by perseverance." Personally, persistence has been one of my strongest attributes, and it has continued to pay big dividends.

Because that's how my health, life's most precious commodity, came back to stay.

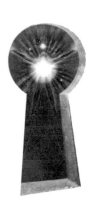

2. Health Now and Forever

T here are many things you can do to stay healthy, and no one can dictate "the right way" for anyone else. I have explored numerous choices over the years, including tools that relieve stress, nourish cells, and improve the body's functioning. In this chapter, I will touch on those that have contributed to my own personal success in living a healthy life.

Feeding the body, mind, and spirit

Yoga: what's it all about?

The meaning of the Sanskrit word *yoga* is "union": union of mind, body, and spirit. Yoga teaches that the union of inside forces can prevail over outside elements. Yoga is said to be the oldest defined practice of self-development in existence—as old as civilization itself. Although archaeological evidence points to the existence of yoga around 3000 B.C. due to the presence of stone seals depicting figures in yoga poses, scholars trace its beginnings to a time long before Stone Age shamanism, and indeed they both share the fundamental approach of encouraging the improvement of the human condition. Yoga is divided into Vedic, pre-classical, classical, and post-classical types. Teachings found in Vedas, the sacred scriptures of Hinduism, for example, are characterized by rituals and ceremonies to overcome limitations of the mind. Similar to Buddhism, yoga stresses the energy and potential of meditation and is considered the strength and core of inner vision.

Supporting this philosophy is India's holy book, the Bhagavad Gita, which expresses many important messages to be adapted to daily life with the goal of self-realization and liberation. The essence of the Bhagavad Gita's message is that to be alive means to be active, or to take action, and that to avoid difficulties in our lives the actions we take have to be benign—that is, exceed the confines and constraints of ego-driven actions. To that end, yoga is instrumental in bringing about positive thinking in conjunction with relaxation, proper exercise, breathing, proper diet, and meditation. Regular practice assists in leading to detoxification, a balanced nervous system, reduction of stress, joint lubrication, and improved muscle tone. It may be hard to believe, but the practice of yoga has been found by many to transform stress, ill health, anxiety, anger, and unhappiness into relaxation, good health, happiness, and selflessness. In essence, it is the practice of helping the body work in total harmony with balance and control. I have personally found this practice of balancing brings peace and tranquility to both my body and mind.

Yoga also helps in mastering the technique of breathing known as *pranayama*. Performing correct postures and body movements while using controlled breathing techniques in this manner is often said to lead to total refreshment of the body and mind. Because the benefits of yoga are not only many, but profound, for our purposes in this book I will share an overview of yoga and its three basic classifications so you will have insight into how helpful this form of practice can really be.

The three yoga classifications are physiological, psychological, and spiritual.

Physiological. One of the physiological benefits of yoga includes a reduction of stress by lowering the level of cortisol, a principal corticosteroid associated with stress production. The cortisol hormone is secreted by the adrenal glands, located on top of the kidneys, and is vital for life. Cortisol helps the body manage stress by maintaining blood pressure, reducing inflammation, maintaining the immune system, and working with the hormone insulin to maintain blood sugar levels. In short, cortisol is the body's natural stress-fighting and anti-inflammatory hormone. It is called the "stress hormone" due to the fact that stress activates cortisol emission and is responsible for the "fight-or-flight" stress-related changes we experience. On the flip side, too much of cortisol's prolonged circulation in the body can also be associated with many health problems, including the development of cancer.

Psychological. The psychological benefits of yoga are well documented. Many people who suffer with depression and/or mood swings and who need psychological treatment find that learning the practice of a specific type of yoga, such as *hatha* yoga, which incorporates various specific postures and breathing techniques, helps them gain calmness and stability of the mind. Other psychological imbalances, such as panic disorders and anxiety attacks, have also been shown to subside with regular yoga practice. At the National Institute of Mental Health and Neuroscience in India, for example, research has shown that treating depression with *sudharshan kriya*, better known as "the healing breath technique" in the United States, has close to a 75% success rate. *Healing breath technique* involves natural breathing through the nose in three distinct rhythms with the mouth closed. Amazingly, these seemingly small movements and exercise regimens have the capacity to improve mood and provide serenity by passing energy through the parts of the body where imbalances exist in the form of anger or grief.

Spiritual. Spiritually, yoga allows us to connect with our sacred self. One type of yoga that brings us closer is *raja* yoga, which concentrates on developing the inner being—the part of us that includes our mental health, morality, and spirituality. This form of yoga is concerned with cultivating the mind using meditation to further one's acquaintance with reality and achieve liberation. Raja yoga helps foster the integration of the intricately woven ingredients of our mind, such as soulfulness and grace, to keep it calm. The Bhagavad Gita describes yoga beautifully when it says, "Equal-mindedness is called yoga; it is skill in the performance of actions." Thus, yoga trains the mind to perform the right action to ultimately improve concentration and provide clarity of thought. Once we start to experience improved psychic control and development, these practices become instrumental in purifying, healing, and rejuvenating our entire being. Ultimately, our body strengthens, our mind calms, and our spirit unites. A united spirit is one which recognizes that the lives of all people are interconnected, and it is when we begin to understand through experience the nature of these revelations that we begin to automatically adopt a kinder, more compassionate, gentler nature. Once we are unified in mind, body, and spirit, we can move forward for our own greater good, as well as for the good of others.

Yoga has been practiced for thousands of years to improve physical and emotional wellbeing, and research suggests far-reaching applications on cancer patients and survivors. For example, studies conducted with cancer patients and survivors have revealed that modest improvements can be made in many areas, including sleep quality, mood, stress, cancer-related distress, cancer-related symptoms, and overall quality of life, and studies conducted in both various patient populations and healthy individuals have shown beneficial effects on psychological and somatic symptoms as well as other aspects of physical function.[1]

It was through learning about yoga that I realized how important it was to introduce consistent physical movement of some kind into my life. But remember, this was the seventies, and yoga classes were nowhere near as commonplace as they are today. So, with no class or instructor in even remote proximity to me at the time, I knew I needed to find another way. I also knew that whatever I found would have to be accessible and relatively simple in order to accomplish similar goals of keeping my mind focused and my body moving.

Regular exercise

I instinctively knew that doing something was far better than doing nothing at all, so I began an exercise program that seemed right for me. I started with running; soon I had added swimming, stretching, walking, and even some occasional weightlifting. Looking back I see that my actions were not all that different from, and in fact seem consistent with, the guidelines that would later be set by the American Cancer Society. The ACS has set aggressive goals for the nation to decrease cancer incidence and mortality, with stress on improving the quality of life for cancer survivors by the year 2015. For this purpose, the ACS publishes the *Nutrition and Physical Activity Guidelines* to affect dietary and physical activity patterns.[2] These guidelines, published every five years, are developed by a national panel of experts in cancer research and prevention. Represented in these guidelines is the most current scientific evidence on dietary and activity patterns relative to cancer risk.

The ACS guidelines recommend adopting a physically active lifestyle, which means engaging in at least 30 minutes or more of exercise five or more days a week. Because the type of exercise each individual ultimately decides to do should be based solely on what he or she feels comfortable doing, the American Cancer Society suggests several levels of activity. "Mild exercise" includes walking, dancing, leisurely bicycling, horseback riding, canoeing, and yoga. "Moderate exercise" includes golfing, baseball, badminton, volleyball, and even activities like the game of horseshoes. Household activities, such as mowing the lawn and vacuuming, also fit in the category of "light-to-moderate" exertion. And, finally, "vigorous exercise" includes jogging, running, fast bicycling, aerobic dancing, martial arts, swimming, and circuit and weight training. The picture is clear: there are endless ways to get the exercise we need to stay in shape.

Food matters

Once we take the plunge and begin incorporating some form of physical activity into our lives, it's only a matter of time before we realize that what we eat is equally as important as how we move. Exercising on a regular basis is great, but if what we ingest defeats our purpose, in the end we lose. What we put into our bodies—in other words, what we eat and how much—needs to be balanced with our level of physical activity. It has become clear, again through research, that being overweight is associated with an increased risk of developing various cancers. In fact, with one third of all adults currently falling into the category of "obese," obesity itself has become a disease. Obesity refers to having an abnormally high proportion of body fat and has been defined by the National Institutes of Health, or NIH,[3] as a Body Mass Index, or BMI, of 30 and above. A BMI of 30, for example, is about 30 pounds overweight. This is important because the disease of obesity tends to lead to other, equally dangerous, health risks.

According to the National Cancer Institute in 2002, 3.2% of all new cancer cases (about 41,000) were estimated to be due to obesity.[4] This research also showed that obesity increases the risk of breast cancer and uterine cancer due to higher exposures to estrogen and insulin. Exercising about 30 minutes a day, however, is now known to be instrumental in reducing the risk of breast cancer by 20%. Scientists further estimate that anywhere from 11,000 to 18,000 deaths per year from breast cancer in women over age 50 in the U.S. might be avoided if women maintained a BMI under 25 throughout their adult lives.[5] Significantly, both men and women with the highest BMIs show higher death rates from all cancers, 52% for men and 62% for women, compared to men and women of normal weight.[6]

The association between obesity and cancer is also thought to have something to do with alterations in sex hormones, such as estrogen and progesterone, insulin, and IGF-1, or Insulin-like Growth Factor 1. We also know that obesity increases the risk of factors that contribute to the risk of cancer, as well as to overall recovery and survival rates.

For example, in one study that has examined the link between obesity and ovarian cancer, it was shown that women who were obese had an increased likelihood for developing ovarian cancer and that those women who had advanced-stage obesity disease saw both shorter recurrence times and shorter overall survival rates.[7] Dr. Andrew Li, the lead study author, states, "This study is the first to identify weight as an independent factor in ovarian cancer in disease progression and overall survival." This comment was based on research revealing that for every one excess unit of BMI a woman's risk of dying from ovarian cancer increased by 5%.

Links between prostate cancer and obesity have also been found. Evidence suggests that diet and weight gain may be important lifestyle factors implicated in prostate cancer, especially in tumor progression. In one study of 526 patients registered at the M.D. Anderson Cancer Center from 1992 to 2001, for example, results revealed that patients who were obese showed higher rates of biochemical failure than those patients of normal weight. Biochemical failure is defined as three consecutive increases in PSA (prostate-specific antigens) following curative treatment of prostate cancer. In this case it was found that men who gained weight quickly experienced these results faster than those who gained weight more slowly.[8]

What's the bottom line? Obesity has a direct relationship to cancer—and obesity is one of the things we can all do something about.

Attending seminars and lectures and going to the library opened up a whole new world for me as I tried to learn everything I could about cancer. It was during this time that I came across an author for whom I have since developed a tremendous amount of respect. Her name is Dr.

Joan Borysenko. Trained in both medicine and psychology, Dr. Borysenko's insights into health through integrative medicine reveal themselves in her books and programs. Dr. Borysenko has gone far beyond her medical training: as co-founder and former director of the mind/body clinical programs at Beth Israel/Deaconess Medical Center in Boston and former instructor in medicine at Harvard Medical School, she has spent years developing a comprehensive understanding in a variety of areas, such as the behavioral sciences, stress, women's health, general wellbeing, and complex spiritual traditions throughout the world. Through her work with many cancer and AIDS patients, Dr. Borysenko has formed the belief that more and more people are becoming "interested in meditation as a way of getting attuned to the spiritual dimension of life. Science, medicine, psychology, and spiritualism need to be together in the service of healing." Dr. Borysenko's observation validates what I believed then and have continued to believe all along: that it is the integration of conventional and complementary ideas, the weaving together of science, psychology, and spirituality to serve the greater good of the whole, that leads to the attainment of health for the mind and body.

The process of healing is a journey of deep personal reflection. During this transformation, change occurs naturally both within us and in the outside world; it is both inevitable and constant. As has often been said, "The only thing that is constant is change," and that couldn't be a truer statement. It is how we react to change that directly affects our health and wellbeing. We all have those days where we seem to react negatively to just about anything that crosses our path. Our feelings and emotions seem heightened when confronted, resulting in feelings of annoyance, anger, or frustration. But we have a choice in how we react to life's challenges, even though we may not think we do. I can't tell you how many times I have had to stop myself when I am in a reactive, agitated state of mind and say, "I need to let this go." I say these words to help stop the pattern of disharmony I am experiencing. In other words, I am releasing my attachment to a situation or thought so I can regain my sense of peace. What I know now is that this ability to step away for a moment and make a conscious, different choice can only come from a grounded core formed by the integrated effort of the mind, body, *and* spirit.

When I began this time of intense learning and pursuit of knowledge, I only knew that I wanted to get my life back, that I needed and wanted to regain those physical, emotional, and spiritual components I felt had been lost in the process of dealing with the very real effects of my cancer. But these sacred components, I have come to learn, are no less important than the surgery, radiation, and IV drip I endured. In fact, they are as critical to replenish as the weight I lost during my treatment process.

It was while reflecting on all this new information that my daydreams started. These daydreams—or fantasies, really—were about the possibility, and ultimately the probability, of creating a "new self." I pictured myself healthy, finishing my college courses, eating nutritious food, getting proper rest, exercising, and quietly reflecting each and every day using the power of my own thoughts and imagination. For the first time, I wasn't focusing so much on locks and latches, but more on handles and hinges. In other words, I stopped thinking about what I didn't have and started to focus on what I wanted. I started to marvel at my mind's ability to imagine what my new self would like and the kind of things I would be doing to help myself continue on the path of health.

It was at this time that I encountered a variety of articles on visual imagery. It has been said that imagination is the mother of invention—that everything we have today is only here because it began in someone's imagination at some earlier point in time. If it is in the realm of imagination, it is in the realm of possibility, and if it is possible, it is attainable—yes, even when it comes to the healing process. There is no doubt that imagination is a potent healer, one that has for too long been overlooked by practitioners of Western medicine. Although imagery may not always be literally curative, it has been found to relieve pain, speed healing, prevent remission, subdue ailments (such as depression, weight gain, and asthma), and has often been shown to be a valuable aid in self-development.

Visual imagery is also known as *visualization* or *guided imagery*, and is a technique that permeates the quiet recesses of the mind with the objective of accomplishing a vividly imagined goal on a deep, subconscious level. Imagery stimulates the brain to communicate to all areas of the body by harnessing the energy of thought and converting it into healing. The action of imagery is simple to do, requires little time, and costs nothing. Spending a few minutes a day in the visual recesses of the mind can assist in bolstering our natural defense mechanisms and subtly shift or reinforce our belief systems about our health. Imagery is used as an adjunct to healing in virtually all cultures and civilizations of the world, both current and ancient, and is considered a vital part of many religions. Aristotle and Hippocrates, for instance, believed that mental images exorcised spirits in the brain which affected the heart and other organs of the body.

The *American Heritage Dictionary* defines imagination as "the ability to confront and deal with reality by using the power of the mind." Albert Einstein has said that imagination is "more important than knowledge. Knowledge is limited, while imagination embraces the entire world." Visualizations can be performed by anyone, including athletes, musicians, inventors, and architects who silently rehearse within before acting on the images held in their mind. Athletes are singularly known for applying mental imagery to "see" their success and perfect their skills. Golfing genius Jack Nicklaus, for example, has admitted to imagining his performance before he hits each shot; that is, imagining the white ball sitting on the green grass and picturing his club tapping the ball into the hole. After that, Nicklaus has said, it is simply a matter of translating the images into reality.

My thoughts continued to be validated on the topic of the effect of thought on the healing process. It made sense, given the fact that the human mind is one of the most powerful and resourceful tools there is. In one 2004 research review I read, for example, relaxation and thermal biofeedback were found to be helpful in the treatment of migraines, while relaxation and muscle biofeedback were found effective in treating tension headaches.[9] In another study, autogenic (self-generating) training was found to reduce the frequency of tension and migraine headaches and the need for medication in its users.[10] We can safely say, therefore, that along with using standard medical treatment, using the mind may provide benefits by reducing pain, decreasing the recurrence of headaches, and eliminating headaches altogether.

Findings of this nature are relevant to cancer treatment as well. For example, guided imagery and relaxation techniques have been shown to be instrumental in improving quality of life and introducing a sense of wellbeing in women undergoing chemotherapy for breast cancer. When the women in this study were separated into two groups, one receiving conventional chemotherapy treatment and the other receiving conventional chemotherapy with relaxation and guided imagery, it was found that the group receiving both treatment types expressed being more relaxed and easygoing throughout the length of the study.[11]

Because all that we create originates from our ability to imagine, it is an asset every single one of us has the option to use for our own benefit. No wonder it has been aptly said that "it is all in the mind." It was while embracing these concepts that I began to use my own visual techniques to reinforce my state of health and wellbeing every day of my life.

The chiropractic approach

As I continued my informational journey about cancer, as well as about health in general, I began learning about chiropractic. After medicine and dentistry, chiropractic is the world's third-largest healthcare system. Chiropractic is derived from the Greek, *cheiro*, meaning "hand," and *prakrikos*, meaning "done by hand." A chiropractor uses his hands to manipulate the spine, to realign vertebrae that are *malpositioned*, or *subluxated*, and that are causing improper joint motion and nerve interference. These manipulations, or "adjustments," are done by applying direct pressure in combination with gentle force in a specific direction for the purpose of realigning the vertebrae. Muscle and joint pain is one way the body has of telling us that something is out of alignment; however, the majority of subluxations go undetected because there is no pain present. Chiropractic care evaluates the patient by doing a physical examination, assessing x-rays, MRIs, EMGs, static palpation, motion palpation, and range of motion, and taking into account the current daily activities and health history of the individual and his family. The tenet of chiropractic is that once the cause of the problem has been determined and corrected by the chiropractor, the body is ready to begin the process of healing on its own.

As a healing art, chiropractic was practiced more than 2,000 years ago, when people with pain were given healing massages which, combined with spinal adjustments, cured their symptoms. In the United States Dr. Daniel David Palmer was responsible for pioneering the formulation of an entire system around chiropractic principles and for establishing the Palmer School of Chiropractic in Davenport, Iowa in 1897. The World Federation of Chiropractic defines chiropractic as "a health profession concerned with the diagnosis, treatment, and prevention of mechanical disorders of the musculoskeletal system, and the effects of these disorders on the function of the nervous system and general health. There is an emphasis on manual treatments, including spinal adjustment and other joint and soft-tissue manipulation."[12]

Doctors of chiropractic are often referred to as chiropractors, or chiropractic physicians, and practice a hands-on, drug-free approach. As I studied chiropractic methods, I became convinced that disease could well be caused by vertebral subluxations, which impair nerve transmission from the brain to all the cells, tissues, and organs of the body. Because nerves of the spine contain sensory, motor, and visceral components, any interference with these nerves can affect sensation, muscle strength, and organ function. The focus of chiropractic is two-pronged: to locate and correct these spinal subluxations, which give rise to many direct and indirect complications in the nervous system, and to improve, regain, and maintain health. Chiropractors diagnose and treat disorders of the musculoskeletal system, including lower back pain, disc problems, headaches related to neurological and muscular problems, arthritis, sciatica, and neck and shoulder pain. I was personally drawn to the practice of chiropractic care because chiropractors aspire towards complete wellness of the whole body—not simply the alignment of bones.

In affecting the path of cancer, radiologists, oncologists, and surgeons work together to cure the disease. Receiving chiropractic care in parallel with this approach can contribute immensely and positively in a non-invasive, non-pharmacological manner. Not only can pain be managed and curtailed, but healing can be promoted by keeping the body's nervous system unobstructed and free-flowing to all cells, tissues, and organs. Chiropractors do not cure cancer; they *do*, however, contribute to many facets of the restorative process toward good health and aid in reducing some of the side effects from other cancer treatments. As Hippocrates said so long ago, "Look to the spine for health and disease."

The stats

Soon my attention turned to further understanding the scope of the disease we call cancer. This is what I found.

Cancer is the second leading cause of death in the United States. The American Cancer Society documents a startling 156 new cancer cases *per hour* in the United States. On a more positive note, cancer research in the United Kingdom reveals that even though cancer cases are on a rise, death rates are falling due to early detection and better treatment.

It was when I began looking at cancer on a broader scale relative to its incidence in the United States compared to the rest of the world that I came across a remarkable research study produced by the British Broadcasting Company (BBC) and Dr. John Toy, Medical Director of Cancer Research UK. Based on his research, Dr. Toy calls cancer "a disease of developed nations."[13] Dr. Toy's research indicates, for example, that only 4% of deaths in Africa are due to cancer, while in Europe the number is 19%. In Canada the percentage is much higher, at approximately 27%; in the United States it is approximately 23%. In his study of 27 different types of cancers throughout the world, Dr. Toy found that lung and breast cancer are the most common of all cancers. Figure 2-1 shows a breakdown of cancer cases per 100,000 in the population.[13] According to this chart, the highest rates of cancer incidence are indeed in developed nations with:

- 301 and above in North America and Canada
- 251 to 300 in Australia, and northern and western Europe
- 201 to 250 in southern Europe
- 151 to 200 in northern Asia, South America, southern Africa, and eastern Africa
- 100 to 150 in Southeast Asia, the Far East, Central America, and central Africa
- Fewer than 100 cases in northern Africa

FIGURE 2-1. Cancer as a disease of the developed nations, as reported by Dr. John Toy, Medical Director of Cancer Research UK, in a study produced by the British Broadcasting Corporation. (Source: *www.news.bbc.co.uk/2/hi/health*)

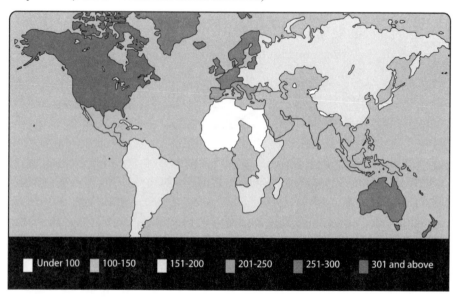

Dr. Toy's comparisons of cancer cases between the years 1975 and 2005 led him to suggest that less-developed nations could learn from developed nations to minimize the incidence of lung cancer by at least substantially curtailing the use of tobacco. Unfortunately, research predicts that the incidence of lung cancer will only continue to increase in less-developed regions, such as eastern Africa, Central America, and Southeast Asia, just as it is increasing in the more developed countries (marked in darker shading on the map in Figure 2-1). That is why campaigns to promote awareness, early detection, and prevention are so very important.

I was relieved to learn through my research that there are actually more cancer survivors than fatalities due to the massive amount of research being undertaken in combination with improved treatment strategies. So, although lung cancer may be on the rise, the *Journal for the National Cancer Institute* reports a decline in both the incidence and the death rates from all cancers combined, in both men and women, for the first time in our nation's history.[14]

FIGURE 2-2. Age adjusted total U.S. mortality rates for all cancer sites, all ages, and all races from 1969 to 2004; age adjusted to the 2000 U.S. standard population. (Source: *www.3.cancer. gov/atlasplus/charts*)

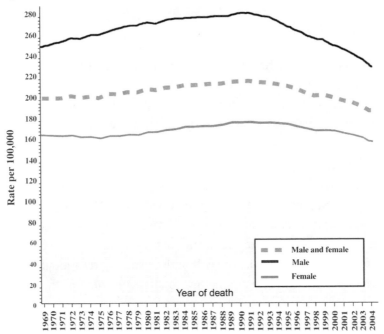

The graph in Figure 2-2 shows the total U.S. mortality rates (age adjusted to the 2000 U.S. standard population) for all cancer sites, all ages, and all races for 1969 to 2004 by gender.

In the U.S., 30% of all deaths are due to heart disease and 23% are due to cancer. Furthermore, a recent statistic reveals that 22% of Americans smoke regularly and that 30% of all cancers and a significant amount of heart disease *are a direct result of smoking.*

In the meantime, according to the World Cancer Report 2008, the annual report published by the International Agency for Research on Cancer (IARC), a division of the World Health Organization, cancer is a growing global crisis, a burden that has doubled over the last 30 years. This report projects that continued growth and aging of the world's population will cause cancer to prevail over heart disease as the world's deadliest disease by 2010 and that if current trends continue, 27 million worldwide could be diagnosed with cancer by 2030. In a press release issued by the IARC, Dr. Peter Boyle, IARC director and co-editor of the report, lamented, "The burden on society caused by cancer is immense in terms of the human suffering of patients and the impact on relatives, friends, and caregivers. The strain cancer produces on health professionals and health systems is substantial and growing rapidly." The report further specified that the greatest number of new cases will occur in developing countries and pointed to the adoption of "Western" habits, such as tobacco use and poor diets, as a driver of these trends.[15]

Acupuncture as a healing tool

I soon came across another practice of healing which the Western world had only just begun to explore, that of using acupuncture as a remedial measure to assist in reducing the side effects of cancer treatment. Acupuncture, a treatment which involves the insertion of very thin metal needles into the skin to balance energy in the body, originated in China about 2,500 years ago.

Two thousand five hundred years is a long time. So you'll understand when I say that it sure took a while before we in the West began to accept the possibility that acupuncture was a valid, if not exceptional, method of healing. It wasn't until 1997, in fact, that the National Institutes of Health Consensus Development Conference came to the conclusion that there was enough consistent scientific evidence to support acupuncture's effectiveness in reducing the side effects of chemotherapy. During my lengthy, grueling treatment so many years ago, I wish I'd known about the use of acupuncture to alleviate some of the consequences with which I struggled. It was at this point in my learning that my world expanded exponentially. It made perfect sense to me that the combination of Eastern techniques and Western treatments would be the consummate approach for combating cancer.

As I continued on my own personal research journey, I consistently came across quotes by Hippocrates, the physician from ancient Greece (ca. 460 BC – ca. 370 BC) who is considered to be one of the most predominant figures in the shaping of medicine. Hippocrates is often referred to as the "father of medicine" in recognition of his lasting contributions, and his insights into health and disease continue to be confirmed today. "The remedy for every illness is to be found in nature," he is known to have said. That basic, "simple" truth is every bit as valid today as it was back in 400 B.C.

Foods of choice

We've been talking for a while about making choices, the kind that can change our lives for the better. And we can't talk about those kinds of choices without including one of the most significant aspects of all: what we eat—that is, the food we put into our bodies.

The good news is that there are foods that absolutely do help in maintaining good health. The not-so-good news is that we may not be as ready, willing, and able as we would like to make the necessary changes for incorporating them into our diet. But the truth is that whenever you're ready is the right time to start, to take the first step. You don't have to be hard on yourself. Each day you make a move in the right direction, know that the step—be it big or small—is a step toward improved health.

What follows is information about the amazing fact that many foods have been shown to be real cancer-fighters by curtailing the growth of cancer and shrinking tumors. Studies done by many researchers, for example, support the evidence that foods such as avocados, broccoli, cabbage, soybeans, and cauliflower have capabilities to combat breast and other cancers. So bear with me as I get a little scientific here.

The protective quality found in these types of foods is mainly attributed to two naturally occurring compounds: namely, indole-3-carbinol, or I3C, and genistein. These phytochemicals stimulate the activity of BRCA1 and BRCA2 genes, or what are now known as the "breast cancer genes." BRCA genes are tumor suppressor genes whose function is to slow down cell division or cause cells to die at the right time. It has been found that although men also get breast cancer, women are more susceptible to it simply due to their gender. In fact, breast cancer is about 100 times more common in women. Furthermore, the chances of getting breast cancer increases as a woman's age increases and about two in three women with invasive breast cancer are above the age of 55 years when the cancer is detected.

Because breast cancer develops when changes occur in the genes of breast cells, it can be said to have a genetic element, as other cancers have. But it's important to recognize that genetic does not mean "inherited." In fact, it is estimated that only 5 to 10% of breast cancer cases result from an inherited ancestral predisposition to the disease. What that means is that more than 90% of all breast cancer cases result from factors that are *not* inherited and are, often, unknown. Furthermore, BRCA1 and BRCA2 are genes that everyone inherits in pairs, one from the mother and one from the father. Functioning normally, these genes work to stop the growth of cancerous cells in the breast. When there are damaged pairs of these genes, however, it can be a indication that cancer may develop, and it turns out that people who inherit a damaged BRCA1 or BRCA2 gene from one parent are at greater risk of developing breast cancer than people who inherit two normal genes.

Although studies can estimate the risk of developing cancer among large numbers of people who have an inherited mutation, they cannot assess the risk for individual women. Between 5 to 10% of breast cancers are suggested to be linked to changes in BRCA1 and BRCA2 genes and it is suggested that close to 80% of women are at risk for breast cancer when they have these gene changes, a risk that increases with age. Recent research in the *British Journal of Cancer* cites that low levels of BRCA are found in cancerous cells, and from this work we may be able to infer that higher levels might well prevent cancer from developing. What is particularly important here, and what brings us full circle and back to my point about cancer-fighting foods, is that due to indole-3-carbinol and genistein's ability to boost BRCA expression, we now know that foods containing these compounds can, at least theoretically, reduce the risk of cancer.[16]

Research performed at the Department of Food Science at Cornell University supports this theory. The Cornell studies reveal that regular consumption of fruits and vegetables is strongly associated with reduced risk of developing chronic diseases, such as cancer and cardiovascular disease. Researchers state that the effects of phytochemicals in fruits and vegetables are responsible for potent antioxidant and anticancer activities and that the benefit of a diet rich in fruits and vegetables is attributed to the complex mixture of phytochemicals present in whole foods.[17]

Grapefruits, oranges, and other citrus fruits have a high vitamin C content, itself a powerful antioxidant in the fight against cancer, and consumption of phytochemical-rich green and yellow vegetables has been associated with reducing the incidence of some cancers. Broccoli, cauliflower, Brussels sprouts, and cabbage, in particular, contain two antioxidants, lutein and zeaxanthin, which stimulate the body's own antioxidant enzymes, such as superoxide dismutase, a naturally occurring enzyme that protects cells from superoxide "free radicals." In doing so, these antioxidants are thought to help decrease the risk for prostate cancer. We will discuss free radicals further in Chapter Four; for now, suffice to say that free radicals are atoms that are highly active, unstable, and prone to attack any cell in the body, and that it is superoxide dismutase that works to catalyze the destruction of free oxygen radicals and thereby prevent further cellular destruction.

There comes a time when we all need to examine our dietary choices, to question whether the choices we're making are helping us or hindering us, increasing or decreasing our risks relative to cancer. The Western diet is generally a high-fat, refined-carbohydrate diet, a diet rich in animal protein and low in fiber, fruits, vegetables, and water consumption. Basically, this is the worst kind of diet for living a healthy life. Consistently choosing this kind of diet over time is likely to result in an overall "dis-ease" in the body. And when the body is in a state of dis-ease—in other words, when it is out of balance—it's not a far leap to increasing the risk for illness and chronic disease. From the perspective of my own experience, and in the words of Thomas Edison, one of this country's greatest inventors, "The doctor of the future will give no medicine, but will interest his patients in care of the human frame, diet, and in the cause and prevention of disease."

Foods that can hurt us

We've already started the conversation about certain foods that can be very beneficial to our health. Given the natural balance of all things, the yin and yang of it, so to speak, we can only expect that the reverse is true: that eating the "wrong" foods can be detrimental if they are eaten consistently over time. Indeed, the American Cancer Society estimates that approximately one third of cancer deaths may be diet related.[18] That is a huge statistic, all the more powerful since diet is one thing (as much as we hate to admit it) that, as adults, we can control.

Trans fats. Let's consider trans fats, or so-called *trans fatty acids*, for instance. Trans fats are used in the cooking process in many commercial food preparations and therefore consistently land on our supermarket shelves. Trans fatty acids form naturally in some foods, such as beef and dairy products, or are created artificially by the food industry. It is the artificial trans fats that wreak so much havoc. Artificial trans fats are formed by hydrogenating vegetable oil and converting it from a liquid to a solid. This type of fat is routinely used to add texture and flavor and to increase the shelf life of the foods that line our grocery shelves. Trans fats are typically found in things like cookies, crackers, icing, potato chips, stick margarine, and microwave popcorn—products most of us love to eat. The process of hydrogenation adds hydrogen gas to liquid, causing the molecular structure to reconfigure into a solid until ultimately it resembles plastic more than an actual food. Due to their unnatural molecular structure, hydrogenated fats can all too easily contribute to clogging of the arteries. Clogged arteries increase the risk of heart disease, stroke, and other diseases.

Nitrates. *Nitrates* are compounds used in preserving meats, but they can also be detrimental to our health. The use of nitrates in food preservation is controversial due to the potential for the formation of *nitrosamines*, well-known cancer-causing agents, when the preserved food is cooked at high temperature. Therefore, the use of nitrates is carefully regulated; in the U.S., for example, the concentration of nitrates and nitrites is generally limited to 200 ppm or lower.

Though research has blatantly shown a higher incidence of cancer in children who consume more preservative-laced, processed, and fast foods, food additives continue to be present in much of the food in the typical American diet. Preservatives are added during the food process to add shelf life—the time it takes to go from the manufacturer to the consumer. Believe it or not, most colorings, flavorings, and preservatives are known to be derivatives of petroleum, and for that reason cannot even be classified as food substances. Synthetic food colorings, also common in processed foods, have been shown to cause DNA changes, even in small doses. And although most fast food restaurants continue to freely lace their cooking oil with preservatives to make the oil last longer, some of these preservatives are well known to promote carcinogenesis in rats.

When the FDA approves the addition of additives to our food supply, we can only assume that those chemical agents are free of risks to human health. Unfortunately, this is not always the case. In one study conducted by the Environmental Toxicology Program of the National Institute of Environmental Health Sciences, for example, Food and Drug Administration-approved food additives were examined for human consumption using rodent testing. In this study of 50 additive samples *that had been approved by the FDA*, 40% were found to be carcinogenic.[19] Researchers of this study stated that if this percentage were extrapolated to all substances added to food in the United States, it would imply that there are more than 1,000 that are potential rodent carcinogens.

Dietary factors are estimated to account for approximately 30% of cancers in Western countries, making diet second only to tobacco as a preventable cause of cancer. The World Health Organization tells us that today's typical Western diet was virtually unknown to humans even a few generations ago. The "affluent" diet today has twice the amount of saturated fat, a third of the daily fiber it had in the past, is high in sugar and salt, low in nutrients, and high in preservatives. The food industry boasts 4,000-plus additives, such as coal tar dyes, emulsifiers, flavor enhancers, and stabilizers. Unaware of—or unconcerned about—both the sheer magnitude of the preservatives in our food, let alone the other additives which can have such deleterious effects, current generations are consuming them on a regular basis—usually daily.

The effects of this lack of concern are significant. For instance, when the Department of Child Health at the University of Southampton examined the relationship of artificial food color and food additives on childhood behavior, it was found that a diet containing both artificial color and food additives resulted in increased hyperactivity in three-year-old and eight- to nine-year-old children in the general population.[20] Paul Stitt has years of experience in American food factories and has written about various food processes in his book, *Beating the Food Giants*.[21] According to Stitt, in order to make the shaped cereals children (and adults!) love so much, the products have to undergo a method of "extrusion," a process that subjects them to very high temperatures and pressure in order to produce the shapes, flakes, and puffed grains. Stitt states that there are two unpublished studies that clearly indicate extruded grains are toxic, particularly to the nervous system. To make matters worse, the cereals that contain these grains are generally high in sugar and low in fiber. To gain a bit more perspective, consider that a small-sized packet of potato chips contains approximately 4 tsp of fat and a 12-oz can of Coke contains about 10 tsp of sugar. Cereals are not excluded from such content. Unfortunately, this is typical of the decisions our food industry continues to make today.

As per the 1958 Food Additives Amendment, added to the Federal Food, Drug and Cosmetic (FD&C) Act of 1938, the Food and Drug Administration is the responsible party for approving the use and safety of all food additives. The FDA must continually monitor foods on the market due to the constant additions in the field. In November of 1973, for example, the FDA established guidelines for nitrates and nitrites (mentioned above), the substances found in packaging mixes and used for curing meat products.[22]

In April, 2002, a conference in Geneva by the World Health Organization confirmed that at that time there were over 100 deep fried, lightly fried, or baked foods in the marketplace that likely contained a chemical compound called acrylamide.[23] Acrylamide, a by-product of the cooking process, has been found to induce tumors in rats and mice at a number of different sites.[23]

After reading these findings and numerous others in the same vein, I came to the conclusion that my health would be better served by avoiding these types of foods whenever I could, and by sticking with things more "natural." The less processed, the less tampered with, the better it would be for all aspects of my health. Consistently working to become educated in order to reduce my risk for the recurrence of cancer has always been my goal. The knowledge that not smoking, eating well, and exercising can lower this risk by almost 65% (according to the National Cancer Institute) is what has continued to motivate me.

In my opinion, more emphasis needs to be focused on all of these health issues in this country—especially diet. "We are what we eat" is a phrase that became popular years ago, and how true it is. Just look at the fact that average Americans today expend far fewer calories through their activities as they did 20 years ago, yet are taking in, on average, about 200 more calories each day.[24]

This is not to say that so-called "natural foods" are free from our concern. The use of pesticides on fruits and vegetables can have a detrimental effect on a person's health as well.

Pesticides. Since 1971, more than 900 chemical agents have been evaluated by the International Agency for Research on Cancer, of which approximately 400 have been identified as carcinogenic, or potentially carcinogenic, to humans. Current levels of pesticides sprayed on produce have been shown to cause cancer, yet many of these pesticides are still in use. In one study, researchers examined the relationship between 45 common agricultural pesticides and prostate cancer incidence in 55,332 male pesticide applicators, workers from Iowa and North Carolina who had no prior history of prostate cancer. Researchers found evidence that the men's work with pesticides increased their risk of prostate cancer, and that this risk was more pronounced in those participants with a family history of the same type of cancer.[25] Other studies have also found a link between exposure to pesticides and childhood cancer, where malignancies linked to pesticides include leukemia, neuroblastoma, Wilms' tumor, soft-tissue sarcoma, Ewing's sarcoma, non-Hodgkin's lymphoma, and cancers of the brain, colorectum, and testes.[26] Researchers have therefore concluded that the potential to prevent at least some childhood cancer exists by reducing or eliminating pesticide exposure. If this is true, then taking the time to wash the produce we buy in order to limit the amount of pesticide residue we ingest may lower our exposure to and risk for cancer.

Doing our part to increase our awareness can only increase the chances that we will ultimately incorporate a healthier diet, a major contributor in preventing illnesses like cancer. That and the promise of new drugs, therapies, and treatments make me confident that we will find ways to finally cure cancer completely in my lifetime. Finding a cure, however, is only half the battle. The other half is teaching people how they can reduce their risk and prevent cancer altogether. Over the past three decades I have been living the second half of the battle as it has slowly unfolded for me, and sharing my experiences and knowledge is my way of helping other people in similar situations. But it has also become obvious to me that funding for lowering cancer risk must be so small as to be virtually non-existent, given the fact that I have never received one email, flyer, ad, or brochure, nor have I seen one television commercial, that focuses on informing the general public for the express purpose of reducing the risk for cancer.

Personally affronted by what I perceived then to be a severe lack in the dissemination of this kind of information, I began my own grass-roots educational "program." I needed to feel I was personally contributing to reducing the risk of cancer through education. Through the years, I began to speak to various groups at organizational meetings and in libraries, and was soon receiving invitations to be a guest lecturer at events sponsored by the American Cancer Society and Cancer Care. Consequently, my already over-burdened office staff has since put in countless hours of typing, photocopying, and collating massive amounts of material to distribute free of charge to the general public. I have found my talks to be well received, as audiences seem to have the same hunger for information as I had 30 years ago, and want to know more so they can do more for themselves. Somehow I have become a voice for the second half of the cancer equation: risk reduction and prevention.

Over time I was gathering and reviewing reams of information and becoming familiar with all of it, yet I was still trying to find clarity. I inherently knew that the most important thing was to dedicate myself to—and stay with—only the things that made sense to me, the things that seemed right. Slowly I began to incorporate those changes into my daily living. I consciously took control to the best of my ability, making the choice to manage the things I could control, which included many aspects of my own health, such as the things I did every day. Since I am currently over 30 years recovered, I can confidently say that my choices have been good ones.

It is true that I was forced into change by circumstance. I certainly had to do things that I would not have ordinarily done. Mark Twain once said, "The only way to keep your health is to eat what you don't want, drink what you don't like, and do what you'd rather not," and that's exactly how I felt. I know I would never have committed to even the small, steady, incremental changes I made unless I had been diagnosed with cancer—in other words, without cancer as the catalyst. I may never have tried to adopt different approaches to food and exercise under any other conditions. Under "normal" circumstances I sincerely doubt a 19-year-old teenager would have woken up at the crack of dawn to go running, taken a few minutes to quietly meditate, made time to eat a healthy breakfast, and used breathing techniques to achieve stress-reduction while studying. Most college students don't think about "positively" socializing with family and friends, don't look forward to weekly visits with the chiropractor, and don't prepare fresh vegetables cooked in a wok at the close of every day. But most college students don't have to deal with the possibility that cancer may return to claim their lives.

It is clear that my life's lesson was to be learned under these circumstances. So, while the transition was at best awkward at first, I stayed with the program. I overcame my daily resistance to sticking with it, and the results far outweighed any and all of my initial resistance to the changes I made. I was determined to NEVER go back to where I had been. Soon I saw myself benefiting both mentally and physically from my choices, and I continue to enjoy the same type of routine to this day. *Health now and forever* has become my mantra, and its pursuit continues to be an integral part of my life.

The seeds of thought planted in the mind of a 19-year-old have been continually growing. These thoughts have converted into experiences, and sharing those thoughts and experiences with others along the way has become a mission. The undeniable truth of research-based evidence has provided an ongoing, ever-changing set of guidelines through which I have been able to help others diagnosed with cancer by sharing information, support, hope, and confidence. It is my preference, and perhaps yours, to think not so much about surviving cancer as about winning over cancer—in other words, living a normal, healthy life in the best way you can.

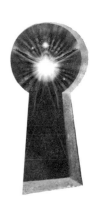

3. The Truth About Cancer

What is cancer?

A brief history

The use of the word *cancer* is credited to the Greek physician we talked about earlier, Hippocrates, who was considered instrumental in lifting medicine out of the realms of magic, superstition, and religion. The word cancer itself is derived from the Greek word *karkinos*, meaning "crab," due to the fact that when malignant tumors spread into adjoining tissue they tend to resemble the claws of a crab. According to the American Cancer Society, cancer is described as "a group of diseases characterized by uncontrolled growth and spread of abnormal cells." Ultimately, if the spread of these "abnormal" cells continues, the body weakens until death ensues. The word "cancer" also serves as an umbrella term for close to 200 other diseases.

The incidence of cancer is not something that has become prevalent solely in recent times. In fact, cancer has afflicted people for many centuries. For example, the bony remains of mummies in ancient Egypt show evidence of *osteosarcoma*, or bone cancer, and the *Edwin Smith Surgical Papyrus*, the only surviving copy of part of an ancient Egyptian textbook on trauma surgery and one of the world's earliest surviving examples of medical literature, describes cases of tumors, or "ulcers" of the breast, for which there was no cure. Apparently, at that time the tumors were actually cauterized with a tool the Egyptians called the "fire drill." The understanding and treatment of cancer has naturally progressed over the centuries due to a greater understanding of the workings of the human body, and it is from this knowledge that new discoveries have been made. Galileo and Newton led the way with groundbreaking objective scientific approaches, and are considered the first advocates for the use of experimental and scientific methods, as opposed to speculation and reason alone.

Scientists began to understand the process of blood circulation from the autopsies performed by Dr. William Harvey in Europe in 1628. By the 1760s, the work of Giovanni Morgagni had revealed, also through autopsies, that anatomical pathological findings were consistent with the illnesses of the deceased. This direct link between human anatomy and illness was said to be the beginning of *oncology*, or the study of cancer. It was in the late 1700s that Dr. John Hunter, a famous Scottish surgeon, proposed the theory that cancerous tumors could be treated and removed through operative procedures if they had not yet spread to other tissues. Almost a century later, Hunter's hypothesis would be proven correct when the advent of anesthesia made it possible to remove cancerous growths with surgical intervention. In the 1800s, the discovery of the modern microscope not only brought us one step further with the study of cellular pathology relative to the clinical course of illness, but the pioneering work of Dr. Rudolf Virchow, considered the "father of pathology," helped oncologists advance in their understanding of the pathology of cancer to the degree that they were now able to treat more specific forms of the disease. These and other advances continue to enable pathologists to aid surgeons in knowing when tumors are isolated or have spread to other areas in the body.

How cancer "works"

Cancer originates within a single cell. This cell will grow and divide as all cells do. It is when cells grow in an "uncontrolled" way that the formation of a tumor is initiated. Normal body cells grow, divide, and eventually die in a process known as *apoptosis*. Cancer cells, on the other hand, grow, continue to divide, and form more and more abnormal cells. Growing out of control and invading other tissues are the attributes that make a cell a cancer cell.

Because every cell in the body contains *deoxyribonucleic acid*, or *DNA*, and this DNA contains the genetic instructions that direct all the functions of our cells, when DNA becomes damaged the human body must have a way to repair it. It turns out that our bodies do indeed have this capability—but only to a point. It is when the damage cannot be effectively repaired that the cell becomes "mutated"; that is, unable to follow the coded instructions it was originally meant to follow. As a result, the cell begins to behave differently. Usually this kind of damage to the DNA is caused by one of two processes. The first is a "mistake" that occurs when a cell copies its DNA in preparation for cell division; the second is due to the effect of an environmental agent, such as ultraviolet light, cigarette smoke, x-rays, or certain chemicals. Though many cancers start with the formation of a tumor or growth, some cancers, such as leukemia, do not. Rather, in leukemia, cancer cells form in the blood and blood-forming organs and then spread to other tissues. Tumors, however, are not always cancerous. Non-cancerous, or *benign*, tumors do not grow in an uncontrolled manner, do not invade surrounding tissues, and do not metastasize. With very rare exceptions these types of tumors are not life threatening.

Classification "cancer"

Cancer can either be classified by the type of cell in which it originates or by the location of the cell in the body. Cancer cells can fragment, seep, or overflow from the primary tumor site and travel through the lymphatic system or the bloodstream to end up in other tissues of the body. This process is called *metastasis*. In such cases, the part of the body where the cancer originated determines the name of the cancer. For example, if cancer spreads from the breast to the liver, it is known as metastatic breast cancer. If cancer spreads from the prostate to the brain, it is considered metastatic prostate cancer. Cancer grows differently in various parts of the body and, as a result, great care is taken in determining the precise type of treatment, which is always distinct relative to the particular type of cancer involved.

Developing an individual treatment plan is crucial for the patient dealing with cancer of any kind. Before treatment can begin, however, the patient's healthcare team must determine if the cancer has spread and, if so, how far. This process is called *staging*. Although staging is time-consuming and involves patience on the part of both patients and families, it helps develop a clearer picture about the most effective treatment protocol. Pathologists then "grade" the cancer cells in terms of abnormality. The type of structural variation involved indicates the rate at which the tumor might grow and spread. Different grading systems are used for different types—and stages—of cancer.

There are various systems of staging. The most utilized is called the TNM system. Each letter provides specific information about the tumor, as follows:

- "T" denotes the tumor
- "TX" means the tumor cannot be evaluated
- "T0" means there is no evidence of the original tumor
- "Tis" means the cancer is *in situ*, or has not spread
- "T1-T4" describes the tumor size and status of the spreading; the higher the number, the more significant the tumor
- "N" denotes the extent to which the cancer has spread to the lymph nodes
- "NX" means the lymph nodes nearby cannot be evaluated
- "N0" means there is no evidence of cancer in the nearby lymph nodes
- "N1-N3" describes the status of the spreading lymph nodes (location, size, and number of lymph nodes involved); the higher the number, the more significant the lymph node status
- "M" denotes whether the cancer has spread, or metastasized, beyond the lymph nodes to different organs in the body

- "MX" means distant spreading cannot be evaluated
- "M0" means there is no evidence of spreading
- "M1" means spreading has been found

Each of these letters may be followed by numbers or letters, which provide more details about the characteristics of the tumor. For example, a "T1, N1, M0" cancer means the patient has a T1 tumor, N1 lymph-node involvement, and no distant metastases. A tumor classified as "T2, N0, M0" means it is slightly bigger than in the first example, with no lymph-node involvement or metastases. Once the TNM system establishes the extent to which the cancer has spread, it can then be grouped under the system of Roman Numeral Staging I-IV, used to reflect the progression of the cancer, with "I" being the lowest and "IV" being the highest.

Who gets cancer?

Theoretically, anyone at any age can get cancer, and it is true that more than a million people are affected by cancer every year. In the United States, one out of every two men and one out of every two women is at risk of getting cancer at some point in their lives, and over 50% of all cancers diagnosed occur in people age 55 and older. The risk factors associated with getting cancer can be environmental, physical, and/or related to lifestyle. Lifestyle trends that can contribute to the risk of getting cancer include use of tobacco and/or alcohol, an unhealthy diet, exposure to some viruses, prolonged exposure to sunlight or ionizing radiation, an overweight physique, and lack of physical activity. These factors play a major role in cancer incidence, but can be controlled to a significant degree.

Most skin cancers, for example, can be highly prevented by taking protective measures against exposure to the sun, and cancers related to viral infections can often be controlled through the use of certain vaccines and through behavioral changes. Avoidance of smoking, limiting alcohol consumption, and eating healthfully are other ways of lowering one's risk. Other factors are not quite as easy to change, such as the physical aspects of age, gender, and family medical history. Environmental factors, such as toxic substances from consumer products, building materials, additives or contaminants in food or drinking water, and pollutants in indoor air and urban environments also continue to play a significant role in cancer risk, not only in this country, but throughout the world.

What, exactly, is a "risk factor"? On the American Cancer Society's website (*www.cancer. org*), a risk factor is defined as "anything that increases a person's chance of getting a disease." Although it is true that having one or more risk factors does not necessarily mean an individual will contract cancer in the future, it is also impossible to eliminate the chances of getting cancer, even when there are no apparent risk factors present.

If an individual does get cancer, the period during which the cancer responds to treatment—that is, when the signs and symptoms of the disease are noticeably reduced—is said to be a time of *partial remission*. If the signs and symptoms of the disease completely recede, the cancer is said to be in *total remission*. Cancer can be in remission from a period of several weeks to many years. If complete remission lasts for several years, meaning any sign of cancer is absent on tests, scans, and examination, then the cancer may be considered to be "cured." However, even after a cure the disease may return after a period of time, and then once again go into remission after further treatment (which may consist of different therapies or a different combination of drugs).

Having lived through the disease of cancer myself, my unwavering desire to know more about it has never abated. Knowing that an otherwise healthy teenager could suddenly get sick taught me that no one is impervious to some degree of risk. On the other hand, all my research—via countless books, journals, and periodicals—and all my conversations with various groups, patients, families, doctors, and social workers have made it perfectly clear that one's risk of getting cancer can be reduced, if not completely avoided. I have come to the conclusion and am of the strong conviction that although some people are more likely to develop cancer than others due to race, social standing, and/or environmental factors, cancer is *not* simply a disease of "genetics." In fact, in most cases, I believe cancer is a disease of lifestyle.

By undertaking this massive search for the truth about cancer, I learned how much research is currently underway by dedicated scientists. Dedicated researchers put in countless hours, eagerly in pursuit of knowledge and cures for life-threatening diseases, including cancer. With the 21st century in full swing, technology has made information available from innumerable sources at the click of a finger, and this has enabled me to access vast amounts of data, leaving me nothing short of awestruck by the number of committed organizations that provide information to the general public. These include the American Cancer Society (ACS, at *www.cancer.org*), the National Cancer Institutes (NCI, at *www.cancer.gov*), Surveillance Epidemiology and End Results (SEER, at *www.seer.cancer.gov*), the Centers for Disease Control and Prevention (CDC, at *www.CDC.gov*), United States Cancer Statistics (UPCS, at *www.apps. nccd.cdc.gov/uscs/*), and Cancer Research UK (at *www.cancerresearchuk.org*), to name just a few. What I have attempted in the pages of this book is to review as many sources as possible, in order to cull the critical information for you. I am compelled to read, learn, and share as much as I can and in as many ways as I can. That is my intention and the goal is simple: to be of service to as many people as possible by sharing what I know about the disease of cancer.

How far we've come

It was in December of 1971 when President Nixon declared a war on cancer and signed the National Cancer Act into existence in his State of the Union address. This act was written to amend the Public Health Service Act and to allow the National Cancer Institute to carry out the national effort against cancer. It was a bold initiative to bring public awareness to what was the second leading cause of death in the United States. Since that time, the federal government and various other organizations and companies have spent roughly $200 billion looking for a cure for cancer, with mixed results. The majority of funding for cancer has gone into the eradication of malignant cells, rather than ways to keep normal cells from becoming malignant. What researchers have realized through this process is that no magic bullet yet exists, as indicated by this statement posted on the NCI website: "The biology of the more than 100 types of cancers has proven far more complex than imagined."

Despite the obvious complex nature of cancer there is some good news on the horizon. The American Cancer Society's *Cancer Statistics 2009* report noted a 19.2% drop in cancer death rates among men from 1990 to 2005, as well as an 11.4% drop in women's cancer death rates during the same period. Overall, cancer death rates fell 2% per year from 2001 to 2005 in men and 1.6% per year from 2002 to 2005 in women. By comparison, between 1993 and 2001, overall death rates declined 1.5% per year in men and, between 1994 and 2002, 0.8% per year in women. Strategic Director for Cancer Surveillance at the American Cancer Society and the report's author, Ahmedin Jemal, reflected on these statistics by saying, "We continue to see a decrease in death rates from cancer in both men and women and this is mainly because of prevention—mostly a reduction in smoking rates; detection, which includes screening for colorectal cancer, for breast cancer, and for cervical cancer; and also improved treatment." These improved mortality statistics are encouraging, but cancer incidence continues to remain powerfully steep. The message? There is much, much more work to be done.

How far we have to go

The World Health Organization's *World Cancer Report* estimates that by 2020, 15 million new cancer cases will be detected globally—an increase of close to 50%![1] And while I understand the great need for the focus on curing cancer, I also feel that with more emphasis on risk reduction this incidence rate could be greatly reduced. How? By educating and informing the general public of the abundant evidence that a healthy lifestyle—consisting of exercise, a low-fat diet, adequate dietary consumption of fruits and vegetables, minimal alcohol consumption, and abstinence from smoking—lowers the risk of developing lung cancer, breast cancer, colon cancer, and prostate cancer, to name only a few of the most common cancers. Research points toward the fact that prevention would avert close to 60% of all cancer development simply through changes in lifestyle, physical activity, and tobacco use. Admittedly, there *has* been a greater effort in recent years to educate people about the health risks of tobacco addiction, and about regular screenings for breast, cervical, colorectal, and prostate cancers. However, as indicated by the staggering statistics cited by the World Health Organization, this effort has clearly not gone far enough.

In general, the overall health status in the United States is improving with regard to most diseases, with the exception of some of the more chronic ones. Studies have shown, for example, that over the past century the nation has defeated many infectious diseases. Improved sanitation, hygiene, vaccines, and better-quality drinking water have made the American life safer. Childhood diseases, such as measles and mumps, and water-borne ailments, such as typhoid and cholera, have, for the most part been eradicated. The major shift is that now most adults are dying from chronic illnesses rather than from infectious diseases; currently more than 60% of all U.S. deaths are now attributed to diseases of the heart, blood vessels, and cancer.

As noted above, national cancer deaths are on the decline. However, cancer is still the second leading cause of death in the United States, and the number of people being diagnosed continues to rise. In fact, it is hard to believe that in the early 1900s the number of cancer and cardiovascular deaths was much lower than it is today. At that time heart disease was the fourth leading cause of death, and cancer was the ninth! Back then, the leading causes of death were pneumonia, influenza, tuberculosis, and gastrointestinal disorders. Now, almost 100 years later, we can see that heart disease is responsible for over 40% of deaths, while cancer is responsible for 25% (see Figure 3-1). That means that an unbelievable 65% of all deaths in this country can be attributed to either heart disease or cancer. But, despite all these changes, life expectancy continues to improve. In 1900, life expectancy was 47.9 years for males and 50.7 years for females; in 2010, life expectancy is projected at an all-time high for both genders: 75.7 years for men and 80.8 years for women.[2,3]

However, while we may be living longer, chronic diseases are now becoming plague-like, both in sheer numbers and in intensity. As discussed, the causes of health problems are many, from physical elements to unhealthy lifestyles to environmental pollutants. Though overall death rates have dropped for some types of cancers, such as breast, leukemia, cervical, stomach, and uterine, the number of people who develop cancer each year has actually increased since 1973. And although leukemia rates have declined in adults, they have not declined in children.

stomach, and uterine, the number of people who develop cancer each year has actually increased since 1973. And although leukemia rates have declined in adults, they have not declined in children.

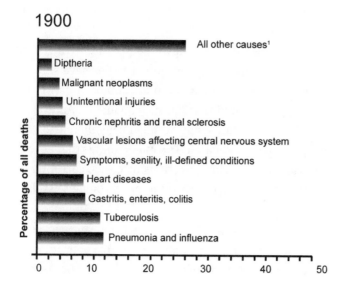

FIGURE 3-1. Causes of death in the United States, 1900 and 1998. (Source: Centers for Disease Control, National Center for Chronic Disease Prevention and Health Promotion. *Unrealized Prevention Opportunities: Reducing the Health and Economic Burden of Chronic Disease,* November, 2000. Data for 1990 from U.S. Bureau of the census; data for 1998 from National Center for Health Statistics.) [1]Other causes may include typhoid fever, measles, homicide, suicide, syphilis, and diabetes. [2]Includes cirrhosis. [3]Other causes may include motor vehicle accidents, AIDS/HIV, septicemia, Alzheimer's and Parkinson's disease.

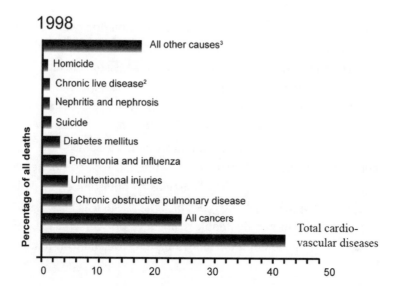

It is very clear from Figure 3-1 that the majority of Americans are threatened with cardiovascular disease as well as any number of types of cancer. In 2007, according to the CDC, there were 2,423,712 deaths registered in the United States. Out of this number, a staggering 616,067 were attributable to diseases of the heart, while 562,875 were due to cancer. Stroke (cerebral vascular disease) caused 135,952 deaths and chronic lower respiratory diseases caused 127,924 deaths. There were 123,706 deaths from accidents, 74,632 deaths from Alzheimer's disease, 71,382 from diabetes, 52,717 deaths from influenza and pneumonia, 46,448 deaths from nephritis, nephrotic syndrome, and nephrosis, and 34,828 deaths from septicemia. Admittedly, as we get older, the odds to contract some of these diseases (or experience related illnesses) increase, particularly after the age of 55.[4]

Cancer has been found to inversely relate to level of education, income, social class, and, in some instances, race, where incidence rates are higher among the poor and less educated. One report, published by the National Cancer Institute, explains the relationship between socioeconomic status and increased incidence of cancer mortality. This report cited that low socioeconomic status was associated with higher mortality, and that minimal leisure, physical activity, poor diet, and a higher incidence of smoking among the lesser-educated and lower-income groups were some of the conditions responsible for the inverse relationship. The report also indicated that certain types of cancers, such as those of the lung, breast, and melanoma, have been documented to be associated with low socioeconomic status, where a lack of insurance, lack of access to care, and lack of information about cancer prevention contributed to an overall increased risk.[5] One British obstetrician as far back as 1902 made the connection between economic status and health when he uncovered the fact that cervical cancer was more prevalent among poor, overworked, underfed, and abused woman. One reported reason for this higher occurrence is that under-educated and low-income groups generally forego regular screenings and see a doctor only in the advanced stages of disease as compared to their more affluent and more educated counterparts. Hence, disease progression is often found to be lower in the group that visits a doctor for regular screenings and early detection. Furthermore, lower-income groups generally have less opportunity for preventive care due to the lack of proper coverage, demands of employment, and limited time relative to child-care concerns.

From 1975 to 1999, accumulated evidence from studies over the years prompted the then director of the National Cancer Institute to state that "poverty is a carcinogen," pointing to the fact that an individual's work environment, which many times is defined by education and social background, can play a role in increasing the risk of cancer due to exposure to occupational carcinogens in the form of unhealthy conditions. Long hours and low wages can also contribute to the potential for an individual to be more physically tired, eat an unbalanced diet, and forego regular check-ups. Cancers of the oral cavity, esophagus, larynx, liver, and bladder specifically have shown a high probability of association with low socioeconomic status and continue to be investigated. A notable exception to these facts is breast cancer, where the incidence is more prevalent in women of higher socioeconomic status. This increased incidence may be due to reproductive patterns, such as delayed childbirth, genetic factors, or dietary factors. Despite the increased incidence, however, affluent women also show above-average survival rates, due at least in part to better access to information, treatment facilities, and early detection.

We see an unequal distribution of cancer not only with regard to education and social status, but also in reference to specific races as well. African Americans have the highest death rate and shortest survival rate of any racial or ethnic group in the U.S. for most cancers. In 2005, the death rate for all cancers combined continued to be 33% higher in African American men and 16% higher in African American women than in white men and women.[6]

The statistics (by number and percentage) in Table 3-1 from the American Cancer Society show the leading sites of new cancer cases and deaths by gender in the United States for the year 2010.[7] Cancer of the prostate, lung and bronchus, and colon and rectum account for an estimated total of 52% of new cancer cases in men. Prostate cancer constitutes a significant percentage at 28%. Among women, the three most common cancers in the year 2010 are breast, lung and bronchus, and colon and rectum, accounting for about 52% of all cases. Breast cancer alone constitutes 28% of all new cases.

In Table 3-2 you will find statistics that reveal the estimated number of *new* cases and deaths of both males and females relative to cancer sites for the year 2010.

TABLE 3-1. Leading sites of new cancer cases and deaths by gender in the United States—2010 estimates.* (Source: American Cancer Society, Surveillance and Health Policy Research 2010, at *www.cancer.org*)

Estimated new cases by site, male*		Estimated new cases by site, female*	
Prostate	217,730 (28%)	Breast	207,090 (28%)
Lung and bronchus	116,750 (15%)	Lung and bronchus	105,770 (14%)
Colon and rectum	72,090 (9%)	Colon and rectum	70,480 (10%)
Urinary bladder	52,760 (7%)	Uterine corpus	43,470 (6%)
Melanoma of the skin	38,870 (5%)	Non-Hodgkin lymphoma	30,160 (4%)
Non-Hodgkin lymphoma	35,380 (4%)	Melanoma of the skin	29,260 (4%)
Kidney and renal pelvis	35,370 (4%)	Thyroid	33,930 (4%)
Leukemia	24,690 (3%)	Kidney and renal pelvis	22,870 (3%)
Oral cavity and pharynx	25,420 (3%)	Ovary	21,880 (3%)
Pancreas	21,370 (3%)	Pancreas	21,770 (3%)
ALL SITES	**789,620 (100%)**	**ALL SITES**	**739,940 (100%)**

(continued on next page)

Estimated deaths by site, male		Estimated deaths by site, female	
Lung and bronchus	86,220 (29%)	Lung and bronchus	71,080 (26%)
Prostate	32,050 (11%)	Breast	39,840 (15%)
Colon and rectum	26,580 (9%)	Colon and rectum	24,790 (9%)
Pancreas	18,770 (6%)	Pancreas	18,030 (7%)
Leukemia	12,660 (4%)	Ovary	13,850 (5%)
Liver and intrahepatic bile duct	12,720 (4%)	Non-Hodgkin lymphoma	9,500 (4%)
Esophagus	11,650 (4%)	Leukemia	9,180 (3%)
Urinary bladder	10,410 (3%)	Uterine corpus	7,950 (3%)
Non-Hodgkin lymphoma	10,710 (4%)	Liver and intrahepatic bile duct	6,190 (2%)
Kidney and renal pelvis	8,210 (3%)	Brain and other nervous system	5,720 (2%)
ALL SITES	**299,200 (100%)**	**ALL SITES**	**270,290 (100%)**

*Excludes basal and squamous cell skin cancers and *in situ* carcinoma except urinary bladder.

TABLE 3-2. Estimated new cancer cases and deaths by gender in the United States in 2010.* (Source: American Cancer Society, Surveillance and Health Policy Research 2010, at *www.cancer.org*)

	Estimated new cases			Estimated deaths		
	Both sexes	Male	Female	Both sexes	Male	Female
ALL SITES	1,529,560	789,620	739,940	569,490	299,200	270,290
Oral cavity and pharynx	36,540	25,420	11,120	7,880	5,430	2,450
Digestive system	274,330	148,540	125,790	139,580	79,010	60,570
Respiratory system	240,610	130,600	110,010	161,670	89,550	72,120
Bones and joints	2,650	1,530	1,120	1,460	830	630
Soft tissue (including heart)	10,520	5,680	4,840	3,920	2,020	1,900
Skin (excluding basal and squamous)	74,010	42,610	31,400	11,790	7,910	3,880
Breast	209,060	1,970	207,090	40,230	390	39,840
Genital system	311,210	227,460	83,750	60,420	32,710	27,710
Urinary system	131,260	89,620	41,640	28,550	19,110	9,440
Eye and orbit	2,480	1,240	1,240	230	120	110
Brain and other nervous system	22,020	11,980	10,040	13,140	7,420	5,720

(continued on next page)

Endocrine system	46,930	11,890	35,040	2,570	1,140	1,430
Lymphoma	74,030	40,050	33,980	21,530	11,450	10,080
Myeloma	20,180	11,170	9,010	10,650	5,760	4,890
Leukemia	44,790	24,690	18,360	21,840	12,660	9,180
Other and unspecified primary sites‡	30,680	15,170	15,510	44,030	23,690	20,340

*Rounded to the nearest 10; estimated new cases exclude basal and squamous cell skin cancers and *in situ* carcinomas except urinary bladder. About 54,010 female carcinoma *in situ* of the breast and 46,770 melanoma *in situ* will be newly diagnosed in 2010. † Estimated deaths for colon and rectum cancers are combined.‡ More deaths than cases may reflect lack of specificity in recording underlying causes of death on death certificates or an undercount in the case estimate. Source: Estimated new cases are based on 1995-2006 incidence rates from 44 states and the District of Columbia as reported by the North American Association of Central Cancer Registries (NAACCR), representing about 89% of the U.S. population. Estimated deaths are based on data from U.S. Mortality Data, 1969-2007, National Center for Health Statistics, Centers for Disease Control and Prevention, 2010. ©2010, American Cancer Society, Inc., Surveillance and Health Policy Research.

As of January 1, 2010 (the most current statistics available), it is estimated that there are 11.4 million cancer survivors in the United States.[7] This represents approximately 3.8% of the population. Among these survivors, 60% are currently 65 years of age and older. Female breast (23%), prostate (20%), colorectal (10%), and gynecologic (9%) cancers were found to be the most common cancer sites of survivors. Approximately 14% of the 11.4 million estimated cancer survivors were diagnosed 20 or more years ago. Table 3-3 shows state-by-state cancer incidence for all sites throughout the United States. California shows the highest incidence rate with 157,320; the District of Columbia shows the lowest with 2,760.

TABLE 3-3. Estimated new cancer cases by state, 2010. (Source: American Cancer Society, 2010, at *www.cancer.org.*)

States	All sites	States	All sites	States	All sites	States	All sites
Alabama	23,640	Illinois	63,890	Montana	5,570	Rhode Island	5,970
Alaska	2,860	Indiana	33,020	Nebraska	9,230	South Carolina	23,240
Arizona	29,780	Iowa	17,260	Nevada	12,230	South Dakota	4,220
Arkansas	15,320	Kansas	13,550	New Hampshire	7,810	Tennessee	33,070
California	157,320	Kentucky	24,240	New Jersey	48,100	Texas	101,120
Colorado	21,340	Louisiana	20,950	New Mexico	9,210	Utah	9,970
Connecticut	20,750	Maine	8,650	New York	103,340	Vermont	3,720
Delaware	4,890	Maryland	27,700	North Carolina	45,120	Virginia	36,410
District of Columbia	2,760	Massachusetts	36,040	North Dakota	3,300	Washington	34,500
Florida	107,000	Michigan	55,660	Ohio	64,450	West Virginia	10,610
Georgia	40,480	Minnesota	25,080	Oklahoma	18,670	Wisconsin	29,610
Hawaii	6,670	Mississippi	14,330	Oregon	20,750	Wyoming	2,540
Idaho	7,220	Missouri	31,160	Pennsylvania	75,260		
U.S. TOTAL	1,529,560						

Figure 3-2 shows how the progression of selected cancers has fluctuated from 1975 to 2002.[8] For men, prostate cancer rose steadily from approximately 90 per 100,000 to close to 240 per 100,000 until the year 1991, after which it declined to about 170 per 100,000 and, in the year 2002, 180 per 100,000.

FIGURE 3-2 (a). Annual age adjusted cancer incidence rates among **women** for selected cancer sites in the U.S. from 1975 to 2002. (Source: SEER Program, Division of Cancer Control and Population Sciences, National Cancer Institute, 2005, at *www.caonline. amcancersoc.org/cgi/content/ full/56/2/106I.*) (right)

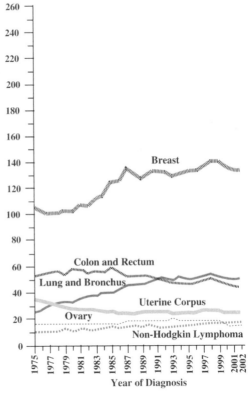

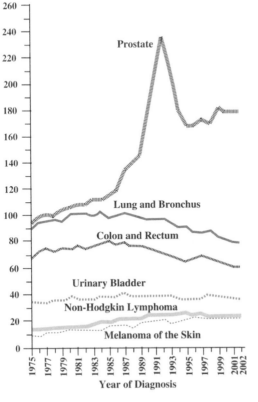

FIGURE 3-2 (b). Annual age adjusted cancer incidence rates among **men** for selected cancer sites in the U.S. from 1975 to 2002. (Source: SEER Program, Division of Cancer Control and Population Sciences, National Cancer Institute, 2005, at *www.caonline. amcancersoc.org/cgi/content/full/56/2/106I.*) (left)

Reviewing the staggering number of new cancer cases throughout the United States, we can calculate that the median age at diagnosis for cancer was 66 years of age. Based on rates from 2005 to 2007, 40.77% of men and women born today will be diagnosed with some type of cancer at some time during their lifetime. Statistically, it appears that 20.59% of men will develop cancer (of some site) between their 50th and 70th birthdays, compared to 15.39% of women.[9]

Geographic variations in cancer incidence and rates are also found between different states. For example, the incidence rate of lung cancer was highest in Kentucky for both men and women; Wyoming had the lowest incidence for men; and Utah had the lowest incidence for women. Tables 3-4 (a) and (b) show the total numbers of cancer cases for both men and women for selected cancer sites in selected areas in the U.S. from 2002 to 2006.[10]

TABLE 3-4 (a). Total cancer cases and average annual age adjusted (2000 U.S. standard) cancer incidence rates[1] for selected cancer sites in selected areas[2] in the United States, 2002-2006, for **males** of all races. (Source: NAACCR *http://www.naaccr.org*)

States	All sites	Bladder	Colon & rectum	Lung & bronchus	Non-Hodgkin lymphoma	Prostate
Alabama	561.2	31.8	61.7	107.8	20.5	154.2
Alaska	529.4	41.6	60.0	84.6	22.6	141.4
Arkansas	562.8	33.0	58.8	111.3	21.8	161.3
Arizona	465.9	35.3	48.9	69.6	18.9	118.9
California	510.1	34.0	52.2	65.1	22.4	149.0
Colorado	501.5	33.6	50.0	60.5	21.0	156.4
Connecticut	591.0	45.4	62.8	81.8	25.8	164.6
Delaware	607.7	42.8	62.0	97.6	23.5	179.9
Florida	537.3	37.4	55.2	89.2	21.6	138.4
Georgia	566.4	32.7	58.7	101.7	20.8	162.4
Hawaii	486.7	26.2	61.3	68.8	19.0	128.6
Idaho	538.4	37.0	49.9	68.7	21.4	165.8
Illinois	579.8	40.7	67.2	92.3	24.1	157.9
Indiana	551.3	37.4	62.8	103.6	22.8	135.9
Iowa	558.9	40.7	64.4.6	89.9	24.4	144.9
Kansas	557.2	36.2	61.3	87.6	24.1	159.6
Kentucky	608.4	39.0	68.0	133.1	23.1	142.5
Louisiana	619.2	35.2	68.5	109.5	23.2	176.8
Maine	620.9	49.4	65.9	99.2	24.5	164.8
Massachusetts	591.8	46.7	63.9	83.7	23.4	164.6
Michigan	597.5	41.9	58.8	93.0	25.2	179.4
Minnesota	567.2	40.1	56.4	69.8	26.4	184.6
Missouri	544.3	35.8	62.3	105.2	21.8	129.3

(continued on next page)

Montana	541.9	40.8	52.5	75.3	22.8	174.5
Nebraska	561.8	37.2	67	84.6	24.7	157.6
Nevada	531.2	40.7	55.2	83.3	22.2	144.2
New Hampshire	584.3	48.0	59.0	82.1	23.5	159.5
New Jersey	603.9	46.2	65.4	79.6	25.6	177.9
New Mexico	480.5	26.7	49.4	57.5	17.9	146.1
New York	577.5	42.3	60.8	79.4	24.7	166.3
North Carolina	553.4	34.9	57.2	101.3	21.2	153.2
North Dakota	549.3	39.6	66.6	74.6	22.7	169.5
Oklahoma	561.4	34.9	60.1	105.6	22.9	150.0
Oregon	529.3	39.2	52.8	79.4	24.4	148.0
Pennsylvania	592.7	44.8	66.1	91.0	25.1	159.7
Rhode Island	608.9	53.1	65.7	92.2	24.8	152.2
South Carolina	587.4	32.4	61.2	102.2	20.7	171.5
South Dakota	547.8	39.1	60.1	78.7	22.1	171.0
Texas	539.6	30.2	57.5	88.3	22.3	144.0
Utah	486.8	28.3	45.3	37.8	22.4	182.2
Virginia	529.5	33.3	55.5	88.5	20.6	155.0
Washington	566.9	41.3	52.6	78.7	27.2	165.3
West Virginia	578.6	39.8	69.5	117.7	22.9	138.6
Wyoming	516.5	42.1	52.0	2.1	21.4	168.0

1 Rates are per 100,000 population and are age adjusted by 5-year age groups to the 2000 U.S. standard population, based on single years of age. Counts and rates are suppressed when fewer than 6 cases were reported for the specific cancer. The suppressed cases, however, are included in the counts and rates for the U.S. combined. Statistics exclude data for AL, LA, and TX from July 2005 through December 2005.

TABLE 3-4 (b). Total cancer cases and average annual age adjusted (2000 U.S. standard) cancer incidence rates1 for selected cancer sites in selected areas in the United States, 2002-2006, for **females** of all races. (Source: NAACCR *http://www.naaccr.org*)

States	All sites	Breast	Colon and rectum	Lung and bronchus	Ovary	Cervix
Alabama	379.6	114.6	42.0	52.9	12.6	8.9
Alaska	417.7	126.4	45.6	64.3	11.8	7.7
Arkansas	383.5	113.1	42.7	59.5	10.9	9.5
California	393.3	122.3	39.2	47.0	13.1	8.4
Colorado	394.1	123.1	39.5	45.2	13.5	6.9
Connecticut	455.5	135.0	46.5	60.1	13.5	6.6
Delaware	440.8	123.9	44.8	70.0	13.5	8.2
Florida	404.2	114.1	41.7	60.3	13.3	9.4
Georgia	392.4	118.5	42.3	53.3	12.6	8.6
Hawaii	383.0	121.4	41.5	40.1	10.7	7.6
Idaho	401.7	117.5	38.0	48.3	12.1	7.2
Illinois	429.1	123.1	48.3	58.8	13.3	9.0

(continued on next page)

Indiana	415.1	115.3	46.4	63.3	12.0	8.2
Iowa	429.2	124.0	49.6	53.1	13.3	7.1
Kansas	417.2	126.1	43.6	53.2	13.0	7.2
Kentucky	446.4	119.8	49.8	76.9	12.2	9.4
Louisiana	409.6	119.6	47.3	57.9	11.8	9.5
Maine	465.8	128.6	48.8	66.0	12.2	7.4
Massachusetts	452.9	132.2	45.7	62.4	13.7	6.1
Michigan	437.9	124.2	44.6	61.5	13.4	7.4
Minnesota	416.4	126.4	42.3	49.5	12.9	6.4
Missouri	417.2	121.9	44.9	63.4	11.9	8.3
Montana	406.3	119.6	40.3	57.4	14.2	6.0
Nebraska	418.2	126.4	47.5	49.3	11.8	7.4
Nevada	412.0	112.1	43.4	69.0	12.6	9.2
New Hampshire	455.3	131.2	44.5	62.7	14.1	6.8
New Jersey	449.5	128.0	48.0	56.0	14.4	9.2
New Mexico	366.1	109.6	35.8	39.0	12.4	8.4
New York	434.4	124.5	45.8	54.1	14.0	8.7
North Carolina	398.1	120.3	41.6	56.0	12.3	8.0
North Dakota	402.7	122.8	43.1	48.0	13.4	6.0
Oklahoma	422.2	127.2	43.7	65.1	13.2	9.0
Oregon	429.7	131.9	41.1	60.4	13.8	6.3
Pennsylvania	444.6	124.5	48.3	56.4	13.8	7.9
Rhode Island	455.3	128.3	46.2	62.2	12.7	7.8
South Carolina	397.5	119.2	44.1	53.0	12.1	8.6
South Dakota	395.3	119.6	44.5	46.3	12.1	6.2
Texas	389.9	114.9	39.7	51.2	12.4	9.7
Utah	346.6	110.0	33.7	23.0	12.5	5.9
Virginia	385.8	120.7	41.8	53.6	12.2	6.8
Washington	443.3	134.8	40.1	59.5	14.3	7.0
West Virginia	437.1	114.7	50.7	70.1	14.1	9.4
Wyoming	392.9	117.8	43.0	47.7	14.3	9.1

1 Rates are per 100,000 population and are age adjusted by 5-year age groups to the 2000 U.S. standard population, based on single years of age. Counts and rates are suppressed when fewer than 6 cases were reported for the specific cancer. The suppressed cases, however, are included in the counts and rates for the U.S. combined. Statistics exclude data for AZ, and from LA, and TX from July 2005 through December 2005.

Cancer worldwide

My questions continued as my research progressed. For instance, was cancer considered epidemic around the world to the same degree it was in this country? I found the following statistics on *www.cancerresearchUK.org*.[11] These worldwide statistics were made available to Cancer Research UK from GLOBOCAN 2008 and published in June 2010. GLOBOCAN is one of the most comprehensive databases available, and provides cancer statistics for all cancers for almost all countries and territories throughout the world.

According to GLOBOCAN, an estimated 12.7 million new cancer cases and 7.6 million deaths occurred in 2008. The most commonly diagnosed cancers worldwide are lung (1.61 million, or 12.7%, of the total), breast (1.38 million, or 10.9%, of the total), and colorectal cancers (1.23 million, or 9.7%, of the total). The most common causes of cancer death are lung (1.38 million, or 18.2%, of the total), stomach (0.74 million, or 9.7%, of the total), and liver cancers (0.69 million, or 9.2%, of the total). GLOBOCAN also provides cancer incidence and mortality projections for the next 20 years. Based on current rates, GLOBOCAN 2008 projects that by 2030, there will be almost 21.4 million new cases diagnosed annually and that there will be over 13.2 million deaths from cancer.

Smoking and cancer

The World Health Organization reports in its *Tobacco Health Toll* publication that globally, one person dies from tobacco use every 6.5 seconds.[12] This translates to the death of approximately 5 million smokers each year, or the equivalent of 13,699 people per day. Cigarettes and other forms of tobacco are addictive, due to the drug nicotine. It is the addition of nicotine to the cigarettes that makes the habit of smoking so hard to break. Smoking has been proven unequivocally to increase the incidence of lung cancer and it is estimated that 85 to 90% of all cases of lung cancer are due to smoking. In fact, smokers are between 20 to 30 times more likely to develop lung cancer than those who are not exposed to tobacco.

Chronic bronchitis, emphysema, and other respiratory diseases are at least 80% related to cigarette smoking. Tobacco use has also been linked to the risk of developing colorectal, liver, pancreatic, and nasal sinuses cancer, as well as leukemia. Long-term and short-term smoking has been found to be associated with a two-fold increase in the risk of certain types of ovarian cancers and is a major risk factor in the development of uterine cervical cancer. Several studies suggest that both passive and active tobacco-smoke exposure cause an increased risk of breast cancer.

Diet

Colon, prostate, and breast cancer cases are found to be more frequent in the United States and other Western countries than in Asia. This is an interesting fact, since we know that compared to Japanese men in Japan, Japanese-American men now have a greater incidence of colon cancer, possibly because they have adopted a Western diet, generally consisting of high animal-protein consumption, fried food, refined grains, high-fat dairy products, and desserts, all of which also create the tendency for weight gain. In general, the Western diet appears to be hazardous for many types of cancers. A diet high in red meat and animal-fat consumption has long been associated with an increase of colon and prostate cancers, for example, and eating an excess of red meat has been linked to DNA damage as well, and an increased risk for bowel cancer. Patients whose diets continue to consist of high amounts of red and processed meats, refined grains, fats, and sugars show a higher recurrence and mortality rate as compared to those whose diets consist mainly of fruits, vegetables, poultry, and fish.[13]

Dana Farber Cancer Center research oncologist Dr. Jeffrey Meyerhardt has suggested that doctors who treat colon cancer patients need to educate their patients about their diets. Meyerhardt says many colon cancer victims seek advice on diet following treatment to improve their outcomes. His advice is to stay away from the "Western dietary pattern" of eating, and he instead recommends a diet rich in fruits, vegetables, whole grains, low-fat dairy, and lean meats. Illustrating this recommendation is a study conducted in the United Kingdom in 2006 with regard to red meat and colorectal cancer. In this case, healthy volunteers who ate various types of diets were studied. When microscopic examination of the cells lining their colons was performed, it was found that the red-meat eaters had a higher level of DNA damage than that of the volunteers on a vegetarian diet. Researchers stated that since red meat increases the endogenous formation of *N*-nitrosocompounds (known to be carcinogenic), diets high in its consumption can be associated with an increased risk for colorectal cancer.[14] While this does not mean that red meat should be avoided altogether, it does suggest that the consumption of anything, including red meat, should be undertaken in moderation.

In 2005, the *Journal of the American Medical Association* published a report in which researchers compiled detailed diet information from almost 150,000 men and women, ages 50 to 74, living in 21 states.[15] A comparison of the data collected in 1982 to that collected in 1992 through 1993 showed that 1,667 of the participants in this study had developed colon cancer. A large sample size and an extended period of data collection supported the fact that consumption of processed and red meat increased the participants' incidence of colorectal cancer. Also noted was that the consumption of poultry and fish over a long period was *inversely* related to the incidence of both distal and proximal colon cancer. So, though red meat alone may not be solely responsible for the development of colon cancer, there is mounting evidence that shows that replacing red meat with fish and poultry can reduce the chances of getting colon cancer—and heart disease as well.

In another study of women's health at Harvard in 2006, it was shown that younger women who consumed red meat regularly had a higher risk of breast cancer.[16] Studying more than 90,000 women, researchers found the consumption of excessive amounts of red meat in their 20s, 30s, and 40s, together with the phases of their naturally occurring hormones, increased the women's risk of developing breast cancer in the next decade. Those women who consumed the most red meat had nearly twice the risk of those who ate red meat infrequently. (Note: This study was found true only for cancers that had receptors for the hormones estrogen and progesterone.)

Pollutants

The National Cancer Institute and the National Institute of Environmental Health Sciences (NIEHS) are two of the 27 institutes that make up the National Institutes of Health. NCI, established in 1937 and the primary agency responsible for cancer research and training, and NIEHS, established in 1966 to reduce illness caused by environmental pollutants, are in agreement that the environment, both natural and man-made, accounts for two thirds of all cancers in the United States. The NIH *10th Report on Carcinogens* lists 228 substances that are either suspected to cause cancer or have been proven to cause cancer.[17] Such environmental factors include tobacco, excessive alcohol consumption, poor diet, lack of regular exercise, viruses, bacteria, pharmaceuticals, hormones, radiation, and environmental chemicals present in the air, water, food, and workplace.

The International Agency for Research on Cancer Monographs identifies environmental factors that can increase the risk of human cancer. These include chemicals, occupational exposures, physical agents, biological agents, and lifestyle factors. Many health agencies in this country and throughout the world use this information to support their cause for preventing exposure to those substances that pose a serious health risk. Since 1971, 400 compounds have been identified as "carcinogenic," "probably carcinogenic," or "possibly carcinogenic" to humans. For example, perchloroethylene, or perc, is the dominant chemical solvent used in the process of dry cleaning. Perc, used by most professional drycleaners because it removes stains and dirt from all common types of fabrics, has been found through IARC research to be carcinogenic in both animal and human studies.[18]

The fibers, fine particles, and dust particles that occur in various manufacturing settings are also associated with increased cancer risk. Asbestos fibers, for instance, are well-known carcinogens which have been shown to cause mesothelioma, a rare cancer of the lung and abdominal cavity. Silica dust, found in workplaces such as coal mines, quarries, mills, and sandblasting operations, is a substance which has been shown to cause lung cancer, and wood dust from sanding and furniture manufacturing has been shown to cause cancer of the sinuses and nasal cavities. Dioxins, the by-products of chemical processing that contain both chlorine and hydrocarbons, are in a class of their own. Over 100 dioxins are found in paper bleaching, manufacturing, smelters, and incineration, as well as in wood preservatives, herbicides, and insecticides. One such dioxin, TCDD (2-, 3-, 7-, 8-tetrachlorodibenzo-p-dioxin), has been found to be extremely carcinogenic and many deaths have been attributed to exposure to TCDD. Furthermore, polycyclic aromatic hydrocarbons (PAHs) cause an increased incidence of cancer of the skin, lung, and urinary system. Not only are PAHs found in the air from burning wood and home fuel, but small amounts of PAHs are also found in smoked, charbroiled, and barbecued food...and even in roasted coffee beans and Coca Cola!

Arsenic, long known for its toxic properties, has been associated with liver, bladder, skin, lung, and kidney cancer, especially when consumed in drinking water. Arsenic is found in wood preservatives, insecticides, pesticides, herbicides, and certain kinds of glass, and is a common pollutant found in our food, air, and water. Lead acetate and phosphate are other well-known carcinogens, which cause both brain and kidney tumors. Lead acetate is found in cotton dyes, metal coating, varnishes, and pigment inks, and can be contacted through the skin, through food consumption, or through the air, and lead phosphate is found in certain kinds of glass and plastic. Diesel exhaust particulate has long been suspected to be carcinogenic as well, due to the reported higher incidence of lung cancer in bus workers, truckers, garage workers, miners, and railroad workers.

The list goes on and on.

My point here is simply that we must do our best to limit our exposure to as many of these cancer-causing substances as possible. Since the reality is that we may not be able to regulate what goes on in the outside world, we can begin to take action inside our own homes. The book *Green This!* by Deirdre Imus is a great start.[19] Imus's book provides sound, environmentally friendly suggestions for cleaning your home in a toxic-free manner. Since most of us spend a lot of time in our homes, learning to reduce our exposure is a good way to exercise some control over our own immediate environment. But, while it is true that cleaning and sanitizing is an effective way of killing germs associated with illness, many of the same household products that are used to maintain and clean our homes are actually as toxic as the substances we are trying to avoid outside. For example, the Environmental Protection Agency has indicated that the air quality inside our homes is often worse than the air quality outside. That's because products like aerosol sprays, moth repellents, abrasives, disinfectants, paint strippers, furniture polish, and carpet cleaners contain volatile organic compounds, or VOCs. VOCs evaporate in the air easily and quickly and thus ease their way into our bodies through the air we breathe. Short-term exposure can cause dizziness, headaches, asthma, skin rashes, allergic reactions, and eye, nose, and throat irritation. Long-term exposure can cause damage to the endocrine system, nervous system, and immune system, and has been shown to cause birth defects and cancer. So, when making choices for your home, look for items that are non-toxic, biodegradable, and natural or citrus-based. Avoid products that are labeled corrosive, irritant, harmful if swallowed, or flammable. Instead, use cleaning products like white vinegar, lemon juice, and baking soda, which are good, inexpensive alternatives to more toxic products, and always make sure there is plenty of ventilation when you use cleaning products of any kind. When it comes to your home's environment, think green!

Cancers declining—and inclining

Some cancers, such as those of the stomach and liver, are on the decline in the United States. Possible reasons for this decline include our decreased consumption of nitrates and nitrites, salt, smoked and pickled foods, and red meat. Other possibilities include the decline in incidence of *Helicobacter Pylori* (a bacterium from contaminated food and water), and the fact that we have marginally reduced our tobacco and alcohol use. In contrast, cancers of the colon, prostate, and breast are on the rise. Breast cancer, for example, has seen a dramatic rise not only in this country but in most countries worldwide over the past few decades. Although the exact causes of breast cancer have not been conclusively established, some risk factors have been identified through extensive research. The factors listed below are from the Susan G. Komen "Risk Factors Table."[20]

- The older a woman is, the more likely she is to get breast cancer.
- Breast cancer is 100 times more common in women than men.
- Certain inherited genetic mutations have been linked to breast cancer. These mutations account for only five to 10% of all breast cancers diagnosed in the U.S.
- Family history is an important risk factor for breast cancer. Having one immediate female relative (mother, sister, or daughter) with breast cancer almost doubles a woman's chance of getting breast cancer compared to that of a woman without a family history.
- Women with dense breasts have an increased risk of breast cancer.
- Proliferative breast conditions, such as hyperplastic breast tissue, indicate an increased risk for getting breast cancer.
- Women with lobular carcinoma *in situ* (LCIS) are seven to 12 times more likely to develop cancer in either breast compared to women without LCIS.

- Breast cancer survivors have an increased risk of getting a new breast cancer, compared to those who have never had breast cancer.
- Exposure to large amounts of radiation early in life is linked to an increased risk of getting breast cancer.

Clearly, there are a number of relevant factors that play a role in increasing an individual's risk of getting cancer at some point: the types of food we eat, race, age, exposure to pollutants, child birth, hormones, and many more. The key word here, however, is *risk,* and that is why common sense dictates that we all need to learn how to reduce the risk factors where we can in order to reduce the odds. Again, none of us can change our genes, age, race, or family history. But the risk factors that we *can* change are easily within the realm of our consideration. As I keep saying—and you'll probably read many more times before you finish this book—aside from not smoking, we can reduce our risk of cancer by maintaining a healthy weight, exercising regularly, and eating as healthfully as possible.

So, let's begin.

Cancer and body weight

To start with, we all need to stay as close as possible to our ideal body weight. What we weigh in relation to our height has a direct relationship to our health. How does each one of us know what our "ideal" weight is? Research points to some accessible calculations to find out.

Body Mass Index, or BMI, is calculated using the following formula* (see Table 3-5).[21]

TABLE 3-5. Calculating BMI (*not applicable to children, athletes, or pregnant/lactating women)

S.I. units	U.S. units	UK mixed units
BMI - mass (kg)	BMI = 703 x weight (lb)	BMI = 6.35 x weight (stone)
height^2(m^2)	height^2(in^2)	height^2(m^2)

An "ideal" body weight can be calculated on the basis of BMI, the measure of body fat based on a person's height and weight (see Table 3-6 on next page).

According to the National Heart, Lung, and Blood Institute, NHLBI, BMI categories are as follows:

- *Underweight:* BMI less than 19.5
- *Normal weight:* BMI between 19.5 to 24
- *Overweight:* BMI of 25 to 29
- *Obese:* BMI of 30 or above

BMI applies to both men and women. Cancer risk has been shown to decrease if an individual's BMI is less than 25. We can keep our weight at an ideal level by exercising, following a diet rich in fruits, vegetables, and whole grains, and limiting processed foods and fat calories.

TABLE 3-6. Body Mass Index chart, based on clinical guidelines on the identification, evaluation, and treatment of overweight and obesity in adults. (Source: NHLBI Obesity Education Initiative, National Institutes of Health, 1998)

WEIGHT lbs.	100	105	110	115	120	125	130	135	140	145	150	155	160	165	170	175	180	185	190	195	200	205	210	215
Kgs.	45.5	47.7	50.0	52.3	54.5	56.8	59.1	61.4	63.6	65.9	68.2	70.5	72.7	75.0	77.3	79.5	81.8	84.1	86.4	88.6	90.9	93.2	95.5	97.7
HEIGHT in./cm																								
5'0" – 152.4	19	20	21	22	23	24	25	26	27	28	29	30	31	32	33	34	35	36	37	38	39	40	41	42
5'1" – 154.9	18	19	20	21	22	23	24	25	26	27	28	29	30	31	32	33	34	35	36	36	37	38	39	40
5'2" – 157.4	18	19	20	21	22	23	23	24	25	26	27	28	29	30	31	32	33	33	34	35	36	37	38	39
5'3" – 160.0	17	18	19	20	21	22	23	24	24	25	26	27	28	29	30	31	32	33	34	35	35	36	37	38
5'4" – 162.5	17	18	18	19	20	21	22	23	24	25	26	27	28	29	30	31	32	33	34	34	35	36	37	38
5'5" – 165.1	16	17	18	19	20	21	22	23	24	25	25	26	27	28	29	30	31	32	33	34	35	35	36	37
5'6" – 167.6	16	17	17	18	19	20	21	22	23	24	25	25	26	27	28	29	30	31	32	33	34	35	35	36
5'7" – 170.1	15	16	17	18	19	20	21	22	23	24	25	25	26	27	28	29	30	31	32	33	34	34	35	36
5'8" – 172.7	15	16	16	17	18	19	20	21	22	23	24	25	25	26	27	28	29	30	31	32	33	34	35	35
5'9" – 175.2	14	15	16	17	18	19	20	21	22	23	24	25	25	26	27	28	29	30	31	32	33	34	35	35
5'10" – 177.8	14	15	15	16	17	18	19	20	21	22	23	24	25	25	26	27	28	29	30	31	32	33	34	34
5'11" – 180.3	14	14	15	16	17	18	18	19	20	21	22	23	23	24	25	26	27	28	28	29	30	31	32	33
6'0" – 182.8	13	14	14	15	16	17	18	19	19	20	21	22	23	23	24	25	26	27	28	29	30	30	31	32
6'1" – 185.4	13	13	14	15	16	17	17	18	19	19	20	21	21	22	23	24	25	26	27	27	28	29	30	31
6'2" – 187.9	12	13	14	14	15	16	16	17	18	18	19	19	20	21	21	22	23	24	25	26	27	28	29	30
6'3" – 190.5	12	13	13	14	15	15	16	16	17	17	18	18	19	20	20	21	22	23	24	25	25	26	27	28

Cancer and exercise

In the words of Dr. Deepak Chopra, "Happiness generates chemicals in our brain that stimulate all cells in our body towards happiness. Exercising regularly to raise the brain's happy chemicals helps in preventing diseases, including cancer." This is why the American Cancer Society recommends exercising 30 minutes a day, five days a week, for cancer prevention.

Estrogen, exercise, and cancer. Estrogen, a hormone involved in the normal development and growth of the breasts and organs important for childbearing, is responsible for controlling a woman's menstrual cycle and is essential for reproduction. Estrogen also contributes to maintaining a healthy heart and bones. However, a woman's risk for breast cancer is associated with that same lifetime exposure to estrogen. Estrogen's role in breast cancer risk may be due to the fact that it stimulates breast cell division, functions during the critical periods of breast growth and development, affects other hormones that stimulate breast cell division, and supports the growth of estrogen-responsive tumors.

We also know through research, such as the study performed at the University of Wisconsin, that recreational physical activity during all periods of life in women with no family history of cancer is inversely associated with invasive breast cancer risk,[22] and that there is also an inverse association between physical activity and breast cancer in postmenopausal American women, as revealed in a study by the National Cancer Institute. In this particular study, it was reported that women with the highest levels of activity had an almost 20% lower risk of breast cancer compared with women who exercised the least. Risk reduction also appeared to be limited to vigorous forms of activity in women of lean or normal weight, compared with overweight women, regardless of their hormone-receptor status.[23]

According to the National Cancer Institute, other types of cancer have also shown incidence reduction with vigorous physical activity.[24] For example, exercise may protect against getting colon cancer through its role in energy balance, hormone metabolism, and insulin regulation, and by decreasing the time the colon is exposed to potential carcinogens. Research also shows that women who are physically active have a 20 to 40% reduced risk of endometrial cancer, with the greatest reduction in risk among those with the highest levels of physical activity, regardless of age. An inverse association between physical activity and lung cancer risk has been seen as well, with the most physically active individuals experiencing an approximate 20% reduction in risk. It has further been shown that regular vigorous activity can: slow the progression of prostate cancer in men age 65 or older by 70%; reduce the risk for colon cancer in people who exercise regularly or have jobs that involve a high degree of physical activity; improve circulation; promote proper skeletal function; and speed up the processes of digestion and bowel movement.

When I first began my study of cancer, it was merely to satisfy my curiosity and understanding. But today, even as I read new research articles and journals daily and continue to broaden my comprehensive knowledge and even with the exorbitant amount of data, statistics, and charts available, I often find myself both overwhelmed and saddened. The reality is that cancer continues to be a disease of epic proportions, not only in the United States but throughout the world.

That is why, while I believe that statistics can be informative and help us gain understanding, I also believe that cancer patients should not get caught up in the numbers. Numbers are just that: numbers. They are not *you*. Let me say that again: *You are not the numbers, and the numbers are not you.* So, when you read statistics in this book or in any other report, understand that they are for informational purposes only. While we may fall into different cancer categories, we are still individuals. The way I see it, statistics provide a foundation for understanding the progress of cancer and for eradicating it. They provide a bottom line so we can note where we are and where we need to go, but much more information and research is needed to understand cancer. You may be inclined toward research and statistics, as I was, or you may not. You may be inspired to delve into scientific research—or not. Either way, you may choose to learn as much as you can about your own experience with cancer.

Types of cancer

In this next section, the types of cancers in the United States with the highest prevalence are discussed. The following statistics relative to the various types of cancers are based on the National Cancer Institute's most current SEER *Cancer Statistics Review* from 2003 through 2007.[25]

Breast cancer. It is estimated that 207,090 women will be diagnosed with breast cancer and 39,840 women will die of breast cancer in 2010. From 2003 to 2007, 60% of breast cancer cases were diagnosed while the cancer was still confined to the primary site, or at the localized stage, 33% were diagnosed after the cancer had spread to regional lymph nodes, or directly beyond the primary site, and 5% were diagnosed after the cancer had already metastasized, in the distant stage. (For the remaining 2% the staging information was unknown.) The corresponding five-year relative survival rates were 98% for localized, 83.6% for regional, 23.4% for distant, and 57.9% for unstaged.

From 2003 to 2007, the median age at diagnosis for cancer of the breast was 61. Approximately 0% was diagnosed under the age of 20; 1.9% between the ages of 20 and 34; 10.5% between 35 and 44; 22.6% between 45 and 54; 24.1% between 55 and 64; 19.5% between 65 and 74; 15.8% between 75 and 84; and 5.6% at 85+ years of age. The age adjusted incidence rate was 126.5 per 100,000 women per year. These rates are based on cases diagnosed from 17 SEER geographic areas. It was found that white women had the highest incidence at 127.8 per 100,000 women. African American women had the second highest, with 118.3 per 100,000. Asian/Pacific Islander women were next at 90 per 100,000, then Hispanic women at 86 per 100,000, and then American Indian/ Alaska Native women, with the lowest incidence, at 76.4 per 100,000. For all races, the incidence was 122.9 per 100,000 women. The same statistics revealed the median age of mortality from breast cancer was 68 years of age, with African American women having the highest mortality at 32.4 per 100,000 and Asian/Pacific Islander women the lowest at 12.2 per 100,000.

Based on rates from 2005 to 2007, 12.15%, or one in eight women born today will be diagnosed with cancer of the breast at some time during their lifetime. The prevalence of breast cancer is high in the United States and as of January 1, 2007, there were approximately 2,591,855 women alive who had a history of cancer of the breast.

Lung and bronchus cancer. In 2010 it is estimated that 116,750 men and 105,770 women, a total of 222,520 for both genders, will be diagnosed with lung cancer, and that 159,300 men and women will die from this type of cancer. From 2003 to 2007, 15% of lung and bronchus cancer cases were diagnosed while the cancer was still confined to the primary site, or in the localized stage, 22% were diagnosed after the cancer had spread to regional lymph nodes, or directly beyond the primary site, and 56% were diagnosed after the cancer had already metastasized, in the distant stage. (For the remaining 8%, the staging information was unknown.) The corresponding five-year relative survival rates were 52.9% for localized, 24.0% for regional, 3.5% for distant, and 8.7% for unstaged.

From 2003 to 2007, the median age at diagnosis for cancer of the lung and bronchus was 71. Approximately 0% was diagnosed under age 20; 0.2% between the ages of 20 and 34; 1.7% between 35 and 44; 8.8% between 45 and 54; 20.9% between 55 and 64; 31.3% between 65 and 74; 29.1% between 75 and 84; and 8.0% at 85+ years of age. The age adjusted incidence rate was 62.5 per 100,000 men and women per year. These rates are based on cases diagnosed from 17 SEER geographic areas. It was found that African American men had the highest incidence of cancer of the lung at 101.2 per 100,000 and African American women had the highest incidence among women at 54.8 per 100,000. White men had the next highest rate of 76.3 per 100,000; white women 54.7 per 100,000. The incidence rate in American Indian/Alaska Native men was 52.7 per 100,000 and in

American Indian/Alaska native women 39.7 per 100,000. Asian/Pacific Islander men had an incidence rate of 52.9 per 100,000 and Asian/Pacific Islander women 28.1 per 100,000. The incidence rates were the lowest among Hispanics at 41.4 per 100,000 men and 25.4 per 100,000 women. For all races, it was found that men averaged a rate of 76.2 per 100,000 and women 52.4 per 100,000. The same statistics utilized during this time revealed the median age of mortality from cancer of the lung and bronchus was 72, with African American men and white women showing the highest mortality at 87.5 per 100,000 for men and 41.6 per 100,000 for women. Hispanics showed the lowest mortality rate of 32.5 per 100,000 for men and 14.4 per 100,000 for women.

Based on rates from 2005 to 2007, 6.95%, or one in 14 men and women born today will be diagnosed with cancer of the lung and bronchus at some time during their lifetime.

In Figure 3-3 the World Health Organization demonstrates the mortality for lung cancer in males and females in five countries: Japan, the United States, the United Kingdom, France, and Italy. This chart shows that in all five countries mortality for lung cancer in men has decreased since the early 1980s. In women this number was on the rise since the 1960s, and began to level off in the early 1990s in some countries, and later in the 1990s in others. In women in the UK and the U.S., mortality rates jumped after 1960 and then stabilized around 1990. Among Japanese, French, and Italian women, mortality was at a lower rate after 1960 and eventually stabilized in the 1990s. In men, the mortality rate of lung cancer showed a rapid increase since 1960 in all five countries.

FIGURE 3-3. Mortality for lung cancer, age standardized rate of various nations. Comparison of cancer mortality (lung cancer) in five countries: France, Italy, Japan, the UK and the U.S. (Source: WHO Mortality Database (1960-2000), Statistics and Cancer Control Division, Research Center for Cancer Prevention and Screening, National Cancer Center; Japanese Journal of Clinical Oncology, 2005. 35(3):168-170)

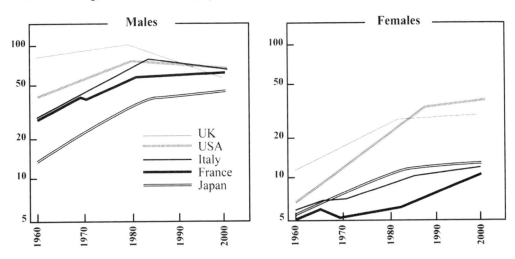

In the early 1960s and 1970s, the mortality rate for men in the United Kingdom and the United States was higher compared with that of Japanese, French, and Italian men. The mortality rate increased until 1970 in the UK and until 1990 in the United States. Recently, the mortality rates in men in all five countries have converged.

Prostate cancer. It is estimated that 217,730 men will be diagnosed with prostate cancer, and 32,050 men will die of cancer of the prostate in 2010. From 2003 to 2007, 80% of prostate cancer cases were diagnosed while the cancer was still confined to the primary site (localized stage), 12% were diagnosed after the cancer had spread to regional lymph nodes or directly beyond the primary site, and 4% were diagnosed after the cancer had already metastasized (distant stage). (For the remaining 3% the staging information was unknown.) The corresponding five-year relative survival rates were: 100% for localized, 100% for regional, 30.2% for distant, and 75.0% for unstaged.

From 2003 to 2007, the median age at diagnosis for cancer of the prostate was 67. Approximately 0% cases were diagnosed under age 20; 0% were between the ages of 20 and 34; 0.6% between 35 and 44; 8.9% between 45 and 54; 29.9% between 55 and 64; 35.3% between 65 and 74; 20.7% between 75 and 84; and 4.6% at 85+ years of age. These rates are based on cases diagnosed from 17 SEER geographic areas. It was found that African American men had the highest incidence at 234.6 per 100,000 men. White males had the second highest incidence at 150.4 per 100,000. The incidence of Hispanic males was 125.8 per 100,000, of Asian/Pacific Islander men 90.0 per 100,000, and of American Indian/Alaskan Native men 77.7 per 100,000, the lowest incidence for all males. For all races, an incidence rate of 156.9 per 100,000 men was revealed. The same statistics during this time revealed the median age of mortality from prostate cancer was 80, with African American men showing the highest mortality at 54.2 per 100,000. Asian/Pacific Islanders men had the lowest mortality rate at 10.6 per 100,000. Based on rates from 2005 to 2007, 16.2% of men, or one in six, born today will be diagnosed with cancer of the prostate at some time during their lifetime.

Ovarian cancer. It is estimated that 21,880 women will be diagnosed with ovarian cancer and 13,850 women will die of cancer of the ovary in 2010. From 2003 to 2007, 15% of ovarian cancers were diagnosed while the cancer was still confined to the primary site (localized stage), 17% were diagnosed after the cancer had spread to regional lymph nodes or directly beyond the primary site, and 62% were diagnosed after the cancer had already metastasized (distant stage). (For the remaining 7%, the staging information was unknown.) Corresponding five-year relative survival rates were reported as: 93.5% localized; 73.4% regional; 27.6% distant; and 27.2% unstaged.

From 2003 to 2007, the median age at diagnosis for cancer of the ovary was 63. Approximately 1.3% were diagnosed under age 20; 3.5% were between the ages of 20 and 34; 7.4% between 35 and 44; 19.2% between 45 and 54; 22.9% between 55 and 64; 19.5% between 65 and 74; 18.4% between 75 and 84; and 7.8% at 85+ years of age. These rates are based on cases diagnosed from 17 SEER geographic areas. It was found that white women had the highest incidence at 13.5 per 100,000. Next were Hispanic women at 11.0 per 100,000. American Indian/Alaska Native women were at 10.9 per 100,000, followed by African American women at 10.2 per 100,000. Asian/Pacific Islander women showed the lowest incidence at 9.8 per 100,000. For all races, the age adjusted incidence rate was 12.9 per 100,000. The same statistics during this time revealed the median age of mortality from ovarian cancer was 71, with white women showing the highest mortality of 8.9 per 100,000 and Hispanic women the lowest, at 6.0 per 100,000.

Based on rates from 2005 to 2007, 1.39%, or one in 72 women born today will be diagnosed with cancer of the ovary at some time during their lifetime.

Pancreatic cancer. It is estimated that 43,140 men and women (21,370 men and 21,770 women) will be diagnosed with pancreatic cancer and 36,800 men and women will die of cancer of the pancreas in 2010. From 2003 to 2007, 8% of pancreatic cancer cases were diagnosed while the cancer was still confined to the primary site (localized stage), 26% were diagnosed after the cancer had spread to regional lymph nodes or directly beyond the primary site, and 53% were diagnosed after the cancer had already metastasized (distant stage). (For the remaining 14% the staging information was unknown.) The corresponding five-year relative survival rates were 22.5% for localized, 8.8% for regional, 1.9% for distant, and 5% for unstaged.

From 2003 to 2007, the median age at diagnosis for cancer of the pancreas was 72 years of age. Approximately 0% was diagnosed under age 20; 0.4% between 20 and 34; 2.3% between 35 and 44; 9.7% between 45 and 54; 19.6% between 55 and 64; 25.6% between 65 and 74; 29.4% between 75 and 84; and 13.0% at age 85+. The age adjusted incidence rate was 11.7 per 100,000 men and women per year. These rates are based on cases diagnosed from 17 SEER geographic areas. It was found that African Americans had the highest incidence of pancreatic cancer, at 16.7 per 100,000 for men and 14.4 per 100,000 for women. White men and women had the next highest incidence, at 13.2 per 100,000 for men and 10.3 per 100,000 for women. Among Hispanics, the incidence rates were at 10.9 per 100,000 men and 10.1 per 100,000 women. Incidence rates for American Indian/Alaska Native men were 10.6 per 100,000 and for American Indian/ Alaska Native women 9.3 per 100,000. Asian/Pacific Islanders showed the lowest incidence rate of 10.2 per 100,000 men and 8.3 per 100,000 women. For all races, it was found that men averaged an incidence rate of 13.3 per 100,000 and women 10.5 per 100,000. The same statistics during this time revealed the median age of mortality from pancreatic cancer was 73 years, with African American men and women showing the highest mortality at 15.4 per 100,000 for men and 12.4 per 100,000 for women. Asian/ Pacific Islander men and women were found to have the lowest mortality rate at 8.2 for men and 6.9 for women.

Based on rates from 2005 to 2007, 1.41%, or one in 71 men and women born today will be diagnosed with pancreatic cancer at some time during their lifetime.

Colorectal cancer. It is estimated that 142,570 men and women (72,090 men and 70,480 women) will be diagnosed with cancer of the colon and rectum and 51,370 men and women will die of this type of cancer in 2010. From 2003 to 2007, 39% of colon and rectum cancer cases were diagnosed while the cancer was still confined to the primary site (localized stage), 37% were diagnosed after the cancer had spread to regional lymph nodes or directly beyond the primary site, and 19% were diagnosed after the cancer had already metastasized (distant stage). (For the remaining 5% the staging information was unknown.) The corresponding five-year relative survival rates were: 90.4% for localized; 69.5% for regional; 11.6% for distant; and 38.3% for unstaged.

From 2003 to 2007, the median age at diagnosis for cancer of the colon and rectum was 70. Approximately 0.1% of cases were diagnosed under age 20; 1.1% between the ages of 20 and 34; 3.8% between 35 and 44; 12.4% between 45 and 54; 19.2% between 55 and 64; 24.4% between 65 and 74; 26.8% between 75 and 84; and 12.2% at age 85+. The age adjusted incidence rate was 47.9 per 100,000 men and women per year. These rates are based on cases diagnosed from 17 SEER geographic areas. It was found that African Americans had the highest incidence of cancer of the colon and rectum, at 68.1 per 100,000 for men and 52.6 per 100,000 for women. White men and women had the next highest incidence at 55.4 per 100,000 men and 40.9 per 100,000 women. Asian/ Pacific Islanders had an incidence rate of 45.5 per 100,000 men and 34.2 per 100,000 women. Among Hispanic men, the incidence was 44.5 per 100,000 and among American Indian/Alaska Native women the rate was 40.4 per 100,000. American Indian/Alaska Natives had the lowest incidence rate for men at 43.4 per 100,000 and Hispanic women had the lowest rate at 31.6 per 100,000. For all races, it was found that men averaged an incidence rate of 55.8 per 100,000 and women 41.7 per 100,000. The same statistics utilized during this time revealed the median age of mortality from cancer of the colon and rectum was 75 years, with African American men and women showing the highest mortality, at 30.5 per 100,000 men and 21.0 per 100,000 women. Asian/Pacific Islanders showed the lowest mortality rate of 13.2 per 100,000 men and 9.9 per 100,000 women.

Based on rates from 2005 to 2007, 5.12%, or one in 20 men and women born today will be diagnosed with cancer of the colon and rectum at some time during their lifetime.

My cancer: Hodgkin lymphoma. It is estimated that 8,490 men and women (4,670 men and 3,820 women) will be diagnosed with Hodgkin lymphoma and 1,320 men and women will die of this type of cancer in 2010. From 2003 to 2007, 19% of Hodgkin lymphoma cases were diagnosed while the cancer was still confined to the primary site (localized stage), 40% were diagnosed after the cancer had spread to regional lymph nodes or directly beyond the primary site, and 35% were diagnosed after the cancer had already metastasized (distant stage). (For the remaining 5% the staging information was unknown.) The corresponding five-year relative survival rates were 90.3% for localized, 91.1% for regional, 74.2% for distant, and 82.3% for unstaged.

From 2003 to 2007, the median age at the time of diagnosis for Hodgkin lymphoma was 38. Approximately 12.0% were diagnosed under age 20; 31.7% between the ages of 20 and 34; 16.3% between 35 and 44; 12.3% between 45 and 54; 9.6% between 55 and 64; 8.6% between 65 and 74; 7.3% between 75 and 84; and 2.3% at age 85+. The age adjusted incidence rate was 2.8 per 100,000 men and women per year. These rates are based on cases diagnosed from 17 SEER geographic areas. It was found that white men and women had the highest incidence at 3.2 per 100,000 men and 2.5 per 100,000 women. African Americans had the next highest incidence with 3.0 per 100,000 men and 2.3 per 100,000 women. Among Hispanics, the incidence rates were at 2.8 per 100,000 men and 2.0 per 100,000 women. It was found that Asian/Pacific Islanders had an incidence rate of 1.5 per 100,000 men and 1.1 per 100,000 women. American Indian/ Alaskan Native males and females were found to have the lowest incidence, with 1.1 per 100,000 men and fewer than 16 cases for women during this time interval. For all races, it was found that men had an incidence rate of 3.2 and women 2.5 per 100,000. The same statistics during this time revealed the median age of mortality from Hodgkin lymphoma was 63 years, with white and black males showing the highest mortality at 0.5 per 100,000 and white females 0.4 per 100,000. American Indian/Alaskan Native males and females were found to have the lowest mortality rate with few recorded cases during this time interval.

Based on rates from 2005 to 2007, 0.23%, or one in 438 men and women born today will be diagnosed with Hodgkin lymphoma at some time during their lifetime.

Stomach cancer. It is estimated that 21,000 men and women (12,730 men and 8,270 women) will be diagnosed with stomach cancer and 10,570 men and women will die of cancer of the stomach in 2010. From 2003 to 2007, 23% of stomach cancer cases were diagnosed while the cancer was still confined to the primary site, or localized stage, 32% were diagnosed after the cancer had spread to regional lymph nodes or directly beyond the primary site, and 34% were diagnosed after the cancer had already metastasized (the distant stage). (For the remaining 11%, the staging information was unknown.) The corresponding five-year relative survival rates were 62.5% localized, 27.0% regional, 3.4% distant, and 17.3% unstaged.

From 2003 to 2007, the median age at diagnosis for cancer of the stomach was 70. Approximately 0.1% of cases were diagnosed under age 20; 1.6% between the ages of 20 and 34; 4.8% between 35 and 44; 11.9% between 45 and 54; 18.1% between 55 and 64; 24.2% between 65 and 74; 27.2% between 75 and 84; and 12.2% at 85+ years of age. The age adjusted incidence rate was 7.8 per 100,000 men and women per year. These rates are based on cases diagnosed from 17 SEER geographic areas. It was found that Asian/ Pacific Islanders had the highest incidence of stomach cancer with 17.5 per 100,000 men and 10.0 per 100,000 women. The next highest incidences were African American men at 16.7 per 100,000 and Asian Pacific Islander women at 10.0 per 100,000. The rate of American Indian/Alaska Native men was 15.5 per 100,000 and of Hispanic women 9.1 per 100,000. Hispanic men had an incidence rate of 14.8 per 100,000 and American Indian/Alaska Native women 7.3 per 100,000. White males and females were found to have the lowest incidence, with 9.6 per 100,000 men and 4.7 per 100,000 women. For all races, it was found that men averaged an incidence rate of 10.9 per 100,000 and women 5.5 per 100,000. The same statistics during this time revealed the median age of mortality from stomach cancer was 73, with African American males having the highest mortality at 10.7 per 100,000, followed by Asian Pacific Islander women at 5.6 per 100,000. White men and women had the lowest rate with 4.6 per 100,000 men and 2.4 per 100,000 women. For all races, it was found that men averaged a mortality rate of 5.3 per 100,000, and women 2.7 per 100,000.

Based on rates from 2005 to 2007, 0.88%, or one in every 114 men and women born today will be diagnosed with cancer of the stomach at some time during their lifetime.

Leukemia. The four most common types of leukemia are chronic lymphocytic leukemia (CLL), with about 14,990 new cases, and acute lymphocytic leukemia (ALL), with an estimated 5,330 new cases likely to occur in 2010. Chronic myeloid leukemia (CML) is estimated to affect an estimated 4,870 individuals and acute myeloid lymphocytic leukemia (ALL) an estimated 12,330 individuals in 2010.

Leukemia/acute lymphocytic leukemia (ALL). It is estimated that 5,330 men and women (3,150 men and 2,180 women) will be diagnosed with acute lymphocytic leukemia and

1,420 men and women will die of ALL in 2010. From 2003 to 2007, the median age at diagnosis for acute lymphocytic leukemia was 13. Approximately 60.7% were diagnosed under the age of 20; 10.3% between the ages of 20 and 34; 6.2% between 35 and 44; 6.5% between 45 and 54; 5.8% between 55 and 64; 5.0% between 65 and 74; 3.8% between 75 and 84; and 1.6% at age 85 and over.

The median age of mortality of acute lymphocytic leukemia is 49. The overall five-year relative survival rate for 1999 to 2006 from 17 SEER geographic areas was 65.2%; however, this number is higher in children at an 85% survival rate of five years and more. Five-year relative survival rates by race and sex were 65.3% for white men, 65.8% for white women, 56.9% for black men, and 63.4% for black women.

According to the Leukemia & Lymphoma Society, about 33% of cancer cases in children age 0 to 14 years are leukemia cancer. Acute lymphocytic leukemia is the most common cancer in children ages one to seven. The incidence of ALL among one- to four-year-old children is nearly eight times greater than the rate for young adults 20 to 24 years. However, as stated previously, survival statistics have improved significantly over the past four decades and most children under 19 with ALL will survive five or more years. The leukemia death rate for children 0 to 14 years of age in the United States has declined 88% from 1969 to 2006. Despite this decline, leukemia causes more deaths than any other cancer among children and young adults under the age of 20.

Leukemia/acute myeloid leukemia (AML). It is estimated that 12,330 men and women (6,590 men and 5,740 women) will be diagnosed with acute myeloid leukemia and that 8,950 men and women will die of this type of cancer in 2010.

From 2003 to 2007, the median age at diagnosis for acute myeloid leukemia was 67. Approximately 6.1% were diagnosed under age 20; 6.5% between the ages of 20 and 34; 6.7% between 35 and 44; 11.3% between 45 and 54; 15.1% between 55 and 64; 19.9% between 65 and 74; 24.5% between 75 and 84; and 9.9% at 85+ years of age. The age adjusted incidence rate was 3.5 per 100,000 for men and women per year. These rates are based on cases diagnosed from 17 SEER geographic areas. It was found that white men and women had the highest incidence at 4.4 per 100,000 men and 3.0 per 100,000 women. African American and Asian Pacific Islander men had the next highest incidence with 3.5 per 100,000, and African American women the subsequent highest at 2.6 per 100,000. Hispanic men had an incidence rate of 3.3 per 100,000. American Indian/Alaskan Native men had the lowest incidence with fewer than 16 reported cases during this time. Asian/Pacific Islanders, American Indian/Alaskan Natives, and Hispanic women had the same incidence rate at 2.6 per 100,000. For all races, it was found that men had an incidence rate of 4.3 and women an incidence rate of 2.9 per 100,000. From 2003 to 2007, the median age at death for acute myeloid leukemia was 72, with white males and females showing the highest mortality at 3.7 per 100,000 for men and 2.2 per 100,000 for women. Male American Indian/Alaskan Natives were found to have the lowest mortality rate at 2.0 per 100,000; female Hispanic and Asian/Pacific Islanders had the lowest rate at 1.4 per 100,000.

Based on rates from 2005 to 2007, 0.38%, or one in 266 men and women born today will be diagnosed with acute myeloid leukemia at some time during their lifetime. The overall five-year relative survival rate for 1999 to 2006 was 23.6%.

Leukemia/chronic myeloid leukemia (CML). It is estimated that 4,870 men and women (2,800 men and 2,070 women) will be diagnosed with chronic myeloid leukemia and that 440 men and women will die of this type of cancer in 2010.

From 2003 to 2007, the median age at diagnosis for chronic myeloid leukemia was 65. Approximately 2.5% were diagnosed under age 20; 7.4% were between the ages of 20 and 34; 10.1% between 35 and 44; 12.3% between of 45 and 54; 15.0% between 55 and 64; 19.0% between 65 and 74; 22.7% between 75 and 84, and 9.9% at 85+ years of age. The age adjusted incidence rate was 1.5 per 100,000 men and women per year. These rates are based on cases diagnosed from 17 SEER geographic areas. It was found that white men had the highest incidence at 2.0 per 100,000. For women, white and African American women had the highest incidence at 1.2 per 100,000. African American men had the subsequent highest incidence at 1.9 per 100,000 and Hispanic women the next highest at 1.0 per 100,000. Asian/Pacific Islander men had an incidence rate of 1.3 per 100,000 and women 0.7 per 100,000. American Indian/Alaskan Native males and females were found to have the lowest incidence with fewer than 16 cases for both men and women during this time interval. For all races, men had an incidence rate of 2.0 and women an incidence rate of 1.1 per 100,000. From 2003 to 2007, the median age at death for chronic myeloid leukemia was 74 years, with African American and American Indian/Alaskan Native males having the highest mortality at 0.6 per 100,000. The rate for white and African American females was 0.3 per 100,000. For males, Asian/Pacific Islanders had the lowest mortality rate at 0.2 per 100,000, and for females, American Indian/Alaskan Natives had the lowest mortality rate, with few recorded cases during this time interval.

Based on rates from 2005 to 2007, 0.16%, or one in 635 men and women born today will be diagnosed with chronic myeloid leukemia at some time during their lifetime. The overall five-year relative survival rate for 1999 to 2006 was 56.8%.

Leukemia/chronic lymphocytic leukemia (CLL). It is estimated that 14,990 men and women (8,870 men and 6,120 women) will be diagnosed with chronic lymphocytic leukemia and that 4,390 men and women will die of this type of cancer in 2010.

From 2003 to 2007, the median age at diagnosis for chronic lymphocytic leukemia was 72 years. Approximately 0.1% were diagnosed under age 20; 0.2% between the ages of 20 and 34; 1.5% between 35 and 44; 9.0% between 45 and 54; 20.0% between 55 and 64; 26.7% between 65 and 74; 29.3% between 75 and 84; and 13.2% at 85+ years of age. The age adjusted incidence rate was 4.2 per 100,000 for men and women per year. These rates are based on cases diagnosed from 17 SEER geographic areas. It was found that white men and women had the highest incidence at 6.1 per 100,000 men and 3.2 per 100,000 women. African Americans had the next highest incidence at 4.4 per 100,000 men and 2.0 per 100,000 women. Hispanics had an incidence rate of 2.4 per 100,000 men and 1.4 per 100,000 women. American Indian/Alaskan Native males had an incidence rate of 1.9 per 100,000 and Asian/Pacific Islander women a rate of 0.7 per 100,000. The lowest incidence rates for men were Asian/Pacific Islanders at 1.3 per 100,000, and for women, American Indian/Alaskan Natives, at fewer than 16 cases during this time interval. For all races, men had an incidence rate of 5.7 and women 3.0 per 100,000. From 2003 to 2007, the median age at death for chronic lymphocytic leukemia was 79, with white males showing the highest mortality at 2.2 per 100,000, and white females 1.0 per 100,000. For men, Asian/Pacific Islanders had the lowest mortality rate at 0.4 per 100,000 and for women, American Indian/Alaskan Natives had the lowest incidence at fewer than 16 cases during this time interval. Based on rates from 2005 to 2007, 0.48%, or one in 210, men and women born today will be diagnosed with chronic lymphocytic leukemia at some time during their lifetime. The overall five-year relative survival rate for 1999 to 2006 was 78.4%.

Brain/nervous system. It is estimated that 22,020 men and women (11,980 men and 10,040 women) will be diagnosed with cancer of the brain and nervous system and that 13,140 men and women will die of this type of cancer in 2010. From 2003 to 2007, 74% of brain and other nervous system cancer cases were diagnosed while the cancer was still confined to the primary site (localized stage), 16% were diagnosed after the cancer had spread to regional lymph nodes or directly beyond the primary site, and 2% were diagnosed after the cancer had already metastasized (distant stage). (For the remaining 8% the staging information was unknown.) The corresponding five-year relative survival rates were: 37.6% for localized; 23.5% for regional; 38.6% for distant; and 34.3% for unstaged.

From 2003 to 2007, the median age at diagnosis for cancer of the brain and nervous system was 56. Approximately 13.0% were diagnosed under age 20; 9.0% between the ages of 20 and 34; 9.7% between 35 and 44; 15.3% between 45 and 54; 18.3% between 55 and 64; 16.3% between 65 and 74; 14.1% between 75 and 84; and 4.3% at age 85+. The age adjusted incidence rate was 6.5 per 100,000 men and women per year. These rates are based on cases diagnosed from 17 SEER geographic areas. It was found that white men and women had the highest incidence at 8.4 per 100,000 for men and 6.0 per 100,000 for women. Hispanics had the next highest incidence at 5.9 per 100,000 men and 4.6 per 100,000 women. African Americans had an incidence of 4.7 per 100,000 men and 3.5 per 100,000 women. Asian/Pacific Islander men had an incidence rate of 4.0 per 100,000 and American Indian/Alaskan Native women 3.4 per 100,000. For men, American Indian/Alaska Natives had the lowest incidence at 3.7 per 100,000 and for women, Asian Pacific Islanders had the lowest incidence rate at 3.2 per 100,000. For all races, it was found that men averaged an incidence rate of 7.6 per 100,000; women averaged 5.5 per 100,000. The same statistics utilized during this time revealed that the median age of mortality from brain and nervous system cancer was 64 years, with white men having the highest mortality of 5.6 per 100,000 and white women 3.8 per 100,000. For men, Asian/Pacific Islanders had the lowest mortality rate of 2.3 per 100,000 and for women, American Indian/Alaska Natives and Asian Pacific Islanders had the lowest rate at 1.6 per 100,000.

Based on rates from 2005 to 2007, 0.61%, or one in 165 men and women born today will be diagnosed with cancer of the brain and nervous system at some time during their lifetime.

Other common cancers. The following information has been compiled from statistics of the American Cancer Society's publication, *Cancer Facts & Figures, 2010.*[26]

Cancer of the endometrium (uterine cancer) is the most common cancer of the reproductive organs. The American Cancer Society estimates there will be 43,470 new cases of cancer of the endometrial lining of the uterus diagnosed in the United States during 2010 and that about 7,950 women in the United States will die from this type of cancer this year. The one- and five-year relative survival rates for uterine corpus cancer are 92% and 83% respectively. The five-year survival rate is 96%, 67%, or 17%, if the cancer is diagnosed at a local, regional, or distant stage, respectively. Relative survival in whites exceeds that for African Americans by more than 8% at every stage of diagnosis. The average chance that a woman will be diagnosed with this cancer during her lifetime is about one in 39.

Skin cancer is a type of cancer that forms in the tissue of the skin. Skin cancer that forms in basal cells (at the base of the outer layer of the skin) is called basal cell carcinoma. Skin cancer that forms in squamous cells (on the surface cells of the skin) is called squamous cell carcinoma and skin cancer that forms in melanocytes (skin cells that make pigment) is called melanoma. Melanoma is considered the most dangerous of the three types of skin cancer and accounts for most skin cancer deaths. The American Cancer Society estimates that about 68,130 new melanomas will be diagnosed in the

United States during 2010. Most of the more than 1 million cases of skin cancer diagnosed yearly in the United States are considered to be related to exposure to the sun.

Diagnosis: Cancer

In the early 1970s, a diagnosis of cancer was often treated as a death sentence by patients and their families. Since then, there has been a significant improvement in both five-year survival and mortality rates due to earlier detection and more effective treatment to combat cancer. With that said, the number of Americans 65 years of age or older will double in next 30 years, and by the year 2030 one in five Americans will be 65 years of age or older. This is important because approximately six of every 10 new cancer cases are diagnosed in this age range. Some types of cancer are more common in the elderly (65 years and older), while some are found more in the younger population. Among men 65 and older, cancer of the prostate, lung, and colon make up around half of all diagnosed cancers. Prostate cancer is around 22 times more frequent among elderly men than among younger men.[27] The corresponding most frequent cancers among women 65 and older, comprising 48% of cases, are breast, colon, lung, and stomach cancer. For all major specific cancer sites except testicular cancer, the incidence rate is significantly higher among the elderly than among any groups of younger and middle-aged persons.[28]

Studies from the National Cancer Institute and the *Journal of Oncology Practice* reveal that the number of Americans diagnosed with cancer, undergoing treatment, in remission, and having completed all therapies will increase by 54%, from 11.8 million in 2005 to 18.2 million, by the year 2020 (see Figure 3-4 (a) and (b)).[29]

FIGURE 3-4 (a). Projected increase in cancer patients in millions, 2005–2020. (Source: National Cancer Institute, *Journal of Oncology Practice*; U.S. Census, July, 2006)

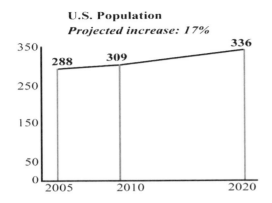
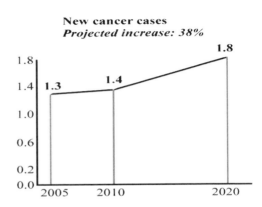

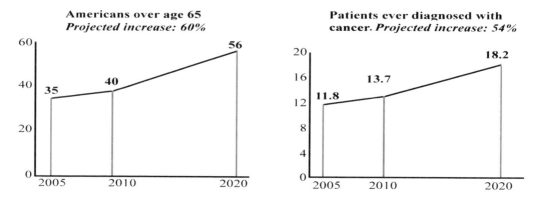

FIGURE 3-4 (b). Projected increase in cancer patients in millions, 2005-2020. (Source: National Cancer Institute, *Journal of Oncology Practice*; U.S. Census, July, 2006)

According to this research, the rise in cancer, which has been called a disease of the aging population, is proportional to the rise in the number of Americans over the age of 65. In the United States, the population that is 65 and older will more than double by 2050, rising from 39 million today to 89 million.

While children are still projected to outnumber the older population worldwide in 2050, the under-15 population in the United States is expected to fall below the older population by that date, increasing from 62 million today to 85 million.[29] This increase is seen worldwide as well. The U.S. Census Bureau reports the world's 65-and-older population is projected to triple by mid-century, from 516 million in 2009 to 1.53 billion in 2050.[30] "This shift in the age structure of the world's population poses challenges to society, families, businesses, healthcare providers, and policy makers to meet the needs of aging individuals," says Wan He, demographer in the Census Bureau's Population Division. Challenges due to this increase in cancer will include a greater need for oncology services to meet the growing needs of the population and studies indicate that demand is expected to rise as much as 48% by 2020.

As a result, the supply of services provided by oncologists during this time is expected to grow more slowly than the demand—approximately 14%, based on the current age distribution; the practice patterns of oncologists and the number of available oncology fellowship positions are also contributing factors to this trend. This course is significant because shortages in the field of cancer-related services translates into significant shortages in the availability of treatment visits and oncologists to treat the growing number of cancer patients.[31] This means that treatment outcomes may also be significantly affected, especially when it comes to having readily accessible oncological care. Pediatric oncology shows us one of the most dramatic examples, where in the developed world cure rates following childhood cancer are approximately 75%, but percentages drop to 10 to15%, or even less, in many low-income countries. It has been calculated that almost 100,000 children who die every year from cancer could have been cured had they received appropriate treatment.[32]

Cancer prevention steps

The Harvard Center for Cancer Prevention, a division of the Harvard School of Public Health, offers various publications, one of which is called *Cancer Causes and Control*.[33] In *Volume I, Cancer Prevention: The Causes and Prevention of Cancer*, by Graham A. Colditz, M.D., David John Hunter ScD. expands on compiled research which explains the causes of cancer, provides evidence-based insight into cancer risk in the United States, and sets forth a series of preventive strategies. *Volume 1* explains the human origins of cancer, and encompasses the potential causes of cancer relating to lifestyle, such as smoking, diet, sedentary lifestyle, occupational factors, viruses, and alcohol. *Volume I* concludes that 65% of all cancer would be preventable if steps were taken for known causes.

What is the bottom line? Cancer is a preventable disease.

The Causes and Prevention of Cancer lists the following relative risk factors:

Cancer Risk Factors	% Cancer Deaths	Cancer Risk Factors	% Cancer Deaths
Tobacco	30%	Reproductive factors	5%
Adult diet/obesity	25%	Alcohol	3%
Sedentary lifestyle	10%	Environmental pollutants	2%
Occupational factors	5%	Radiation	2%
Family history of cancer	5%	Prescription drugs;	
Virus/biologic factor	5%	medical procedures	2%
Perinatal factors/growth	5%	Food additives/contaminants	1%

Perinatal/growth factors form the link between an individual's weight and the risk of breast cancer—and possibly other cancers as well. For example, a higher birth weight has been associated with some cancers, such as breast and prostate cancer, later in life. *Reproductive factors* are explained by the influence of early-age menarche, late maternal age, late age of menopause, birth weight, and multiple births as causes of cancer. Again, most of the risk factors expressed in this report pertain to lifestyle choices that can be modified to prevent the incidence of cancer.

How cells become cancerous

As we discussed earlier, many things in our daily living can generate free radicals and cause damage to the genetic material, or DNA, in normal cells. These genetic blueprints contain instructions which tell the cell what role it will perform in the body, so that any alteration to the code can alter the role that cell will play. This can be better understood from Figure 3-5, which shows the steps involved in how a normal cell becomes a cancerous cell.

FIGURE 3-5. Tumor development model, demonstrating developmental steps of cancer. (Source: *http://ecam.oxfordjournals.org/cgi/content/full/1/3/233*)

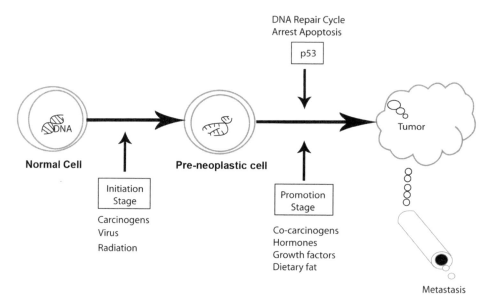

Looking at this chart, we can see that damage to our DNA can initiate the formation of preneoplastic cells, precursors to tumor development. Huge sections of the population naturally carry a number of preneoplastic cells in their body, however, so having them does not automatically imply a link to cancer. This is because normally the damaged DNA signals "p53" genes to initiate repairs or puts the cell cycle "on hold" so the cell does not divide. On the other hand, if the process does *not* work, either because the p53 gene is defective or suppressed by some other factor or factors, then the damaged cell is directed to perform apoptosis, or "programmed cell death," due to the irreparable DNA damage.

The fact that cancer is so prevalent in the United States obviously means that not all preneoplastic cells destruct following the genetic instructions of programmed death. In reality, approximately half of all cancer cases show defective p53 genes, but generally only at the end-stage of the disease. Even in the early stages of prostate cancer, however, the p53 gene is suppressed from acting. Because we know that co-carcinogens can impede the normal action of p53, and that when the p53 gene is unable to perform its action of destroying preneoplastic cells the result is that the cells will continue to divide, we also know the consequence will be the ultimate formation of a tumor.

The finances of cancer

The Organization for Economic Co-operation and Development (OECD) is a group that brings together the governments of countries from around the world that are committed to democracy and the market economy in order to support economic growth and financial stability, create employment, raise living standards, and contribute to worldwide trade. The OECD compares policy experiences, seeks answers to common problems, identifies good practice, and coordinates domestic and international policies. For more than 40 years OECD has been one of the world's largest and most reliable sources of comparable statistic and economic social data. In its "2009 Written Statement to Senate Special Committee on Aging," OECD reported that the United States spends more on healthcare than any other industrialized nation. In fact, the United States spent 16% of its national income (GDP), or $7,290 per person, on healthcare in 2007. This is by far the highest number provided in the report, both in terms of GDP and per person cost, compared to that of other OECD countries. Statistically it is more than seven percentage points higher than the 8.9% average of other countries.

Interestingly, OECD states that this cost is not due to the fact that Americans are more likely to be sick than people in other developed nations. OECD further contends that the very high rate of overweight and obesity in the United States is already costly and will drive health spending higher in the coming decades. We know that having a higher than normal body weight has been shown to increase the incidence of many diseases, including cancer. Given this fact, it is estimated that in the future 75% of the nation's healthcare spending will be in the area of chronic diseases.[34]

The pharmaceutical industry has always been on the forefront of researching cures for many diseases, including cancer. The Pharmaceutical Research and Manufacturers of America (PhRMA), this country's organization of leading pharmaceutical research and biotechnology companies, is devoted to developing medicines that allow patients to live longer, healthier, and more productive lives. In 2008, PhRMA members alone invested an estimated $50.3 billion in discovering and developing new medicines, and industry-wide research and investment reached a record $65.2 billion. A report by PhRMA, in response to President Obama's call for "a cure for cancer in our time," has revealed that America's pharmaceutical research and biotechnology companies are currently testing a record 861 new medicines and vaccines in their quest to find the cure for cancer.[35]

The country stands united in the war against cancer; however, efforts do not come without a cost. The National Institutes of Health estimates that the overall cost of cancer in 2008 was $228.1 billion, comprised of $93.2 billion for direct medical costs (total of all health expenditures); $18.8 billion for indirect morbidity costs (cost of lost productivity due to illness); and $116.1 billion for indirect mortality costs (cost of lost productivity due to premature death).[36]

The National Cancer Institute is the nation's principal agency for cancer research. Its mission statement reads, "The National Cancer Institute coordinates the National Cancer Program, which conducts and supports research, training, health information dissemination, and other programs with respect to the cause, diagnosis, prevention, and treatment of cancer, rehabilitation from cancer, and the continuing care of cancer patients and the families of cancer patients." NCI reports that its total budget for fiscal year 2007 was $4.79 billion; for 2008, $4.83 billion; for 2009, $4.97 billion; and that its total budget in 2010 was $5.15 billion. In 2011, the NCI is seeking an increase of 163 million, or approximately 3.2%, over the 2010 budget. NCI has proposed this budget increase to fulfill two components, the first being the maintenance of current levels of operations and the second to expand and broaden existing initiatives. In the year 2008, NCI spent about 68% of its budget on researching cancer, 14% on resource development, 9% on program management and support, and 9% on cancer prevention. It is also worth mentioning here that, in real numbers, only $472 million of the $4.83 *billon*-dollar budget was spent on cancer prevention and support.[37]

Table 3-7 illustrates NCI spending for the most common types of cancer studied in the United States. NCI's budget for Fiscal Year 2009 was $4.97 billion, excluding the additional $1.26 billion received by the Institute from the American Recovery and Reinvestment Act, or ARRA (an economic stimulus package enacted by the 111th United States Congress in February 2009), for spending in FY 2009 and FY 2010.

Table 3-7. NCI spending in FY, 2007, 2008, and 2009 for the 10 most common types of cancer in the United States, excluding basal cell and squamous cell skin cancers. The cancers are listed in decreasing order of incidence; that is, from the highest number of new cases each year to the lowest. (Source: NCI, Office of Budget and Finance (OBF) at *www.cancer.gov*)

Cancer type	2007 spending (in millions)	2008 spending (in millions)	2009 spending (in millions)	2009 ARRA spending (in millions)
Lung	$226.9	$247.6	$246.9	$48.0
Prostate	$296.1	$285.4	$293.9	$47.0
Breast	$572.4	$572.6	$599.5	$85.5
Colorectal	$258.4	$273.7	$264.2	$44.5
Bladder	$ 19.8	$ 24.1	$ 25.9	$ 2.8
Melanoma	$ 97.7	$110.8	$103.7	$17.6
Non-Hodgkin lymphoma	$113.0	$122.6	$130.9	$14.0
Kidney	$ 35.2	$ 43.4	$ 45.2	$ 7.2
Leukemia	$205.5	$216.4	$220.6	$33.9
Pancreas	$ 73.3	$ 87.3	$ 89.7	$10.7

With its updates, statistics, research, and articles consistently providing well-rounded, clear information, the NCI is doing a great job meeting the goals expressed in its mission statement. I wonder how many of us are aware of the time, money, and effort spent compiling the vast database available on cancer. I, for one, feel fortunate to have all this information at my disposal. I also believe that we will succeed in the war against cancer when everyone works together in concert to spread cancer awareness and to ensure that healthy lifestyles are maintained, regular screening occurs, prompt treatment is obtained, and proper follow-up care is adopted.

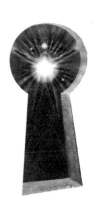

4. Physical Facets of Health

"Lack of activity destroys the good condition of every human being, while movement and methodical physical exercise save it and preserve it."

- Plato (427 B.C.–347 B.C.)

Staying well

What does it take to stay healthy—to stay well? I have always felt that the health of every form of life depends on how well it is able to adapt to both external and internal challenges. Adaptation is the ability to change or respond in ways that will improve the chances of survival in any given environment. Adaptation allows any organism to meet any condition that presents itself. It is when we lose some of these adaptive qualities that the loss of health generally ensues.

Adaptation can be structural, behavioral, or physiological. Healthy structural adaptations are physical changes of the body that help it meet its daily demands, such as our Body Mass Index, muscle strength, muscular endurance, and flexibility. Healthy behavioral adaptations are actions we can take in response to our environment. Examples of behavioral adaptations include stress reduction, meditation, dietary choices, and smoking cessation. Lastly, healthy physiological adaptations are the biochemical responses that occur inside the body and are designed to protect us from harm, such as those in the form of the immune response, detoxification, and DNA repair.

In general, organisms that have adapted to their environment are able to:

- obtain light, water, food, and nutrients
- cope with physical conditions, such as temperature, light, and heat
- defend themselves
- reproduce
- respond to changes around them

For our overall wellbeing, working toward supporting and maintaining the adaptive process is the key to health. When we give our bodies the basic daily attention they need, we can continually adapt to stay healthy. *Health needs to be our number one responsibility: to take a proactive stand to be, and stay, disease-free.* Taking a stand in this case most certainly involves change as well, since the actions of the past have most likely not served us as well as they should. As most of us know already, change of any kind is often met with discomfort, so taking consistent action toward a healthier self is bound to meet up with some form of resistance through procrastination, doubt, or even guilt. But facing these walls of resistance and working through them is a sure way to receive considerable health dividends.

Where do we begin? The first step is gaining a basic understanding of the physical components that make up the human body. Expanding our knowledge about the different systems of the body heightens our awareness of how we are able to adapt. Once we gain an appreciation of our bodies and how they work, we can examine what we can do to support all the various systems of the body. This knowledge will ultimately allow us to be more adaptable.

When we have a body that exists in a weakened state, we can become easy prey to disease. Comprehending the basic mechanisms of how our body works invites us to make positive changes in our lifestyle, to "adapt" in ways that will ultimately improve the quality of our lives.

Systems of the human body: an overview

There are eleven major organ systems in the human body. They are:

1. The *digestive system*, for absorption of nutrients and excretion of waste
2. The *skeletal system*, for support, movement, and blood cell production
3. The *muscular system*, for support, movement, and production of heat
4. The *nervous system*, for mental activity and for integration and coordination through electrochemical signals
5. The *endocrine system*, for integration and coordination through hormones
6. The *cardiovascular system*, for internal transport
7. The *respiratory system*, for elimination of CO_2 and absorption of O_2
8. The *reproductive system*, for production of offspring (procreation)
9. The *integumentary system*, for covering the body
10. The *lymphatic system*, for regulation of fluids and immunity
11. The *urinary system*, for excretion of nitrogenous waste and maintenance, or homeostasis, of electrolytes

The digestive system

The digestive system (see Figure 4-1) consists of a set of hollow organs joined by a flexible tube. It commences at the mouth, continues at the stomach and intestines where food is processed, and terminates at the anus. The entire length of the digestive system is lined with a mucosal layer of cells capable of secreting a soft, jelly-like substance called *mucus*. In the mouth, the stomach, and the small intestine, the *mucosae* have tiny glands that produce juices which aid in digesting food. Both the liver and pancreas form a part of the digestive system in their capacity to secrete hormones and digestive juices into the intestine.

FIGURE 4-1. The digestive system.

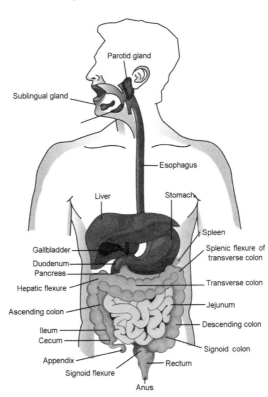

The food we eat needs to be broken down into a form that allows for the absorption of nutrients. *Digestion* is a process which facilitates that absorption, helping our body derive the nourishment it requires for proper functioning. As a first step, the food is mixed with the saliva in the mouth, which breaks down the larger carbohydrates into relatively smaller molecules when we chew. Saliva is secreted by the parotid glands, submandibular glands, and sublingual glands.

Swallowing pushes this substance into the stomach, where it is further acted upon by digestive enzymes. Swallowing is actually the first major muscle movement of digestion and although we swallow voluntarily, once we have initiated this act the rest of the digestive process is under involuntary control. The stomach churns the food substance with a large dose of digestive juices, which consist of acid and a protein-digesting enzyme. After processing the food, the stomach slowly empties its content into the small intestine.

Once in the small intestine, the partially digested food substance is mixed with secretions from the pancreas and liver, allowing further digestion to occur. All of the nutrients, i.e., the vitamins, minerals, water, and the digested molecules of food, are absorbed through the intestinal walls. Most of the absorbed material then enters the cells that line the intestine and is carried off into the bloodstream to supply other parts of the body, either for storage or for immediate use. The waste products of this process include undigested food particles, roughage, fiber, and aged cells. These materials are propelled into the colon and then expelled by the bowels. The entire process of digestion is controlled by two main factors: hormones and neural impulses.

Hormonal regulators. When the presence of food in the stomach has been sensed, hormones are produced by the cells of the stomach and small intestine to aid in the digestive process. The two major hormones are gastrin and secretin. Gastrin stimulates the secretion of acid in the stomach for dissolving and digesting the food and is required for the maturation and growth of the cells lining the stomach. Secretin, found in the mucosal cells of the duodenum, stimulates pancreatic, pepsin, and bile secretion, while inhibiting gastric acid secretion.

Other hormones are also involved in digestion. Cholecystokinin, or CCK, is a hormone that stimulates the pancreas to release digestive enzymes. Ghrelin, produced in the stomach and upper intestine, stimulates appetite in the absence of food. Produced in the digestive tract in response to a meal, peptide YY is the hormone that inhibits our appetite. Together, ghrelin and peptide YY exert an influence on the brain and control our intake of food.

Nerve regulators. Digestion is controlled by two neural networks, which also serve as regulators in the digestive process. Our extrinsic neural pathways come from the outside, specifically the brain and the spinal cord. The chemicals these nerves release are acetylcholine and adrenaline. Acetylcholine increases the secretion of the digestive juice and causes the muscles of the digestive system to squeeze. This, in turn, helps to "push" the food and the juice through the digestive tract. Adrenaline has the opposite effect in that it relaxes the muscles of the stomach and intestine and decreases the flow of blood to these organs; in this way the digestive process is either slowed or stopped. Our intrinsic nerves constitute a dense network in the walls of the esophagus (throat), stomach, small intestine, and colon. These nerves are triggered when the walls are stretched by food.

Together, nerves, hormones, the bloodstream, and the organs of the digestive system conduct the complex tasks of digesting and absorbing nutrients from the foods and liquids we consume everyday.

The musculoskeletal system

The primary feature that characterizes all life forms is motility, or the ability to move. How the organism achieves this capability depends on how developed the organism is. Unicellular (single-celled) organisms, such as some bacteria, propel themselves by means of long, spindle-shaped "wires" called *flagella*, while more advanced life forms, such as human beings, are able to move through the use of their muscles and skeleton, or musculoskeletal systems.

The skeletal system, which forms the body's framework and helps us maintain an erect posture, consists of bones, ligaments (that attach bone to bone), cartilage (the protective, jelly-like substance that covers the joints and forms the intervertebral discs in the spinal column), and tendons (that attach muscle to bone).

Bones possess cavities that are filled with a soft, flexible tissue, called *marrow*, which is responsible for generating fresh red blood cells along with most of the white blood cells and other cells required by the immune system. The skeletal system forms an outer cage that protects our lungs and heart, as well as the thick, bony, outer covering that protects our brain and spinal cord. The skeletal system also plays a huge role in maintaining the concentration of minerals at its optimum level in the blood, a process called *mineral homeostasis*.

Our musculoskeletal system (see Figure 4-2) has 206 bones and more than 600 muscles. These muscles, which are attached to the skeletal system, allow us to move. Bones and muscles both contribute to our physical strength. Muscles also act as storehouses for *glycogen*, the secondary short-term energy source for cells. When we exercise, for example, and energy is required, glycogen becomes mobilized and metabolizes to generate the energy we need.

FIGURE 4-2(a). The musculoskeletal system (frontal view).

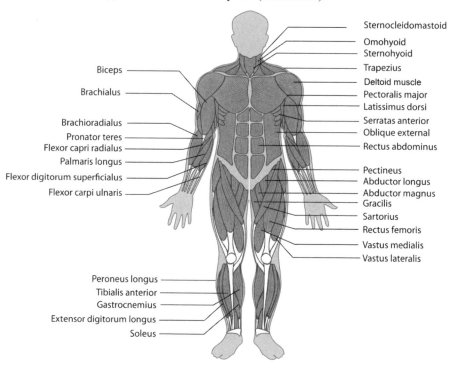

Biceps
Brachialus
Brachioradialus
Pronator teres
Flexor capri radialus
Palmaris longus
Flexor digitorum superficialus
Flexor carpi ulnaris

Sternocleidomastoid
Omohyoid
Sternohyoid
Trapezius
Deltoid muscle
Pectoralis major
Latissimus dorsi
Serratas anterior
Oblique external
Rectus abdominus

Pectineus
Abductor longus
Abductor magnus
Gracilis
Sartorius
Rectus femoris
Vastus medialis
Vastus lateralis

Peroneus longus
Tibialis anterior
Gastrocnemius
Extensor digitorum longus
Soleus

FIGURE 4-2(b). The musculoskeletal system (back view).

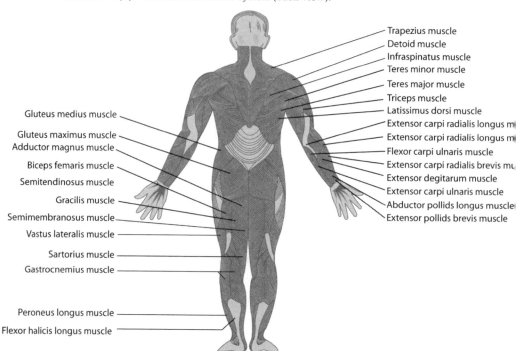

Gluteus medius muscle
Gluteus maximus muscle
Adductor magnus muscle
Biceps femaris muscle
Semitendinosus muscle
Gracilis muscle
Semimembranosus muscle
Vastus lateralis muscle
Sartorius muscle
Gastrocnemius muscle
Peroneus longus muscle
Flexor halicis longus muscle

Trapezius muscle
Detoid muscle
Infraspinatus muscle
Teres minor muscle
Teres major muscle
Triceps muscle
Latissimus dorsi muscle
Extensor carpi radialis longus m
Extensor carpi radialis longus m
Flexor carpi ulnaris muscle
Extensor carpi radialis brevis mu
Extensor degitarum muscle
Extensor carpi ulnaris muscle
Abductor pollids longus muscle
Extensor pollids brevis muscle

There are three types of muscles: skeletal, or striated muscles help the body move; smooth, or unstriated muscles are found inside the linings of the stomach and intestine; and cardiac muscle is found in the heart.

Based on the type of action performed, our muscles are broadly classified into two types: voluntary and involuntary. Voluntary muscles, whose actions can be controlled, include those muscles found in the extremities, such as the arms (see Figure 4-3). Involuntary muscles comprise the heart, pupils, and digestive system: all muscles that are not directly controlled at will (see Figure 4-4). When we wish to walk we move with the help of the muscles attached to the bones in our legs. The skeletal muscles produce movement by bending the skeleton at specific movable joints. Joints are the points where two bones meet. The joints bend because the muscles attached to the bones contract and shorten in length, pulling the bones closer together. Skeletal muscles can move only in one direction and reversing the bend requires contraction of a different set of muscles with the simultaneous stretching of the first group.

FIGURE 4-3. Voluntary muscles.

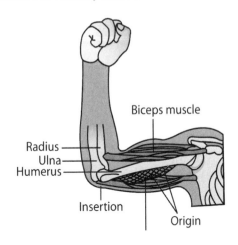

FIGURE 4-4. Involuntary muscles.

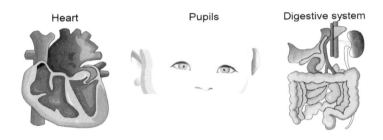

Movement, therefore, is essentially a function of two groups of muscles acting, in a sense, opposite to each other. When one set contracts, the other stretches itself and is ready to reverse that state when required. For example, when our biceps, or muscles of the upper arm, contract, the action pulls the lower arm toward the shoulder. For this action to take place, the muscles on the opposite side, the triceps, must relax. Alternately, the triceps, or the muscles on the underside of the arm, need to contract to straighten out the arm. This then requires the biceps to relax, so the triceps can perform this action. All movements of the body—walking, nodding the head, carrying, and so on, are due to the contraction and relaxation of skeletal muscles, and the skeletal muscles always work in pairs. Voluntary movements from various muscle groups allow us to perform all types of physical exercise; exercising the muscles can increase both their strength and endurance.

When it comes to our involuntary muscles, we are generally not even aware of their constant, smooth functioning. These muscles work without our having to think about them, and are controlled by hormonal systems and neural inputs. These smooth muscles are the "housekeepers" of the body, and include: the involuntary contraction of the intestinal wall, pushing food through the body; the involuntary contraction of the bladder and expelling of urine; and the involuntary contraction of the pelvic muscles, facilitating childbirth. In the same way, the pupil of the eye shrinks due to the involuntary contraction of the pupillary sphincter muscle, in response to bright light.

The nervous system

The nervous system is the body's master control center and network for communication (see Figure 4-5). It is one of the earliest systems of the human body to develop, usually beginning to form during the third week of fetal growth. It is made up of the brain, spinal cord, cranial nerves, and spinal nerves. The nervous system has three basic functions:

1. to receive information from the sensory receptors through sensory neurons;
2. to transfer and process impulses through interneurons; and
3. to send appropriate impulses/instructions to perform an action through motor neurons.

FIGURE 4-5. Map of the nervous system.

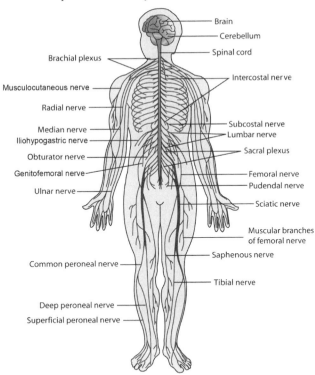

Brain
Cerebellum
Spinal cord
Intercostal nerve
Brachial plexus
Musculocutaneous nerve
Radial nerve
Subcostal nerve
Median nerve
Lumbar nerve
Iliohypogastric nerve
Sacral plexus
Obturator nerve
Genitofemoral nerve
Femoral nerve
Pudendal nerve
Ulnar nerve
Sciatic nerve
Muscular branches
of femoral nerve
Saphenous nerve
Common peroneal nerve
Tibial nerve
Deep peroneal nerve
Superficial peroneal nerve

The two major components of the nervous system are the central nervous system (CNS), made up of the brain and spinal cord, and the peripheral nervous system (PNS), made up of the cranial and spinal nerves. The central and peripheral nervous systems, while different, are always in constant communication with one another. The autonomic nervous system (ANS), comprised of three other systems, the sympathetic, parasympathetic, and enteric, is that part of the peripheral nervous system which controls the visceral functions of the body. For example, the enteric nervous system is a meshwork of nerve fibers that innervate the visceral organs, such as the intestine, gall bladder, and pancreas. It is the job of the ANS to monitor and assess the internal environment and then send its assessment to the central nervous system. The CNS processes this information and then responds by regulating the functions of the internal environment. The parasympathetic system can be summed up as the "rest and digest" system, as it is concerned with the conservation and restoration of energy, the reduction of heart rate and blood pressure, the facilitation of digestion, the absorption of nutrients, and the excretion of waste products. In contrast to the parasympathetic system, the sympathetic system enables the body to be prepared for "flight or fight." Sympathetic responses include increased heart rate, blood pressure, and cardiac output; increased blood flow to skeletal muscle; increased pupil size and respiration; and decreased gastric motility. What follows is an overview of the nervous system.

The structure of a nerve cell. A *neuron* is a cell that is specialized to conduct nerve impulses. Typical neurons, or nerve cells, have long, root-like projections on one end called *dendrites*, a cell body, or *soma*, and an *axon*, the primary transmission line that conducts electrical impulses. Axons of some neurons can be split up into about 150 parts, each part signaling more than one cell. The smallest neuron is about four microns wide (1 micron = 1/1000 mm). Some of the largest neurons are about 100 microns wide. The axon is covered by a protective layer, predominantly made up of fats, called the *myelin*, or *medullary*, *sheath*. The main function of the myelin sheath is to facilitate the transfer of nerve impulses along the axon. This sheath protects the neuron to a certain extent and acts like the insulation around a wire. While other cells are replaced when they die, a neuron is never replaced when it becomes nonfunctional. That is why the number of our functional neurons tends to decrease as age advances.

The brain has approximately 100 million neurons. Our brain weighs less than 2.5% of our body weight, but consumes about 20% of the total energy when our body is at rest. It burns 10 times more glucose and oxygen than the other organs. The brain receives and sends information in the form of nerve impulses. The spinal cord is a thick bundle of nerves originating at the base of the brain and running down the middle of the back inside the bony spinal column. There are 31 pairs of spinal nerves that branch off and exit the spinal cord like branches from a tree. The neurons are present in all the parts of the body, from the soles of the feet to the surface of the scalp, and are found below the skin, extending to internal organs. If you stretch the nerves supplying the skin end to end, they are likely to reach almost 45 miles! In fact, the length of a single nerve cell can range from a fraction of an inch to more than two feet. The sciatic nerve, which runs from the base of the spine to the tip of a toe, is estimated to average around three feet in length. A neuron transmits the nerve impulses at a speed of 250 miles per hour, or at roughly one third the speed of sound traveling through the air.

Neurons communicate with each other through an electrochemical process. When a stimulus is received by the dendrite of the neuron, it passes it along the cell body to the axon. The axon then empties a neurotransmitter, a chemical substance, into the *synapse*, or the junction between two neurons. When the neurotransmitter is in the junction, a response is elicited. An interesting quality relative to the transmission of nerve impulses is that it is an "all-or-nothing effect." This means that either the nerves fire and transmit the impulse, or they do not. There is no weak nerve transmission. A noteworthy fact about the human nervous system is that it is the only system in the body completely encased by bone. The skull envelops the brain, and the spinal cord is protected by the vertebral column: both are hard coverings which act as shields to protect the brain and spinal cord. This protective design again stresses the overall importance of the nervous system.

The endocrine system

The endocrine system consists of an arrangement of glands and the hormones secreted by these glands (see Figure 4-6). Hormones (from the Greek word *hormaein*, "to excite," or "to stir up") are chemical messengers carried through the blood to exert a functional effect on another part of the body. The glands that secrete hormones are known as *endocrine glands*. Endocrine glands (from the Greek *endo*, "within," and *krinein*, "to separate") are notable in their difference from the other glands of the body, such as sweat and sebaceous (oil-secreting) glands, in that the hormone molecules of these glands are secreted directly into the bloodstream, where the other glands are not. The endocrine system regulates growth and development, mood, the reproductive cycle, the immune system, and metabolism.

> **Glands.** A *gland* is an organ of specialized cells that synthesizes a substance for release. In this case, that substance is a hormone. The main endocrine glands in our system are: the pituitary, adrenals, thyroid, parathyroid, pancreatic islets, gonads (both testes and ovaries), and placenta. In some cases, hormones are also synthesized by certain neurons. For example, vasopressin and oxytocin are synthesized by the supraoptic and paraventricular nuclei of the hypothalamus. Some hormones identified in the brain have been found to function as neurotransmitters; others are secreted by cells that are not exactly organized into glands, but function in "clusters." For example, gastrin and secretin regulate the gastrointestinal function and are secreted by cells present along the walls of the intestine.

FIGURE 4-6. Location of the endocrine glands in the body.

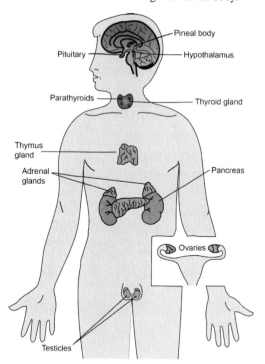

The pituitary gland. The pituitary gland is located at the base of the brain. It is called the "master gland" since it secretes most of the hormones that regulate the secretions from other endocrine glands. Pituitary secretions are sensitive to both emotional and seasonal changes. The pituitary is under the control of the hypothalamus, which is considered the master gland's master. The hypothalamus is the primary functional player in the neuroendocrine system. It is the portion of the brain that secretes neurohormones, which stimulate or inhibit the release of pituitary hormones.

The pituitary is divided into two main lobes, anterior (in front) and posterior (in back). There are six major anterior pituitary hormones, one intermediate lobe hormone, and two posterior pituitary hormones. The anterior pituitary lobe controls the thyroid, adrenal, and the reproductive glands and produces the following hormones:

- GH, the "growth hormone," responsible for growth and development of bone and other tissues and mineral homeostasis
- Prolactin, important in the generation of milk in breastfeeding mothers

- TSH, the thyroid-stimulating hormone, which controls the normal functioning of the thyroid gland
- ACTH, the adrenocorticotrophic hormone, which controls the adrenal glands and stimulates the secretion of glucocorticoids
- LH, the lutinizing hormone, and FSH, the follicle-stimulating hormone, which control the production of sex hormones (estrogen and testosterone), as well as sperm and egg maturation and release

The posterior lobe of the pituitary produces ADH, the antidiuretic hormone called vasopressin, and is responsible for maintaining the water balance in the body; oxytocin is the hormone responsible for the contraction of the uterus during childbirth.

Melanocyte-stimulating hormones (MSH) regulate the production of melanin, a dark pigment, by melanocytes in the skin. MSH is found in the intermediate lobe of the pituitary gland.

The thyroid gland. The thyroid gland is a butterfly-shaped gland located in front of the neck, just below the *larynx,* or "voice box." It releases the iodine-containing hormones, thyroxine (T4) and triiodothyronine (T3). These hormones are responsible for the rate at which the body burns up food nutrients for energy. An increase in thyroid hormone concentrations increases the body's metabolic rate. Thyroid hormones are also responsible for the development of bones in growing children.

The parathyroid glands. The parathyroid glands are attached to the thyroid glands. These glands release the parathyroid hormone, which regulates the secretion of calcitonin, a hormone secreted by the thyroid gland to maintain calcium levels in the body.

The adrenal glands. The adrenal glands are located on top of the kidneys. They have two parts: the outer adrenal cortex and the inner medulla. The adrenal cortex produces corticosteroids, which control the body's use of fats, proteins, and carbohydrates, suppress inflammatory reactions, and affect the immune system. They also produce hormones that control the water and salt balance in the body, and they have some effect on male sexual development and function. The adrenal medulla releases catecholamines, such as adrenaline or epinephrine, and noradrenaline or norepinephrine, in response to stress. This action increases heart rate and blood pressure.

The pineal gland. The pineal gland is located in the brain and secretes melatonin, which controls the sleep-wake cycle.

The gonads. The gonads release the sex hormones. In males, *testes* secrete androgens, most importantly, testosterone. These effect changes in the body during puberty and the appearance of secondary sex characteristics, such as growth of body and facial hair, deepening of the voice, increase in muscle growth, and strength and production of sperm. In females, the *ovaries* produce estrogen, progesterone, and the eggs for fertilization. Estrogen is associated with the development of female secondary sexual characteristics, such as breast development and redistribution of fat around the hips and thighs. The ovaries are also involved in the regulation of the menstrual cycle and pregnancy.

The pancreas. The pancreas produces the hormones insulin and glucagon, which work to maintain the blood's glucose level at a steady state. They also function to mobilize stored fats and carbohydrates for energy purposes.

Hormones can elicit their effects on target cells at a distance by traveling in the bloodstream. This effect is called the *telecrine function*. When hormones target cells in their immediate vicinity it is called the *paracrine function*. Other hormones transported in the blood are bound to proteins that function as hormone carriers. The target cells have receptors for these hormones. The hormone-receptor complex activates a series of sequences within the cell and thus carries out the intended chemical process. Once the desired hormone levels and effects of those hormones have been achieved, the process shuts down and inhibits further secretion. For example, once the thyroid hormone and its effects have reached a certain level, the pituitary cells are acted upon to immediately turn off the secretion of the thyroid-stimulating hormone. Similarly, parathyroid hormones increase the calcium levels in the body. The parathyroid hormone secretion turns off when there is sufficient calcium. This kind of regulatory mechanism is called *negative feedback control*.

On the other hand, *positive feedback control* occurs during lactation, for example, where the more a baby nurses, the more milk is produced, and in childbirth, where more oxytocin is released into the bloodstream as contractions occur, further stimulating more contractions. Another example is blood clotting. In this case, feedback is initiated when injured tissue releases chemicals that activate platelets in the blood. Once the platelets are activated they release chemicals to activate more platelets, causing a rapid formation of aggregated platelets to form a blood clot.

Although the endocrine glands are our main hormone producers, some non-endocrine organs, such as the kidneys and thymus, also produce hormones. The kidney produces the hormone renin, which plays a role in the body's water balance, while the thymus secretes thymosin, required for producing the cells of the immune system.

Though the roles of each system of the body are clearly delineated by their functions, there is always constant communication among them. For example, when we feel thirsty it means the body's circulating fluid level is low. To counteract this sensation, we turn to drinking water, or a liquid beverage, to replenish our fluid level. Normally, about 60% of our body is made up of water. The thirst sensation is felt when this fluid volume drops 0.5 to 1% below normal. This is accomplished when specific receptors located in the brain's hypothalamus detect the decrease in fluid volume. These receptors then exert control over the release of the antidiuretic hormone, *ADH*, or vasopressin, from the pituitary gland, also located in the brain. ADH then initiates the reabsorption of water in the kidney to conserve fluid volumes in the body. Drinking lots of water, more than what is required or utilized by the body, decreases ADH secretion; all excess water is eliminated in the urine. Aldosterone, another hormone, assists in maintaining the body's water balance, with increased concentrations of potassium ions in the extracellular fluid as the stimulus. Aldosterone is sensitive to potassium concentrations as well as to angiotensin II of the renin-angiotensin system. These physiological responses by the body help restore the electrolyte-fluid balance.

This is a highly simplified version of the complex mechanism of maintaining the body's overall fluid composition, especially when we consider that just about all the systems of the human body—the kidneys and the adrenal glands (forming the renal system), the nervous system, the cardiovascular system, the lungs and the nasal cavity (constituting the respiratory system), the gastrointestinal tract (comprised of the stomach and the intestine), and even the skin (covering the entire body and forming the integumentary system)—are all players in balancing the body's fluid levels. In fact, each and every physiological function, regardless of where it occurs in the body, is communicated by way of hormones or nerve impulses.

The major point I want to make here is that there is an active dialogue, a constant communication, among all of the various organ systems within the body. The different systems of the human body depend on each other for functioning efficiently and working in perfect synchronicity to achieve the desired result through mutual cooperation.

This is especially apparent when we look at the relationship between the nervous system and the endocrine system. The endocrine system secretes its hormones, or chemical messengers, through the body. Each is synthesized by a particular gland and then released into circulation. Hormones attach to receptors exactly the way a correct key fits into its matching lock, and the binding of hormones to receptors triggers a series of events that elicit the desired response. For example, when an individual is frightened suddenly, the brain instantly contacts the adrenal glands to release the hormone adrenaline. This hormone switches on a state of alert throughout the body and immediately a whole series of responses are activated: the heart starts to beat rapidly, the breath quickens, the digestive system slows down to allow more blood flow to the muscles, and the eyes dilate to allow more light for proper vision. This fight or flight reaction is in response to the neural impulses set off by the initial release of adrenaline. Physiologists often call this branch of study interconnecting the nervous and the endocrine systems *neuro-endocrinology*.

The cardiovascular system

The heart. Can you name the most tireless worker in the human body? The heart, of course: the origin of our primary life-sustaining force. The human heart starts beating around day 22 of fetal development. What initiates the first heartbeat is still an unanswered question, but technically at least, it appears that the electrical impulses needed to stimulate the heartbeat arise from the cells of the developing heart, or cardiac myocytes. The input from the central nervous system only serves to modify the rate at which the heart beats and does not play a part in the initiation of the heartbeat. Scientists have actually been able to demonstrate that random heart cells cultured in the laboratory beat sporadically, but when a group of such cells come in contact with each other they begin to beat in cooperative fashion.

In the adult human body the heart is only the size of a fist, yet along with the associated *blood vessels*, *arteries*, *capillaries*, and *veins*, it is responsible for keeping nearly 5 liters (l), or 5.28 quarts (qts) of blood in constant flow (see Figure 4-7). The heart does this very effectively through a steady pumping action. From the moment it starts to work, the heart beats 100,000 times each day and about 35 million times a year. Over an average lifetime, the heart pumps an estimated 2.5 billion times without "skipping a beat." The heart has four chambers: two upper chambers and two lower chambers. The upper chambers are called *atria*; the lower chambers are *ventricles*. Blood enriched with oxygen and nutrients leaves the left side of the heart through a large blood vessel called the *aorta*. The aorta branches into smaller vessels, to the arteries and eventually the *arterioles*, which further branch into *capillaries* to supply the oxygen and nutrients to the tissues. This extensive network of arteries, arterioles, and capillaries is estimated to be 50,000 to 60,000 miles long.

Waste products and carbon dioxide are picked up from the tissues and carried back to the heart through the veins. These are channeled toward the clearing organs, mainly the lungs, liver, and kidney. Carbon dioxide is then expelled through the lungs, and the blood is loaded with oxygen once again for another cycle.

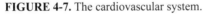
FIGURE 4-7. The cardiovascular system.

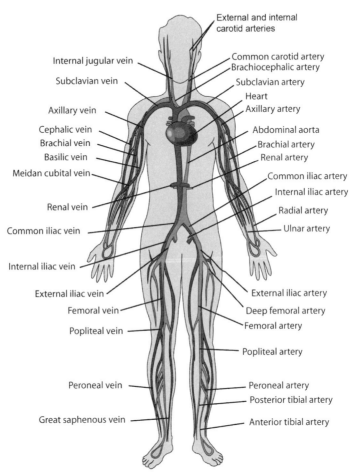

One heartbeat is a complete cardiac cycle, consisting of the contraction and relaxation of the upper chambers, then the subsequent contraction and relaxation of the lower chambers, and then a short gap. The upper and lower chambers contract alternately. At rest, the heart beats about 72 times a minute, though this can vary, depending on an individual's age and physical condition. When the ventricles (lower chambers) contract, blood pressure in the arteries increases due to the pumping action of the heart, known as the *systolic pressure*. Blood pressure during relaxation is known as the *diastolic pressure*. Blood pressure is measured in terms of millimeters (mm) of mercury, and is expressed as the ratio between the systolic and the diastolic pressure. Under normal conditions, adults have a systolic pressure of 120 mm and a diastolic of 80 mm, written as a blood pressure of 120/80.

The volume of blood expelled out of the heart after a single ventricular contraction is called the *stroke volume*. Cardiac output is a function of the stroke volume per the number of times the heart beats in a minute, or: *cardiac output = stroke volume x heart rate*.

For example, suppose the heart ejects about 73 ml of blood for each beat and at rest beats about 72 times. In this case, cardiac output can be calculated as: *cardiac output = 73 x 72 = 5.25 l per minute*.

At rest, men's bodies typically circulate about 5 l (or 5.28 qts) per minute; women typically circulate about 20% less. During exercise, due to an increase in heart rate or number of times the heart beats per minute, cardiac output can increase up to 30 l (or 31.7 qts) per minute. Cardiovascular response to exercise is a tremendous contributory factor to cardiac conditioning. Aerobic, or endurance training exercises, such as swimming, biking, and walking, produce more cardiovascular conditioning than weight training by increasing stroke volume as well as heart rate.

The respiratory system

The respiratory system consists of the gas-exchanging organs, the lungs, and a pump which helps the lungs (see Figure 4-8). This pump consists of the chest wall, the muscles around our chest that contract and relax to increase or decrease the size of the cavity inside our chest, and the area of the brain which controls the process. When we are at rest, we breathe about 12 to 15 times per minute. In every breath we take in 500 ml (or 0.53 qts) of air and an almost equal amount is expired. Our lungs handle 6.3 to 8.5 qts of air per minute.

The air we inhale is composed of 20.95% oxygen, 0.03% carbon dioxide, 78.09% nitrogen, and 0.93% other inert gases, such as argon and helium. When air enters our nose dust particles are filtered out by the tiny hairs inside the nostril. Any irritation at this stage in the process usually results in a more forceful response: a sneeze! During inhalation the air is moistened by the mucus in the nose. We also breathe in air through the mouth, which helps condition the inspired air. From there the air continues to travel down the nasopharynx, larynx, and trachea to finally reach the bronchial tubes, which direct the air into the two lungs. The bronchi divide several times in the lungs and form smaller bronchioles. Each bronchiole ends in a small, spongy chamber, or air sac. These are called the *alveoli*. The alveoli form the actual site where gasses are exchanged. The walls of the alveoli contain the blood vessels and capillaries. Capillary walls are so thin that it is possible for the oxygen and the carbon dioxide to pass through freely to enter the bloodstream. What drives the exchange forward and what makes us selectively take in oxygen and expel carbon dioxide? The answer is in the difference in the concentration, or amount, of the gases in relation to one another. The air that enters the alveoli is rich in oxygen when the oxygen-deficient blood reaches the capillaries lining the alveoli. The oxygen simply takes the place of the carbon dioxide, and the carbon dioxide diffuses into the alveoli to be exhaled. One indication of just how well this system works is that the air we exhale has roughly 100 times more carbon dioxide than the air we breathe in. The oxygen-enriched blood is then delivered to the heart, which supplies the different organs and tissues by its ceaseless pumping action. What's this complex process called? That's right: *breathing*.

FIGURE 4-8. The respiratory system.

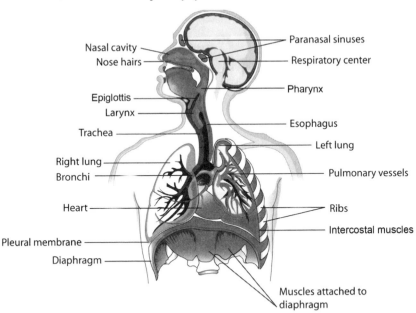

The diaphragm. One of the most important respiratory muscles is the diaphragm. This is the muscle that separates our chest cavity from our abdominal organs. During deep, quiet breathing, there is an increase in the size of the cavity in the chest. This is caused by the downward movement of the diaphragm. During normal breathing, our diaphragm moves down about 1 cm, and it moves as much as 10 cm during deep breathing or strenuous exercise. The lungs, along with the blood vessels leading to and from the heart, are collectively called the *pulmonary system*.

The integumentary system

The integumentary system is comprised of the external covering of the body, which includes skin, hair, nails, sweat, mucus, and sweat glands (see Figure 4-9). In animals, this covering serves to cushion, to protect, to excrete waste, to regulate temperature, and even to waterproof.

FIGURE 4-9. The integumentary system.

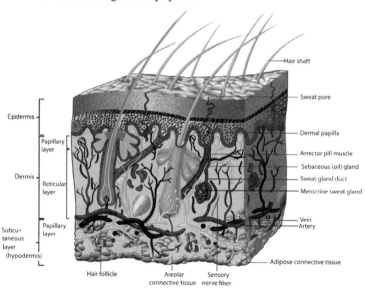

Skin. There are three layers of skin, or *cutis*, namely: *epidermis*, *dermis*, and *subcutaneous tissue*. Epidermis is the thin, outer layer of the skin that contains the melanin, which gives skin its color. The skin also contains the protein *keratin*, which contributes to the flexibility and strength of the epidermal tissue. Our fingernails and toenails are made of keratin as well.

Dermis is the bottom-most thick layer of skin, and includes blood vessels, connective tissue, nerves, lymph vessels, sweat glands, and hair shafts. Dermis is divided into two layers. The upper papillary layer contains the touch receptors that communicate with the central nervous system. This layer is also responsible for the skin's friction ridges that occur in patterns—otherwise known as fingerprints. The skin's lower, reticular layer is made of thick elastic fibers that house the hair follicles, nerves, and glands. Subcutaneous tissue, often called the *subcutis*, is the layer of tissue directly under the cutis. Its functions include insulation and storage of nutrients.

The above three layers together play a vital role in helping to maintain the body's proper internal environment. The skin has an enormous task of protecting the body, as it is the body's first line of defense against temperature, infections, and all other environmental factors. Some of the skin's most important functions are:

- to protect internal living tissues and organs
- to protect against infectious organisms
- to protect from dehydration
- to protect from temperature and environmental changes
- to aid in excretion through perspiration
- to store water, fat, and vitamin D
- to help us to feel touch, pressure, pain, heat, cold, wetness, and so on.

The urinary system

The urinary system consists of the kidneys, ureters, urinary bladder, and the urethra (see Figure 4-10). The main functions of the urinary system are to maintain the body's fluid volume and composition and to filter and eliminate waste products from the cellular metabolism through the urine. The actual filtering mechanism, present in the kidney, is called a *nephron*. One kidney contains nearly 1 million nephrons. Each nephron has a ball-shaped network of capillaries, called a *glomerulus*, where the blood is filtered and where some of the water and nutrients are reabsorbed. This process is controlled by hormones, in particular, the antidiuretic and adrenal hormones. About 1 to 2 l (or 1.06 to 2.11 qts) of urine are produced over a typical 24-hour period, although actual amounts depend on the measure of water and fluid intake. The kidneys also regulate the amounts of minerals (calcium, potassium, and sodium), hydrogen ions, and urea, a byproduct of protein metabolism, which are excreted.

Urine is emptied into the ureters every 10 to 15 seconds. The urine passes through the ureters, which are about eight to 10 inches in length, from the kidney and is then collected in the urinary bladder. The bladder is a hollow organ that can hold up to 500 ml (17 fl oz) of urine for two to five hours. Apart from regulating the fluid homeostasis in the body, the kidneys are involved in the production of red blood cells by secreting the hormone erythropoietin, and are also important for maintaining blood pressure by secreting the enzyme renin.

FIGURE 4-10. The urinary system maintains the body's fluid balance.

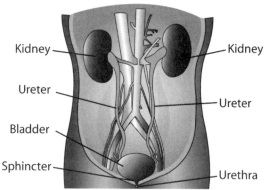

The immune system

The immune system is composed of many interdependent organs and cell types. These components combined create the two types of immunity: cell-mediated immunity and humoral immunity (see Figure 4-11). Cell-mediated immune response is activated by the cells of the immune system and does not involve any antibody or any type of complement. Humoral immune response is facilitated by the secretion of antibodies that bind to antigens (harmful/foreign substances), and in doing so, signal them for destruction. The objective of both responses is to protect the body from bacterial, parasitic, viral, and fungal infections and to combat against the growth of tumor cells. Some of these cell types have unique functions, such as overcoming bacteria, exterminating parasites, or even destroying viral-infected cells. To understand this combined effort of immunity, it helps to understand how the system is designed to protect our body from invaders.

FIGURE 4-11. Cell-mediated and humoral immunity.

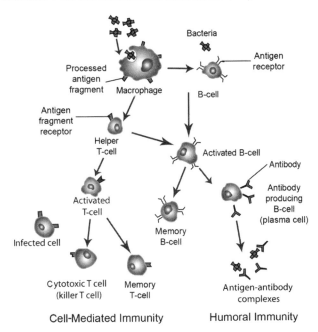

The immune system consists of the following organs: bone marrow, the thymus, the spleen, and lymph nodes.

Bone marrow. All the cells of the immune system originate in our bone marrow, formed through a process called *hematopoiesis*. During this process, the bone marrow–derived stem cells differentiate into mature cells of the immune system and migrate out of the bone marrow for maturation elsewhere. The production of B-cells, natural killer cells, granulocytes, immature thymocytes, red blood cells, and platelets takes place in the bone marrow.

Thymus. The thymus produces mature T-cells. The maturation and release of beneficial T-cells into the bloodstream and elimination of detrimental T-cells are its principal functions.

Spleen. The spleen functions to filter the blood. It is comprised of B-cells, T-cells, dendritic cells, red blood cells, and natural killer cells. It captures antigens from the blood when they pass through the immune response complex, beginning when the dendritic cells deliver the antigen to the right B- or T-cells for elimination. Old red blood cells are destroyed in the spleen, while B-cells become activated to produce antibodies. From this description, you can see why the spleen is rightly called the "immunological conference center."

Lymph nodes. Body fluid, called *lymph*, is filtered through the lymph nodes, which are present throughout the body. Lymph nodes are compiled of T-cells, B-cells, dendritic cells, and macrophages. Antigens are filtered from the lymph in the lymph node and then returned to circulation for elimination. As in the spleen, macrophages and dendritic cells capture the foreign antigens and deliver them to the T- and B-cells to begin the immune response.

The cells of the immune system, the T-cells described above, are a vital component in the adaptive immune response. The adaptive immune response is highly specific to the particular pathogen with which these cells come in contact. The function of this immune response is to destroy any invading pathogens. Because these responses are destructive, it is crucial that they be made only in response to that which is foreign to the body and not to the body itself. The ability to distinguish what is *foreign* from what is *self* in this way is a fundamental feature of the adaptive immune system. It is this adaptive process that provides us with long-lasting protection.

T-cells are subdivided according to their specific function and identification. The various subsets of these T-cells, as well as other cells which contribute to the immune response, are listed below:

Helper T-cells. The function of T-, or helper cells is to support the adaptive immune response. The secretion of small proteins, called *cytokines*, effectively regulate this response.

Cytotoxic T-cells. Cytotoxic T-cells are vital, as their name suggests, in directly destroying parasites, virally infected cells, and tumor cells. These cells are found throughout the body and are often as dependent on the secondary lymphoid organs as they are on the sites where the activation takes place. They are also, however, found in other organs, such as the liver, lungs, blood, intestines, and reproductive areas.

Memory T-cells. Memory cells, yet another subset of T-cells, remain indefinitely after an infection has concluded. Memory cells grow in numbers to become effector T-cells if they are again exposed to the same antigen. This process provides the immune system with a "memory" against past and future infections by the same antigen.

Natural killer T-cells have the ability to combine the adaptive and innate immune response to directly kill tumors, such as melanoma, lymphoma, viral-infected cells, herpes, and cytomegalovirus-infected cells. Killer cells destroy these tumors, or targets, without conferring in the lymphoid organs as other T-cell subsets do.

Gamma Delta T-cells comprise the smallest T-cell subset of cells with a T-cell receptor on the surface. Found in large numbers in the digestive mucosa, these cells are unique in that they respond quickly to metabolic bacterial byproducts.

Regulatory T-cells are considered the "brakes" of the cell-mediated immune response. Their role is to halt the T-cell response at the end of the immune reaction to ensure no damage comes to the body as a result of the event.

B-cells play a role in the humoral immune response rather than in the cell-mediated immune response, which, as seen above, is led by the T-cells. The primary function of B-cells is to manufacture antibodies against antigens. *Antibodies* are specialized proteins that bind and neutralize foreign bacteria, viruses, and tumor cells. These antibodies help direct the appropriate immune response toward any foreign object with which they come in contact.

Granulocytes or polymorphonuclear leukocytes. Defined by granules in the cytoplasm, this group of white blood cells is composed of three cell types: neutrophils, eosinophils, and basophils. Neutrophils are the most abundant and are phagocyte-eating, engulfing any invader they contact. Eosinophils contain granules that are toxic to parasites and enhance destruction of tumor cells. Basophils, the least common, have granules containing histamine, peroxidase, and platelet-activating factor. When basophils are damaged, they release histamine, which stimulates the inflammatory response.

Macrophages. From the Greek meaning "big eaters," macrophages are white blood cells produced from monocytes. Their role is to engulf and digest cellular debris and pathogens. Macrophages help to initiate the immune response with their front-line defense capabilities.

Dendritic T-cells are immune cells that function in an antigen-presenting capacity. This means that they present a foreign antigen on the surface to attract T-cells that have a receptor complex. Dendritic cells have the widest range of antigen presentation. Once activated, they are found in the structural compartment of the lymphoid organs, where they interact with T-cells and B-cells to initiate the immune system response.

The immune response is the body's way of recognizing and defending against bacteria, viruses, and harmful and foreign substances, or antigens. Antigens are molecules, usually proteins and polysaccharides, on the surface of cells, viruses, and fungi, or bacteria. Even nonliving substances such as toxins, chemicals, drugs, and foreign particles can be antigens.

Innate immunity is immunity that naturally occurs in us when we are born, and is comprised of nonspecific barriers with the means to keep harmful materials from entering the body. These barriers are our first line of defense in the immune response. The enzymes in stomach acid, skin, mucus, tears, skin oils, and the cough reflex are all part of that system of barriers. If an antigen does get past this primary protective external barrier, we are born with organs and immune system cells that will generally be capable of destroying it.

Acquired immunity is immunity that develops upon exposure to various antigens. It occurs when the immune system builds a defense specific to an antigen or antigens.

Passive immunity involves antibodies produced in a body other than our own. Infants have passive immunity because they are born with antibodies that are transferred through the placenta from the mother. These antibodies generally disappear between six to 12 months of age. The transfusion of antiserum, containing antibodies that are formed by another person or animal, is another example of passive immunity. Although this type of antibody provides immediate protection against an antigen, the protection is generally not long lasting.

The inflammatory response

The inflammatory response, or inflammation, occurs when tissues are injured by bacteria, trauma, toxins, heat, or any other cause. The damaged tissue releases chemicals, such as bradykinin, histamine, and serotonin, which are responsible for causing blood vessels to leak fluid in the tissue. This leakage causes swelling, which then isolates the foreign substance from further contact with body tissues. The released chemicals attract the white blood cells, or phagocytes, which eat bacteria and dead and damaged cells, in a process called *phagocytosis*.

The lymphatic system

The lymphatic system consists of a network of organs, ducts, and nodes that transport the watery clear fluid (the lymph) through thin tubes, much like blood vessels of the circulatory system (see Figure 4-12). These tubes, called *lymph vessels* or *lymphatic vessels*, are present throughout the body, except in the superficial layers of the skin, muscles, central nervous system, and bone. The parts of the body *not* traveled by the lymphatic vessels consist of an alternative system, called *prelymphatics*, or *cerebrospinal fluid*, as in the central nervous system.

FIGURE 4-12. The lymphatic system.

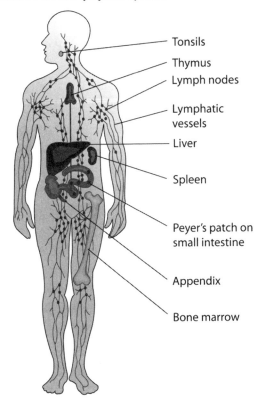

Tonsils

Thymus

Lymph nodes

Lymphatic vessels

Liver

Spleen

Peyer's patch on small intestine

Appendix

Bone marrow

The main functions of the lymphatic system are:

- to collect and transport tissue fluids from intercellular spaces of all tissues back to the bloodstream

- to help in the absorption of fat and its transport to the circulatory system
- to produce immune cells, such as *lymphocytes* and *monocytes*, and antibody-generating cells, such as plasma cells

Lymph fluid consists mainly of the plasma component of blood, and is made up of proteins, fats, and white blood cells. Plasma diffuses out of the capillaries to bathe the surrounding tissues. This fluid around the tissues is called the *interstitial fluid*. Most interstitial fluid re-enters the blood vessels; the excess fluid drains into the lymph capillaries. The ends of the lymph capillaries contain overlapping sets of cells which form a valve-like structure, an opening inside the capillary. Once the fluid enters the capillaries it can only move forward to drain into the lymph node because the valves are structured in such a way as to prevent backflow. These valves are located every 0.15 inches within the lymphatic system. The lymph is then further filtered by the lymph nodes and returned to the circulatory system.

The thymus, spleen, lymph nodes, Peyer's patches (the aggregation of lymphatic tissue found in the ileum section of the small intestine), tonsils, appendix, and bone marrow are individual tissues that constitute the lymphoid organs in the body.

These organs are responsible for maintaining the circulating B- and T-lymphocytes and other immune cells, such as macrophages and dendritic cells. When foreign organisms attack the body or when the body encounters other antigens, such as nonmicrobial pollen, the antigens are transported from tissue and forced to move forward to the lymph nodes through the lymph capillaries. There are about 500 to 600 lymph nodes distributed throughout the body, with clusters found in the underarms, groin, neck, chest, and abdomen. Lymph nodes filter the fluid and remove the foreign material, which can consist of nonmicrobial particles, viruses, parasites, bacteria, or cancer cells. The macrophages will either directly engulf the particles or the dendritic cells will present them to the other lymphocytes for destruction. When these pathogens are recognized, the lymph nodes enlarge and more immune cells are produced to help resist the infection. When cancer is present, lymph nodes serve as effective indicators in determining the degree of infection or the stage of the cancer. Approximately 68 to 101 oz (or 2 to 3 l) of lymph is filtered by the lymph nodes every day.

Exercise

"All parts of the body which have a function, if used in moderation and exercised in labours in which each is accustomed, become thereby healthy, well-developed, and age more slowly, but if unused and left idle they become liable to disease, defective in growth, and age quickly."

- Hippocrates (460–377 B.C.)

When I first looked for the definition of *exercise* in my table dictionary and on the Internet, I was overwhelmed by the number of definitions. The term seems to mean many different things to different people, where some consider playing a sport exercise and others talk about joining a gym. Regardless of the interpretation, most everyone concurs that exercise means undertaking some form of physical activity. I did find a couple of definitions that seem to do justice to its meaning in a holistic sense, so these are the ones I've chosen to use here: Exercise is an activity which "requires physical or mental exertion, especially when performed to develop and maintain fitness," and is "the activity of exerting muscles in different ways to keep fit." But what do these definitions mean to us?

Physical activity is significant for so many attributes and health benefits that it is hard to know where to begin. A few of these benefits include weight management, muscle maintenance, strong bones, stress reduction, and proper sleep. In addition, physical activity has been shown to reduce the risk for many diseases, such as cardiovascular disease, diabetes, and cancer.[1]

Exercise is a huge category, but for our purposes it can easily be broken down according to purpose and type. There is cardiopulmonary exercise, gymnastic exercise, kickboxing, step-up exercise, aerobic exercise, anaerobic exercise, muscle and body building exercise, isometric exercise, isotonic exercise—well, you get the idea. Even simple stretching and yoga are forms of exercise, and it is not stretching the truth to say that any form of exercise is beneficial. Even a simple neck rotation or a stomach crunch is beneficial to some degree.

On being physically fit

There is more and more evidence to support the fact that being physically fit, a state partially due to regular physical activity, is vitally important for our health and wellbeing, no matter what age we are. There is no one who cannot benefit in some way from exercise of one kind or another.

Regular physical activity can improve health and reduce the risk of premature death by:

- reducing the risk of developing coronary heart disease (CHD) and of dying from CHD, and reducing the risk of stroke and of having a second heart attack (in people who have already had one)

- lowering both total blood cholesterol and triglycerides, increasing high-density lipoproteins (HDL, or the "good" cholesterol), and reducing the risk for high blood pressure
- reducing blood pressure in people who already have hypertension
- lowering the risk of developing non-insulin-dependent (type 2) diabetes mellitus and colon cancer
- helping to achieve and maintain a healthy body weight
- reducing depression and anxiety; promoting overall psychological wellbeing and reducing stress
- building and maintaining healthy bones, muscles, and joints (particularly in older adults)

Unfortunately, despite these benefits, Americans tend to be relatively inactive. On the plus side, however, according to the Centers for Disease Control, the proportion of the U.S. population that reported they undertook no leisure-time physical activity decreased from about 31% in 1989 to about 28% in 2000, and fell even further to about 24% in 2007. "No reported leisure-time physical activities" is defined as not performing "any physical activities or exercises (such as running, calisthenics, golf, gardening, or walking) in the previous month" (see Figure 4-13).[2]

FIGURE 4-13. "No Leisure-Time Physical Activity Trend Chart." Data reported from 36 participating states from 1988 to 2005. (Source: Centers for Disease Control, 1988–2005)

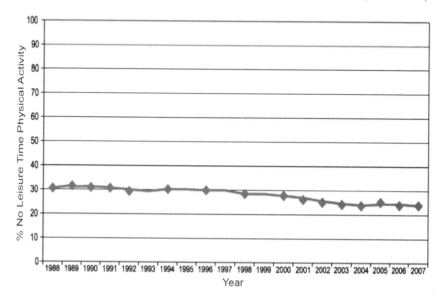

Defining *physical activity*. The CDC recommends that adults engage in "moderate-intensity physical activity for at least 30 minutes on five or more days of the week," or "vigorous-intensity physical activity for at least 20 minutes on three or more days of the week" because consistent physical activity over time promotes physical fitness. Physical fitness has been defined as "a set of attributes that people have or achieve that relates to the ability to perform physical activity." These recommendations have been made because the CDC recognizes that lack of physical activity is a risk factor for many diseases and conditions, including cancer. The five main components for overall fitness are: cardiorespiratory endurance, muscular strength, flexibility, muscular endurance, and body composition. We'll touch on each of these components briefly.

Cardiorespiratory endurance. According to the authors of *Fitness for Life*, "Cardiorespiratory endurance is the ability of the body's circulatory and respiratory systems to supply fuel during sustained physical activity."[3] In order to improve cardiorespiratory endurance, activities that keep the heart rate elevated at a safe level for a sustained length of time—such as walking, swimming, or bicycling—are the ones to try. Activities do not have to be strenuous; starting slowly with an enjoyable activity and gradually working up to a more intense pace is always advisable.

Muscular strength. In *Physiology of Sport and Exercise*, the authors describe muscular strength as "the ability of the muscle to exert force during an activity."[4] The key to increasing muscle strength is to work the muscles against resistance, either with weights or the force of gravity.

> *Muscle action.* There are four types of muscle action that contribute to muscle strength: *isometric, isotonic, isokinetic,* and *eccentric.*

> - **Isometric exercise.** In this type of strength-training exercise, the joint angle and muscle length do not change during muscular contraction. When these exercises are performed they are done in static positions, rather than through range of motion. To perform these exercises in a static position, the joint and muscle fibers are held either against an immovable force or in a static position in opposition to a force. Examples of isometric exercise involve the body's own muscle to cause the resistance, such as when pressing opposing fingertips of each hand against one another. Other examples include pushing a muscle against a structural area, such as a wall, or holding free weights or an elastic device in a fixed position.

- **Isotonic and isokinetic exercise.** Isotonic exercise moves a body part to shorten or lengthen the muscle. Free weights are the preferred (and classic) form of isotonic exercise, although sit-ups, push-ups, and pull-ups are also considered isotonic. Isokinetic exercise controls the speed of contraction within the range of motion and is generally performed with machines (such as Cybex and Biodex).
- **Eccentric contraction.** Eccentric contraction is the opposite of isotonic, where as the muscle lengthens it gains tension. An example of this type of contraction is when someone tries to pull your arm straight, while at the same time you attempt to keep your arm locked in the bent position. Eccentric exercises are much less common than the other exercises discussed, and are not considered as beneficial as isotonic exercises.

Muscular endurance. "Muscular endurance is the ability of the muscle to continue to perform repetitively without fatigue."[5] Having endurance is the key to perform everyday activities. Walking, repetitive weightlifting, and swimming are all excellent ways to improve muscle endurance.

Flexibility. Flexibility is the ability to move the joints of the body through the range of motion that is specific for that joint. One of the main goals of stretching through flexibility exercises is to elongate connective tissue and muscle fibers. Stretching has many benefits, such as increasing flexibility, improving range of motion, improving circulation, promoting better posture, and helping to prevent injury. Although stretching doesn't offer the dramatic overall benefits of aerobic or resistance exercise, regular stretching helps maintain the body's mobility and freedom of movement, particularly as we age.

Body composition. Body composition refers to the relative amount of muscle, fat, bone, and other vital parts of the body. Although a person's total body weight (what we see on the bathroom scale) may not change over time, this is not necessarily an accurate assessment of how much of that weight is fat and how much is lean mass (muscle, bone, tendons, and ligaments).

Exercising too much and/or too soon is the most common source of injury when undertaking physical activity. Even if you consider yourself to be in relatively good shape, start any new exercise slowly and gradually increase your level of exertion over a number of weeks. "No pain, no gain" is a myth; rather, pain is an indicator, a warning that you are doing something incorrectly or overdoing it.

Exercise and cancer

The Department of Health and Human Services states, "Each person must understand the value of physical activity for his or her health and wellbeing and commit to a lifestyle that is truly active."[6] The American Cancer Society recommends regular exercise as an important part of any cancer prevention program, and research suggests that exercise modifies some risks associated with certain types of cancer as well.[7] Obesity, for example, has been linked to cancers of the female reproductive system and breast.

Any kind of physical activity can have remarkable effects on various functions of the body, which in turn can influence the risks of getting or not getting cancer. These effects may vary according to the method, duration, frequency, and intensity of the activity. Various modes of exercise may effect positive changes in cardiovascular and pulmonary capacity, bowel motility, endogenous hormones, energy levels, immune function, antioxidant defense, and even DNA restoration. Research emphasizes the importance of maintaining an ideal body weight (or avoiding significant weight gain) to avoid cancer. Unfortunately, our global current lifestyle trends have led the majority of people toward obesity, thereby increasing the general population's overall risk of cancer.

This is a good time to explore exactly how exercise can actually lead us away from cancer. Until as recently as a few years ago, it was still being debated whether or not exercise contributed positively as a preventive measure or whether it should only be considered beneficial during and after cancer treatment. To answer that question, let's look at some research findings.

Exercise and prostate cancer. A study performed at Stanford University revealed that exercise showed an average risk reduction ranging from 10 to 30% for getting prostate cancer. Because exercise affects hormone levels, prevents obesity, enhances immune function, and reduces oxidative stress, these physiological mechanisms have all been hypothesized to explain why exercise reduces the risk of getting prostate cancer.[8] In another study at the Durham Veterans Affairs Medical Center involving 190 men who underwent prostate biopsy, it was shown that men who reported nine or more metabolic-equivalent task hours per week of exercise were significantly less likely to have cancer. For men with malignant biopsy results who reported moderate exercise (three to 8.9 metabolic-equivalent task hours weekly), a lower risk of high-grade disease (that is, a Gleason score of seven or greater) was also seen.[9] In a research study published in the *Archives of Internal Medicine* in 2005, it was found that older men who exercised regularly had a lower risk of dying from prostate cancer. In a *Health Professionals Follow-up Study,* 47,620 men were followed over a 14-year period. In this case, researchers observed that a lower risk of prostate cancer was found in men 65 years or older who had the highest level of vigorous activity.[10]

Colon cancer (cancer of the large bowel). Cancer of the large bowel is the most common cancer linked directly to levels of physical activity. Physically active men and women experience less than half the risk for this particular cancer when compared to those who lead a sedentary lifestyle. One reason may be that physical activity affects the colon's transit time and the time it takes for the bowel's contents to be eliminated. Physical activity has been shown to increase the bowel's transit time, which as a result, leads to the reduction of time that waste residue, parasites, and foreign bacteria remain in contact with the walls of the colon.

Based on current research, the American Cancer Society suggests increasing physical activity and maintaining one's ideal body weight to prevent colon cancer. For example, when 17,148 Harvard alumni between the ages of 30 to 79 years were studied for occurrence of colon cancer and rectal cancer, it was found that alumni who were "highly active" had 50% the risk of developing colon cancer relative to those who were inactive.[11]

We've all heard about "good" and "bad" cholesterol. In this case, exercise is known to increase the levels of high-density lipoprotein (HDL), or good cholesterol, which has been shown to reduce risk of cardiovascular disease. Evidence also indicates that high levels of insulin may actually advance the growth of tumors.[12]

Another study of patients with stage 3 colon cancer reviewed 832 patients who had undergone surgery and chemotherapy. In this case it was found that patients who exercised the most had higher survival rates by at least 45% than those who did not exercise consistently.[13]

Knowing the benefits of exercise on reducing cancer risk, you might think the temptation to sit on the couch and watch television would diminish. Unfortunately, it does not. According to the CDC, more than one third of U.S. adults—more than 72 million people—and 16% of U.S. children are obese. Since 1980, obesity rates for adults have doubled and rates for children have tripled. The CDC also analyzed data from its Behavioral Risk Factor Surveillance System survey and found that physical inactivity is more common among women than men, African American and Hispanic adults than whites, older than younger adults, and less affluent than more affluent people.[14]

Who hasn't heard of Herbert Spencer's phrase, "the survival of the fittest"? Exercise is a sure way to help us become and stay fit. In the case of breast cancer, for example, exercise has added new meaning to the lives of patients who have been diagnosed. More and more women are trying to exercise more often to increase their flexibility as well as to develop their arms, chests, and backs to build strength. In doing so, they are also increasing their lean body mass and becoming more physically fit. In the *Breast Cancer Survivor's Fitness Plan*, the authors have indicated that breast cancer survivors who exercise regularly also enjoy happier moods, experience higher self-esteem, and tend to ward off many conditions that shorten lives.[15] In one study involving 201 breast cancer patients receiving chemotherapy, half the participants incorporated exercise as part of their treatment and half did not. When the women were asked to fill in questionnaires after a six-month period to compare quality-of-life assessments, it was observed that the group reporting regular aerobic and resistance exercise also reported better patient-rated outcomes, including a better quality of life. Furthermore, patients reported reduced anxiety and better self-esteem during this time.[16]

In another study examining the relationship between post-diagnosis recreational physical activity and risk of breast cancer death in 4,482 women (ages 20 to 79 with a previous invasive breast cancer diagnosed between 1988 and 2001), it was found that the women who engaged in greater levels of activity had a significantly lower risk of dying from breast cancer.[17] While this study assessed a number of specific activities, it did not qualify any particular kind of physical activity which should be undertaken. Research results, however, do suggest that regular aerobic exercise not only reduced the risk of breast cancer mortality but the risk of death from any cause.

According to one study in the journal *Cancer*, exercise was found to improve the participants' oxygen-carrying capacity and to maintain the levels of red blood cells, the body's principal means of delivering oxygen to our tissues via the blood, during radiation treatment.[18] In this case, aerobic activity was shown to preserve red blood cell levels both during and after radiation therapy. In this particular study, researchers concluded that moderate aerobic exercise was safe, effective, and economical for improving physical fitness and maintaining levels of erythrocytes (red blood cells) in women undergoing radiation therapy for breast cancer.

It has also been found that intense physical activity can have an effect on *in situ* breast cancer. This research, published in the *Journal Archives of Internal Medicine*, looked at a study of 110,599 teachers in California, where it was confirmed that *in situ* breast cancer risk and invasive breast cancer risk was inversely associated with long-term strenuous activity.[19]

The type of treatment received relative to cancer can also play a role in one's ability to exercise. For example, survivors of childhood leukemia comprise one group that has often been found to be less physically active than the general United States population. In one study in 2007, researchers found that adult survivors who received cranial radiotherapy (CRT), or whole brain radiation, as children had overall lower activity levels as adults, suggesting that some of the therapy administered might be responsible for impairing their physical activity levels later in life.[20] This subsequent level of inactivity is posited to increase adult risk for cardiovascular diseases, osteoporosis, and various other cancers.

Physical activity and acute lymphoblastic leukemia (ALL). Another study, undertaken at Sloan-Kettering Cancer Center in New York, examined the relationship between survivors of childhood acute lymphoblastic leukemia who received cranioradiotherapy and obesity. In this case it was found that among young adult ALL survivors, CRT is a risk factor for elevated total, abdominal, and visceral adiposity levels, elevated metabolic risk levels, and altered IGF-I and leptin levels.[21] Cranioradiotherapy was also shown to be associated with an increased prevalence of obesity in females as compared to males who have been treated at a young age.[22]

On the plus side, research conducted at the Department of Rehabilitation Services at St. Jude Children's Research Hospital in Tennessee has found positive effects related to physical therapy and children with ALL. For example, in one study 28 children, ages 4 to 15 years were randomly assigned to an intervention or control group. The intervention group received five sessions of physical therapy and was instructed to perform a series of individualized exercises at home, consisting of ankle-dorsiflexion stretching, lower-extremity strengthening, and aerobic exercise. After four months the children in this group who received physical therapy intervention had significantly improved ankle-dorsiflexion in terms of active range of motion and knee-extension strength, both important elements for a normal gait. Based on studies like this, researchers surmise that therapy programs that emphasize endurance activities and are initiated early on during maintenance chemotherapy treatment may improve stamina and quality of life.[23]

Definitive scientific research indeed supports the fact that exercise helps prevent cancer. This message is underscored by the ACS Advisory Committee on Nutrition and Physical Activity, which cites numerous studies in its *Guidelines on Nutrition and Physical Activity for Cancer Prevention: Reducing the risk of cancer with healthy food choices and physical activity.* These guidelines state, "For the great majority of Americans who do not use tobacco, weight control, dietary choices, and levels of physical activity are the most important modifiable determinants of cancer risk."[24]

Furthermore, in many cases of chronic disease, physical activity levels have been found to be inversely related to mortality; in other words, when the level of activity increases, the death rate decreases. Although the relationship between physical *fitness*, which can be measured objectively, and physical *activity* is still subjective by nature, evidence continues to support that the more activity, the better. For example, researchers studied 13,344 men and women who were given a treadmill exercise test. Based on treadmill performance, age, and sex, each participant was assigned to one of five physical fitness training categories and then tracked for more than eight years. At the end of the tracking period, death rates were calculated for each level of fitness training. Results of this study showed clearly that low physical fitness was an important risk factor in increasing death rates for both men and women. (Other risk factors taken into consideration were smoking, cholesterol level, blood pressure, blood sugar, and family history of heart disease.) Furthermore, two specific conditions, heart disease and cancer, showed lower death rates in participants who were assigned to the higher fitness categories. Again, these results show a strong, inverse relationship between physical fitness and death, where even moderate levels of physical fitness can protect against early death.[25]

Given that physical activity is good for us, why are so many of us reticent to institute regular exercise programs? A benchmark study performed in Canada attempted to answer this question about physical activity habits by compiling data from the 1981 Canadian Fitness Survey and the 1994 National Health Population Survey from the Lifestyle Research Institute. What researchers found is that there are actually several common barriers that keep people from following active exercise programs.[26] Below are some of the most prevalent reasons for avoiding exercise, along with some suggestions for overcoming them.

No time. Most of us can relate to the common complaint of having little or no time to exercise. However, the half hour a day you spend exercising will not be felt so acutely if you make it a regular part of your daily routine. If necessary, further splitting up the half hour into sessions of 10 minutes can make the undertaking virtually painless. How about taking the stairs instead of the elevator, or walking to the office and back home again instead of taking the car or bus? This kind of effort pays off nicely with a renewed sense of vigor and energy when you arrive at your destination.

No energy. Prior to exercising regularly, it is not uncommon to feel a decided lack of energy. That's why the best feature about regular physical activity is that it significantly increases energy levels. If you feel especially tired on a particular day, however, there's no reason to push yourself unduly; tomorrow is another day to get started. When you begin your physical activity, no matter how little or how much, no matter what kind, you will be amazed by how quickly feelings of fatigue can be reversed. As I've said, I always felt that a little something is better than nothing. Take a simple walk around the block or stretch your calves, knowing that your efforts will refresh both your body and mind.

No motivation. Do you suffer from a lack of motivation? Does simply watching others exercise make you break into a sweat? Being part of a group exercise program or partnering with an exercise buddy is a great way to find your incentive. It's always easier to do something with a friend when the emphasis is on the fun of being together. As Johann Goethe, the German writer and philosopher, once wrote, "A joy shared is a joy doubled."

No money. While it's true that fitness gyms can be expensive, it doesn't cost much—if anything—to follow a regular exercise program. For example, comfortable sneakers and clothing are all that you need to initiate a walking program. An inexpensive set of dumbbells can be used for a variety of exercises, and the vast array of workout DVDs available for home exercising boggles the mind.

No facilities. Again, joining a gym in order to exercise is not always an option, but there is no reason you have to join a gym to exercise. Most forms of exercise, such as walking, stretching, lifting dumbbells, or running, are great workouts that do not require any facilities at all. If finances allow, there is always the possibility of purchasing exercise equipment to use at home, too.

No skill. There are many forms of exercise that do not require special skills. After all, we all know how to walk. If there are specific types of exercise you want to try, but feel you have insufficient skill to attempt, join a class or access the wealth of information available. There are books, DVDs, magazines, and websites to help you with everything from cardio-respiratory training to stretching.

Remember, resistance is universal! The brain is a smart operator. It can motivate us or indulge in mental trickery or rationalization to keep us from staying physically fit. It can convince us we don't have the time, the energy, the money, the skill, or the wherewithal. But this kind of resistance is not yours alone. In fact, it's been found to be noticeably widespread. What I mean by this is that all the reasons *not* to exercise as cited above in the Canadian research are familiar pitfalls, pitfalls many of us fall into at some time or another. The important thing to remember is that SOME degree of physical activity is definitely far better than NONE at all.

One of the interesting attributes of physical activity is that the more we do, the better we feel. Exercise is known to be a great destressor and is a time-tested antidote for depression. Why then, if it is often just what we need to help us feel motivated, do we continue to put it off? Sometimes we need to get going...*to get going*.

Researchers believe that exercise increases the body's levels of *opioid peptide* hormones, protein molecules in the brain that include the endorphins we hear so much about. Endorphins offset the effect of adrenaline, the stress hormone, and this results in our experiencing a "feel good" state, like the one runners talk about when they describe a "runner's high." As an effective stress buster, exercise does a good job of breaking up cycles of pessimistic thoughts that can control our minds. What's the upshot? Exercise just plain feels good.

Because exercise also comes in many forms, it need not necessarily be a tough, huffing-and-puffing type of activity that makes you want to collapse at the end of it. For physical wellbeing, moderate activity may be all you need. As I mentioned, a brisk 30-minute walk, a game of basketball with your kids, or taking the stairs instead of the elevator are all ways to get your heart pumping, raise your endorphins, and help you feel better. Remember to check with your physician before you embark on any exercise program.

Aerobics

Irrespective of age, it is a good idea to follow a fitness plan. Plans can vary in terms of how often you exercise and how long and how hard you exercise, depending upon your ability and motivation. As exercise has gained popularity, people have come to understand two common forms: *aerobic* and *anaerobic*. Originally, these terms were used by biologists as a means of classifying microorganisms, where aerobic microorganisms require oxygen or air for their survival. Other microorganisms, like bacteria, are able to survive even in the absence of oxygen. These are called anaerobic.

An aerobic exercise is any brisk physical activity that requires the heart and lungs to work harder to meet the body's need for increased oxygen, hence aiding the circulation of oxygen through the blood. By conditioning the heart and lungs, and thereby allowing for higher levels of activity, aerobic exercise is known as exercise that improves "functional ability," or the capacity to perform activities of daily living. Performing aerobic exercises simply implies you are breathing, or using oxygen.

During aerobic activity the body uses a great deal of oxygen, which is transported by the blood. At the same time, glucose, also found in the bloodstream, is utilized to create energy for performance activity. If quick energy is needed, glycogen, made up of glucose molecules, is immediately released by the liver and muscles, where it is made and stored. As energy demands continue due to the exercise being performed, more glycogen is broken down to meet these demands.

Anaerobic exercises, on the other hand, are carried out for the most part "without oxygen." Obviously, breathing does not literally cease during anaerobic exercise, but anaerobics focus on activities like weightlifting, which use alternate oxygen-dependent processes to produce energy.

Below are some of the most common ways to integrate a regular aerobic exercise into your daily routine.

Walking. Convenient for many reasons and possible to do anywhere, walking is probably one of the simplest and cheapest aerobic exercises available to absolutely everyone who has the capacity for mobility. All you need is a pair of good sneakers and breathable clothing. You can walk outdoors, indoors, at malls, or at a track. You can use the treadmill at home or at the gym, and can walk even when you're traveling for work or pleasure. It is a good, safe way to begin your exercise regime.

Cycling. Cycling is another type of aerobic exercise with wide appeal. Many consider outdoor cycling more fun than indoor, where fresh air is the added bonus, but even a stationary bike fulfills the purpose of staying fit. Cycling helps the functioning of the cardiorespiratory system without putting stress on any particular body part or parts, such as the back, hips, knees, or ankles, the way other forms of more strenuous exercise might.

Exercise machines: stair-climbers, steppers, and ellipticals. These are machines or devices that provide good aerobic workouts in a controlled setting, without the inconvenience of possible weather changes.

Swimming. Swimming is an excellent aerobic exercise. Swimming tones the entire body as it simultaneously provides a great cardiovascular workout. It strengthens the heart, muscles, and lungs, and improves oxygen delivery to the muscles. Water aerobics and water-walking have also caught on as highly enjoyable sports. The buoyancy provided by the water eases stress on the body's joints and helps prevent injury. as well as general wear and tear.

Jogging and running. The continuum that begins with walking ends with running. Jogging is in between the two. In essence, jogging occurs at a pace slower than running, but faster than a walk. Running is faster than both walking and jogging and can be identified when the runner has both feet in the air at the same time. All that you need to begin are comfortable sneakers with proper foot and ankle support, and breathable clothing. Always stretch fully before running (or performing any exercise) and cool down afterwards.

Professionally managed aerobic exercise classes. As per our definition above, aerobics is a collection of exercises that increase the intake of oxygen and boost the circulatory system. Professionally managed aerobic classes are conducted by trained instructors, who guide participants through rhythmic exercising of all their muscles and body parts. Generally, music with a good strong beat plays in the background, which motivates exercisers and boosts energy levels. You can choose from either low-impact or high-impact aerobics, depending on your stamina and current capabilities. For beginners, low-impact aerobics are the best way to start because they are less "impactful," as one foot stays stationed on the floor at all times. High-impact aerobics are exercises in which both feet leave the ground with more jumping and balancing moves. Aerobics has so many variations that I'll name just a few: step aerobics, abdomen or Ab Blast, kickboxing, Zumba®,[27] spinning, dancing, jazzercise, and core ball.

Step aerobics. Step aerobics are high impact workouts performed by stepping up and down on "steppers," impact-absorbing platforms of various sizes and heights. Step aerobics provide a vigorous cardiovascular workout. Different sports companies sell steppers for all levels, from beginner to professional. It is always important to work out on a stepper suitable to your capabilities to avoid injury.

Abdomen or Ab Blast. "Ab Blast" ("ab" is short for "abdomen") includes, as the name suggests, 20 minutes or so of intense abdominal workout combined with aerobic movement to work all the abdominal muscles. Working out under a trainer's guidance with this kind of exercise is a good idea in order to avoid any injuries to the lower back.

Kickboxing. Kickboxing refers to the sport of using martial-arts-style kicks and boxing-style punches to "defeat an opponent." Unlike other types of kickboxing, aerobic-style cardio kickboxing does not involve physical contact between competitors. It is a physically active cardiovascular workout that is done while listening to your favorite dance mixes. Kickboxing increases flexibility, stamina, strength, and concentration, and it also generates confidence and releases stress.

Spinning. Spinning exercise (also called "spot" or "studio" cycling) to rhythmic music has caught on with exercise fans as an excellent way to keep fit. Spinning bikes have weighted flywheels in the front to contribute to the feeling of riding a real bicycle. Spinning bikes allow you to adjust the tension to keep pedaling within a comfortable range for your fitness level. This type of exercise strengthens the heart and tones the glutes, calves, and thighs, in addition to slimming the legs. It is important to maintain a correct back posture as well as the position of the arms and legs to get the maximum benefit from spinning.

Zumba®. Zumba® fuses Latin rhythms and easy-to-follow moves to create a dynamic workout. Routines feature fast and slow rhythms and resistance training. This Latin-inspired fitness program boasts 20,000 trained instructors worldwide in 35countries.[27]

Dancing. Dancing has always been a popular pastime, but dancing as a form of exercise has been gaining momentum over the years, making it an interesting and beneficial workout combination. "Dancing your way to health" has become a popular saying with dancers who combine jazz, salsa, ballet, and funk, thereby adding health to enjoyment. Dancing is an excellent way to achieve a vigorous cardiovascular workout for the whole body.

Jazzercise®. Jazzercise® is typically a 60-minute class of cardio, strengthening, and stretching moves for a total body workout. Jazzercise® hip hop, yoga, Pilates, jazz, kickboxing, and resistance training are all combined into that one hour. Jazzercise® provides a welcoming and competitive environment to burn calories and have fun!

Core ball. Core ball is an exercise ball workout that not only strengthens the abs but puts many other muscles to work as well. It improves balance and overall coordination by working on a variety of muscle groups. Undertake core ball exercise with a trained instructor, as this kind of exercise includes a powerful workout of abdominal, chest, and back muscles.

Water aerobics. Water aerobics is aerobic exercise performed in shallow water. Water aerobic workouts use a variety of techniques, including walking or running backward and forward, performing jumping jacks, and using flotation devices. Water adds resistance to the training, which improves aerobic capacity, strength, and endurance.

Again, remember to consult your physician before embarking on any of these—or other—forms of exercise.

Exercise and your heart rate

Your heart rate can be a good indicator for monitoring your exercise quotient. *Heart rate* is a term used to describe the number of resting contractions of the heart, or heart beats, in a one-minute interval. This measurement is expressed as beats per minute, or BPM. In general, the resting heart rate for both men and women is between 60 and 80 BPM. A maximum heart rate is the highest number of times the heart is able to contract per minute. This rate is *not* the level one should sustain while exercising, but rather serves as a basis to determine your "target" heart rate, the preferable range to be reached during the peak of your aerobic exercise to receive the maximum heart and lung benefit. Maximum heart rate can be expressed as your age subtracted from 220, if you are male, and 206 minus 88% of your age if you are female. The desired target heart rate for an ideal exercise regimen is 70% of the maximum heart rate. For example, for a 35-year-old male the target rate equals (220–35) x 70%, or 130; for a 35-year-old female, the target rate equals (206–31) x 70%, or 122. Maintaining your heart rate at this level is the desired outcome during exercise.

We can check the rate of our heartbeat during aerobic activity by using simple watch-like devices called heart rate monitors. This is an excellent way to monitor the intensity of our exercise. Heart rate monitors measure heart rate, time spent in target zones, and how many calories are burned during the exercise period. These devices range in price between 30 and 50 dollars. A less high-tech method, which costs nothing, is to monitor your heart rate by taking your pulse, since pulse rates are identical to heart rates. Taking your pulse is easy, as explained below. Although pulse-taking requires no special equipment, a watch with a second hand or digital second-counter is helpful. This method is from the National Emergency Medical Association's (NEMA) website.[28]

1. Turn the palm side of your hand facing up.
2. Place your index and middle fingers of your opposite hand on your wrist, approximately one inch below the base on the side of the thumb (the radial artery). You can also place your index and middle fingers at the neck area below the angle of the jaw (carotid artery), where the pulse can also be felt strongly.
3. Press your fingers down in the groove between your middle tendons and your outside bone. The throbbing you feel indicates you have located your pulse.
4. Count the number of beats for 10 seconds, then multiply this number by six. This will give you your heat rate for one minute.

Example: If you count **12 beats** in the span of **10 seconds,** multiply **12 x 6 = 72.** This means your heart rate or pulse is **72,** or 72 beats per minute.

Lack of physical activity

It is clear from all we now know that little or no physical activity keeps us from staying fit and in optimal health. A lack of fitness often brings with it a marked reduction in musculoskeletal performance, pulmonary and cardiovascular efficiency, neuromuscular function, and/or psychological wellbeing—all of which contribute to a sure prescription for poor overall health. It was in 1970 that Dr. Alan Cooper published his book, *The New Aerobics*, which began to popularize aerobics as a "new" form of exercise for staying fit,[29] and it didn't take long before video releases and television shows promoted by celebrities such as Jane Fonda and Richard Simmons further capitalized on the market for aerobic exercise programs.

Since then, literature has supported the conclusion that aerobic exercise has a positive health impact by not only making us feel good, but by having a constructive influence on our immune system as well. Four out of six studies report statistically significant improvements in a number of cancer-related immune system components as a result of exercise.[30] (While the authors of these studies concede there are limitations involving the samples, designs, physical exercise interventions, physical fitness assessments, and immunologic assessments used, results are promising and further research is being undertaken.) In 2007, for example, principal investigators researched the relationship between physical activity and *immunosenescence*, a change found to occur in the process of aging. Immunosenescence, or the dysregulation of the immune system, impacts both innate and adaptive immunity, and leads to increased incidences of infectious disease morbidity and mortality as well as heightened rates of other immune disorders, such as autoimmunity, cancer, and inflammatory conditions. The researchers of this study suggest that physical activity may be an effective and logistically easy strategy for counteracting immunosenescence, based on their findings which showed that long-term, moderate physical activity in geriatric populations appeared to be associated with several benefits, including reduced risk for infectious disease, increased rates of vaccine efficacy, and improved physical and psychosocial aspects of daily living. Researchers further suggested that exercise may represent a viable therapy for patients for whom pharmacological treatment is unavailable, ineffective, or inappropriate.[31]

The effects of exercise on infections of the respiratory tract and the common cold have also been examined. In this study, lead researcher Dr. David Neiman of the Department of Health and Exercise Science at Appalachian State University states, "Research has shown that during moderate exercise several positive changes occur in the immune system. Although the immune system returns to pre-exercise levels very quickly after the exercise session is over, each session represents a boost that appears to reduce the risk of infection long term."[32]

Other studies have demonstrated the beneficial effects of aerobic exercise on cancer as well. For example, regular physical activity has been shown to increase the performance status in breast cancer patients treated with conventional chemotherapy,[33] aerobic exercise programs have been shown to improve the physical performance of patients undergoing bone marrow transplantation,[34] and the link between reduced lung cancer risk and aerobic exercise has been established in a large 1997 Norwegian study of 53,242 men over 19 years of age.[35]

Epidemiological studies have further suggested the strong association between physical activity and the risk for prostate and other cancers in American and European men. In a review of epidemiological studies undertaken in 2001, investigators reported that 14 out of 28 studies showed a reduction in the risk for prostate cancer by 10 to 70% with occupational or leisure-time activity,[36] and that aerobic exercise was shown to reduce the risk of breast cancer by 30% in 26 of 41 studies.

According to researchers of a study published in the *Journal of Nutrition* in 2002, the most definitive evidence for an association between physical activity and cancer exists for colon cancer. Of 51 studies on colon or colorectal cancer, 43 demonstrated a reduction in risk in the most physically active men and women with an average reduction of 40 to 50% and values as high as 70% for the most physically active.[37]

Aerobic exercise interventions have also consistently exhibited a powerful effect on cancer-related fatigue. In studies reported, significant differences have been seen between experimental and control groups, where fatigue levels are approximately 40 to 50% lower in exercising subjects.[38] In studies cited by the National Cancer Institute, even light to moderate walking programs have shown improved physical energy, appetite stimulation, enhanced functional capacity, improved outlook and sense of wellbeing, enhanced sense of commitment, and the ability to meet the challenges of cancer and cancer treatment.[39]

Anaerobic exercise

While aerobic exercises are based on endurance activities, anaerobic exercises are comprised of strength-based training. Anaerobic exercise increases muscle strength and enhances the ability to be involved in "sustained action." Anaerobic exercise consists of high-intensity movements over a short period of time lasting up to two minutes, such as lifting weights, in order to work the various muscle groups.

As mentioned earlier, anaerobic exercises are activities performed without oxygen—on a molecular level—that is, where energy is produced not by the breathing of the body, but by other means. Because during anaerobic activity there is insufficient oxygen to meet the demands of the muscles, a non-oxygen-dependent process is required to produce the same energy. Two types of energy systems act in this capacity in the absence of oxygen: the *creatine phosphate system*, the body's main energy source, and the *lactic acid*, or *anaerobic glycolysis*, system, which uses glucose, or glycogen.

Resistance training and cancer

Many studies are being performed to examine the effects of resistance training on cancer. In one study, published in the journal *Cancer* in 2006, 86 women who had survived breast cancer were divided into two groups, four to 36 months post treatment. While one group was recruited into a resistance (weightlifting) training program, the other group underwent no resistance training program. Researchers of this study observed that the women who exercised not only showed improved body composition and increased strength, but also a greater improvement in their quality of life.[40]

Another study in 2009 reviewed and evaluated the research of a number of previous studies which focused on using resistance training in the post-treatment phase of breast and prostate cancer patients. In this case, investigators found that positive training effects were observed for cardiopulmonary and muscle function, with significant increases in peak oxygen uptake.[41] Yet another study followed 54 healthy women, 30 to 50 years of age, who engaged in strength training twice a week. In this study, several risk factors for colon and breast cancer were assessed according to components such as body fat, waist circumference, fasting insulin, fasting glucose, insulin-like growth factor I (IGF-I), and several IGF-binding proteins. Results of this study indicated that strength training produced favorable changes in several of the proposed cancer risk factors.[42]

Stretching

Stretching is an act of lengthening muscles to increase muscle flexibility. Stretching is probably the least recognized part of an exercise program, and very often its importance is overlooked. Stretching serves to elongate the muscles and promote flexibility, ultimately improving range of motion of the joints. Because most strength-training programs cause our muscles to contract and tighten, stretching offers a way for us to relax our muscles and regain a sense of balance. Mostly, however, it just feels great.

Stretching increases flexibility. Flexible muscles improve our daily lives by enabling us to have a higher level of performance. Difficult tasks, such as lifting packages, bending for shoelaces, or even hurrying to get to a train or a bus, all become easier when our motions are more fluid and comfortable.

Stretching improves motion. Stretching benefits our joints with increased fluidity in range of motion. Our sense of balance can also improve considerably, something which ultimately helps prevent injury at any age, but especially as we get older.

Stretching improves circulation. Stretching increases blood flow to the muscles, and increased blood flow makes for healthier muscle tissue.

Stretching promotes good posture. Were you told to "stand up straight" when you were growing up? Well, it turns out there is a good reason. Not only do we look better when we stand up straight, but an erect posture prevents the muscles from becoming tight. Posture is considered a true "window" to the spine. This means that if we are out of balance in any way, we can be sure that our spine will reflect that imbalance. Since imbalance of any sort puts an unhealthy pressure on the body's nervous system, correcting the imbalance with proper posture through stretching can help minimize any aches and pains we may experience.

Stretching relieves stress. Stretching relaxes tense muscles, bringing about a feeling of balance and relaxation.

Different types of stretching methods are outlined below.

Ballistic stretching uses the momentum of a moving body or a limb in an attempt to force it beyond its normal range of motion. This high-force, short-duration type of stretching uses the stretched muscles as a spring to pull you out of the stretched position. One example of ballistic stretching is to bounce down repeatedly to touch your toes with straight knees or diagonal leg lunges. Some consider this type of stretching less than optimal and recommend it only for the most advanced athletes.

Dynamic stretching involves moving parts of the body and gradually increasing reach, speed of movement, or both. It incorporates gradual, controlled movements performed to the limit of the individual's range of motion. Steady arm and leg swings, neck-bending, and side-to-side movements performed to range-of-motion limits are examples of this type of stretching.

Active stretching involves stretching the *antagonist* muscle, using only the tension in that muscle. One example is the stretch performed by holding your leg out in front of you and as high as possible. In this case, the hamstring muscle is the antagonist being stretched, while the hip *flexors* and *quadriceps* are the "primary movers," or *agonists*, holding up the leg. Many of the movements (or stretches) found in various forms of yoga are active stretches.

Passive stretching. Passive stretching involves assuming a position and holding it with another part of the body with the assistance of a partner or apparatus to complete the stretch. Passive stretching is also referred to as slow, relaxed stretching. Passive stretches are often used to cool down after exercise because they can help reduce post-workout muscle tiredness and ache. One example of a passive stretch is to bring the leg up high and then hold it in the resultant position with the hands.

Static stretching. Static stretching involves stretching to the farthest possible point and then holding the stretch. Static stretching is often used as both a warm-up and a cool-down before and after many exercises. An example of a static stretch is a calf stretch, where one stands with one leg in front of the other, pushes the hands against a wall, and presses the heel of the back leg into the floor. Another example is to bend down to touch the toes, holding the position for about 10 seconds.

Isometric stretching. Isometric stretching involves the resistance of muscle groups through isometric contractions of the stretched muscles. An isometric contraction is a contraction which, as discussed previously, does not change in length. Isometric stretching is one of the fastest ways to develop increased static flexibility. An example of this type of stretching is to hold onto the ball of your foot to keep it from flexing, while using the muscles of your calf to try to point your toes. Another example is attempting to force your leg down to the ground, while a partner provides resistance by holding your leg up high and keeping it in that position.

PNF stretching. PNF stretching is a combination of passive stretching and isometric stretching. PNF stands for "proprioceptive neuromuscular facilitation." PNF stretching is an effective way to increase static flexibility. PNF stretching refers to any technique in which a muscle group is alternately passively stretched, and then contracted isometrically against resistance while still in the stretched position. Most PNF stretching techniques employ isometric agonist contraction/relaxation, where the stretched muscles are contracted isometrically and then relaxed. Some PNF techniques also employ antagonist contraction, where the antagonists of the stretched muscles are contracted. PNF stretches begin after an initial passive stretch. The muscle being stretched is then isometrically contracted for seven to 15 seconds, briefly relaxed for two to three seconds, and then immediately subjected to a passive stretch, which stretches the muscle even farther than the initial passive stretch. This final passive stretch is held for 10 to 15 seconds. The stretched muscle is then relaxed for 20 seconds before the performance of another PNF technique is undertaken.

The following guidelines are usually recommended for stretching:

1. *Warm up.* Warming up prior to stretching is essential to avoid injury. A warm muscle makes for easier flexibility and movement. Warm-ups can be done by walking or gently moving your body for a few minutes.

2. *Target major muscle groups.* When stretching, focus on the muscle groups used the most. This may include the muscles of the calves, thighs, hips, lower back, neck, and shoulders.

3. *Hold stretches.* Stretching muscle safely takes time, relaxation, and patience. Stretch until you feel a mild tension, then hold. It is best to hold stretches for a minimum of 10 seconds and a maximum of 60 seconds. Regardless of the duration, even a single stretch benefits the involved muscle area.

4. *Relax and breathe.* Try to relax through the stretches being performed, as relaxing helps to alleviate any tension held in the muscle. Always try to breathe normally and do not hold your breath while stretching.

How often you stretch is totally up to you; however, the general rule is to add stretching to every exercise regimen. If you are not currently involved in an exercise program on a regular basis, stretching at least three times a week, if not more often, is a great way to stay flexible and contributes to a sense of overall wellbeing.

Some simple whole-body stretching exercises have been outlined here for you to follow (see Figures 4-14, I–III). Move slowly while performing these exercises until you feel a gentle stretch. The durations mentioned for these exercises are approximations. Start slowly and increase the intensity gradually and according to your body's signals. Normally, it is good to begin with a set of eight to 10 repetitions. Repetitions can be increased over time as your muscle tone improves. While performing stretching exercises it is important to concentrate; in other words to be "mindful," by thinking, feeling, and being aware.

FIGURE 4-14. Illustrations depict muscles worked during stretching exercises.

I. *Neck and shoulder stretching exercises.* Movements should be slow and gentle.

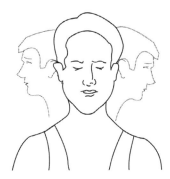

I(a) Head Turn: Turn head to one side and hold for 10 seconds. Repeat, changing the side. (left)

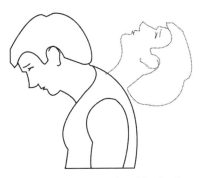

I(c) Head Tilt: Face forward, tilt and lower the head towards one shoulder. Hold for 10 seconds and repeat on the other side. (right)

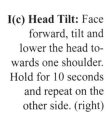
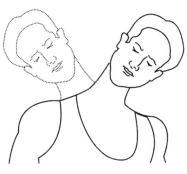

I(b) Head Lift: Raise chin slowly (extension) and hold for 10 seconds. Lower chin towards chest (flexion) and hold for another 10 seconds. (above)

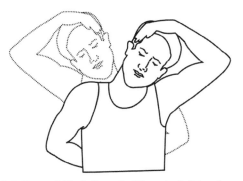

I(d) Lateral Neck Stretch: Place the left hand on the opposite side of the head near the ear and gently pull towards the left shoulder. Hold for 10 seconds and release. Then switch to the other side. Repeat again after you are done with the other side. (above)

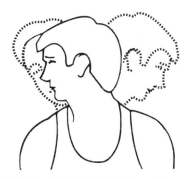

I(e) Head Roll: Start with the chin moving forward and downward. Slowly and gently move the chin and the neck in circular motions. Once you come back to your starting point, change direction and repeat. (above)

II. *Shoulder and upper back stretching exercises.* Movements should be slow and gentle.

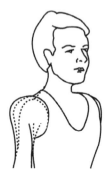

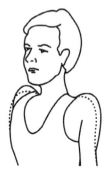

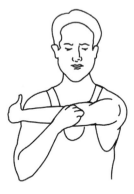

II(a) Shoulder Rolls: Roll the shoulder in a circular motion and repeat in the opposite direction. (above)

II(b) Shoulder Shrugs: Elevate both shoulders and hold for 20 seconds. (above)

II(c) Shoulder Stretch: Keep arms at shoulder height and grasp your elbow and pull it across your chest as far as you comfortably can. Hold for 20 seconds and release. Repeat after side change. (above)

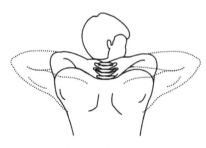

II(e) Arm Circles: Stretch out arms sideways at shoulder height; rotate in small circular motions. Repeat in the opposite direction. Gradually increase the arc of the arm circles. (below)

II(d) Shoulder Blade Squeeze: Clasp hands behind the base of the head. As you inhale, slowly press the shoulder blades together. Hold for 5 seconds, exhale, and release. (above)

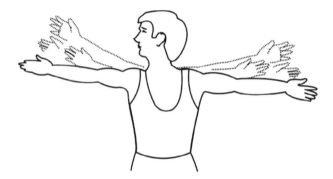

III. *Mid- and lower-back exercises.* Feel an easy stretch in your mid back, lower mid back, hips, and abdominal muscles. Movements should be slow and gentle.

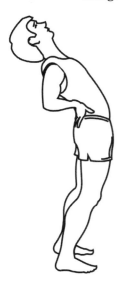

III(a) Abdominal Extensions: Place both hands in the small of your back. Keep head facing forward with knees slightly bent. Gently extend the upper body backwards and hold for 15 seconds. (left)

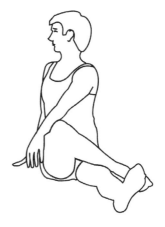

III(b) Seated Rotation Stretch: Sit on a firm surface with legs straight in front of you. Bend your right leg at the knee and place foot on the floor against the outside of your left knee. Place your left elbow against your right knee and slowly rotate your body towards the right. Hold for 15 seconds and repeat on the opposite side. (above)

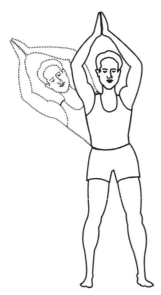

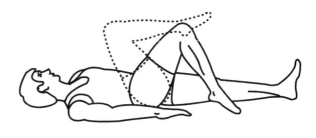

III(c) Side Stretch: Reach overhead and clasp hands together. Slowly, lean to one side and hold for 20 seconds. Repeat after side change. (above)

III(d) Knee Pull: Lie on your back with knees bent, feet flat on the floor, and arms relaxed at the sides. Bring one knee up to your chest and hold for 20 seconds. Release the knee slowly, extending the leg. Resume the start position and repeat with opposite knee. (above)

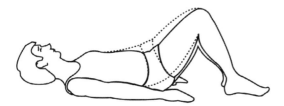

III(e) Bridging: Lie on your back with knees bent and arms at the sides of your body. Raise your hips and buttocks slightly. Hold for 15 seconds and slowly release. Tighten your stomach muscles when you raise your hips. (above)

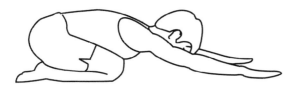

III(f) Cat Stretch: Starting on all fours, round your back towards the ceiling and slowly start to sit back on your heels while extending your arms directly in front of you. Hold for 15 seconds, release, and move back into a cat-like arching position. (above)

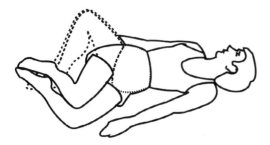

III(g) Rotation: Lie on your back with bent knees, feet flat on the floor, and arms at the sides of your body. Slowly drop your knees to one side. Hold for 15 seconds. Resume start position and repeat on the opposite side. (above)

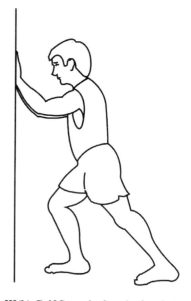

III(h) Calf Stretch: Stand a few feet from a wall or a fixed support. Place one foot forward. Bend at the knee and stretch the other foot backwards with the heel planted firmly on the ground. Push against the wall with your hands and slowly lean towards the wall at the same time.
Hold for 20 seconds and repeat with the opposite leg. (above)

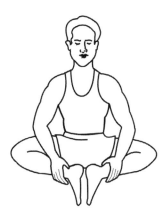

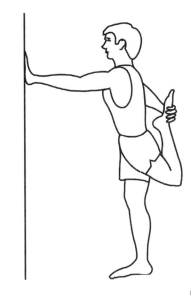

III(j) Quadriceps Stretch: Holding onto a firm surface with one hand, grasp the opposite ankle and pull the foot behind the body. Hold for 20 seconds. (left)

III(i) Groin Stretch: Sit on the floor straight-backed, shoulders relaxed, and heels together. Gently pull your upper body forward. Hold for 20 seconds and release. (above)

III(k) Hip Flexor Stretch: Stand in a forward lunge position with your back leg straight in back of you and your front leg bent at the knee. Put your hands on your hips. Hold for 20 seconds. Repeat after side change. (right)

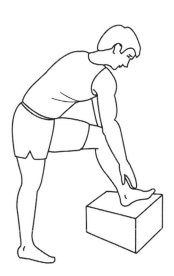

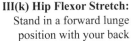

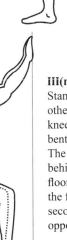

III(l) Hamstring Stretch: Stand with one foot firmly on the ground and place the other foot (heel) upon a flat, firm surface no higher than the hip level. With both hands try to reach towards your ankle as far as is comfortable. Hold for 20 seconds. (above)

III(m) Lunges Modified: Stand with one leg in front of the other as in mid-stride. Bend one knee and move forward till it is bent 90° directly over the ankle. The other leg is outstretched behind, with foot resting on the floor. Hold the position and lower the front of the hips. Hold for 20 seconds and release. Repeat with opposite leg. (left)

Physical activity guidelines

Physical activity guidelines in the U.S. have been expressed by two primary agencies in two formats: the U.S. Department of Health and Human Services (HHS) "2008 Physical Activity Guidelines for Americans," and the American College of Sports Medicine (ACSM) guidelines for healthy adults under 65 years of age. To achieve substantial health benefits, HHS recommends that adults participate in one of the following: at least two and a half hours a week of moderate intensity aerobic activity; one hour and 15 minutes a week of vigorous intensity aerobic activity; or an equivalent combination of moderate and vigorous intensity aerobic activity. The aerobic activity performed should be undertaken in episodes of at least 10 minutes spread throughout the week. Adults are also recommended to perform muscle-strengthening activities of moderate to high intensity, which involve all major muscle groups, on two or more days a week.[43] The American College of Sports Medicine recommends the following: moderately intense cardiovascular exercise 30 minutes a day, five days a week, or vigorously intense cardiovascular exercise 20 minutes a day, three days a week, along with eight to 10 strength-training exercises and eight to 12 repetitions of each exercise twice a week (see Table 4-1).[44]

TABLE 4-1. Physical Activity Guidelines as of 1999. (Source: CDC/ACSM Physical Activity Guidelines, 1999.)

Moderate activity plus 3.0 to 6.0 METs* (3.5 to 7 kcal/min)	Vigorous activity plus greater than 6.0 METs* (more than 7 kcal/min)
Walking at a moderate or brisk pace of 3 to 4.5 mph on a level surface inside or outside • Walking to class, work, or the store • Walking for pleasure • Walking the dog • Walking as a break from work • Walking downstairs or down a hill • Race-walking (less than 5 mph) • Using crutches • Hiking • Roller-skating or in-line skating at a leisurely pace	Race-walking and aerobic walking (5 mph or faster) • Jogging or running • Wheeling your wheelchair • Walking and climbing briskly up a hill • Backpacking • Mountain climbing, rock climbing, rappelling • Roller-skating or in-line skating at a brisk pace
Bicycling 5 to 9 mph, level terrain, or with few hills Stationary bicycling, using moderate effort	Bicycling more than 10 mph or bicycling on steep uphill terrain Stationary bicycling, using vigorous effort
Aerobic dancing—high impact Water aerobics	Aerobic dancing—high impact Step aerobics Water jogging Teaching an aerobic dance class

(continued on next page)

Calisthenics—light • Yoga • Gymnastics • General home exercises, light or moderate effort, getting up and down from the floor • Jumping on a trampoline • Using a stairclimber machine at a light-to-moderate pace • Using a rowing machine with moderate effort	Calisthenics—push-ups, pull-ups with vigorous effort Karate, judo, tae kwon do, jujitsu Jumping rope Performing jumping jacks Using a stair climber machine at a fast pace Using a rowing machine with vigorous effort Using an arm cycling machine with vigorous effort
Weight training and bodybuilding using free weights, Nautilus- or Universal-type weights	Circuit weight training
	Boxing, in the ring, sparring Wrestling, competitive
Ballroom dancing Line dancing Square dancing Folk dancing Modern dancing, disco Ballet	Professional ballroom dancing, energetically Square dancing, energetically Folk dancing, energetically Clogging
Table tennis, competitive Tennis, doubles	Tennis, singles • Wheelchair tennis
Golf, wheeling or carrying clubs	
Softball, fast pitch or slow pitch Basketball, shooting baskets Coaching children's or adults' sports	Most competitive sports • Football game • Basketball game • Wheelchair basketball • Soccer • Rugby • Kickball • Field or rollerblade hockey • Lacrosse
Volleyball, competitive	Beach volleyball, on sand court
Playing Frisbee Juggling	
Curling Cricket, batting and bowling Badminton Archery (non-hunting) Fencing	Handball, general or team Racquetball Squash
Downhill skiing with light effort Ice skating at a leisurely pace (9 mph or less) Snowmobiling Ice sailing	Downhill skiing, racing or with vigorous effort Ice-skating, fast pace or speed-skating Cross-country skiing Sledding Tobogganing Playing ice hockey

(continued on next page)

Swimming—recreational Treading water, slowly, moderate effort • Diving, springboard or platform • Aquatic aerobics • Waterskiing • Snorkeling • Surfing, board or body	Swimming—steady, paced laps • Synchronized swimming • Treading water, fast, vigorous effort • Water jogging • Water polo • Water basketball • Scuba diving
Canoeing or rowing a boat at less than 4 mph Rafting, white water Sailing, recreational or competition Paddle boating Kayaking, on a lake, calm water Washing or waxing a powerboat or the hull of a sailboat	Canoeing or rowing, 4 or more mph Kayaking in white water rapids
Fishing while walking along a riverbank or while wading in a stream, wearing waders	
Hunting deer, large or small game Pheasant and grouse hunting Hunting with a bow and arrow or crossbow—walking	
Horseback riding, general • Saddling or grooming a horse	Horseback riding, trotting, galloping, jumping, or in competition • Playing polo
Playing on school playground equipment, moving about, swinging, or climbing • Playing hopscotch, 4-square, dodge ball, T-ball, or tetherball Skateboarding Roller-skating or in-line skating, leisurely pace	Running Skipping Jumping rope Performing jumping jacks Roller-skating or in-line skating, fast pace
Playing instruments while actively moving; playing in a marching band; playing guitar or drums in a rock band Twirling a baton in a marching band Singing while actively moving about, as on stage or in church	Playing a heavy musical instrument while actively running in a marching band
Gardening and yard work: raking the lawn, bagging grass or leaves, digging, hoeing, light shoveling (less than 10 lbs/min), or weeding while standing or bending:	Gardening and yard work: heavy or rapid shoveling (more than 10 lbs/min), digging ditches, or carrying heavy loads:
• Planting trees, trimming shrubs and trees, hauling branches, stacking wood • Pushing a power lawn mower or tiller	• Felling trees, carrying large logs, swinging an ax, hand-splitting logs, or climbing and trimming trees • Pushing a non-motorized lawn mower
Shoveling light snow	Shoveling heavy snow

(continued on next page)

Moderate housework: scrubbing the floor or bathtub while on hands and knees, hanging laundry on a clothesline, sweeping an outdoor area, cleaning out the garage, washing windows, moving light furniture, packing or unpacking boxes, walking and putting household items away, carrying out heavy bags of trash or recyclables (e.g., glass, newspapers, and plastics), or carrying water or firewood	Heavy housework: moving or pushing heavy furniture (75 lbs or more), carrying household items weighing 25 lbs or more up a flight or stairs, or shoveling coal into a stove Standing, walking, or walking down a flight of stairs while carrying objects weighing 50 lbs or more
Putting groceries away—walking and carrying especially large or heavy items less than 50 lbs	Carrying several heavy bags (25 lbs or more) of groceries at 1 time up a flight of stairs Grocery shopping while carrying young children and pushing a full grocery cart, or pushing 2 full grocery carts at once
Actively playing with children, walking, running, or climbing while playing with children • Walking while carrying a child weighing less than 50 lbs • Walking while pushing or pulling a child in a stroller or an adult in a wheelchair • Carrying a child weighing less than 25 lbs up a flight of stairs	Vigorously playing with children, running longer distances or playing strenuous games with children • Race-walking or jogging while pushing a stroller designed for sport use • Carrying an adult or a child weighing 25 lbs or more up a flight of stairs
Child care: handling uncooperative young children (e.g., chasing, dressing, lifting into car seat), or handling several young children at one time Bathing and dressing an adult	Standing or walking while carrying an adult or a child weighing 50 lbs or more
Animal care: shoveling grain, feeding farm animals, or grooming animals • Playing with or training animals • Manually milking cows or hooking cows up to milking machines Handling or carrying heavy animal-related equipment or tack	Animal care: forking bales of hay or straw, cleaning a barn or stables, or carrying animals weighing over 50 lbs
Home repair: cleaning gutters, caulking, refinishing furniture, sanding floors with a power sander, or laying or removing carpet or tiles	Home repair or construction: very hard physical labor, standing or walking while carrying heavy loads of 50 lbs or more, taking loads of 25 lbs or more up a flight of stairs or ladder (e.g., carrying roofing materials onto the roof), or concrete or masonry work
General home construction work: roofing, painting inside or outside of the house, wallpapering, scraping, plastering, or remodeling	

(continued on next page)

Outdoor carpentry, sawing wood with a power saw	Hand-sawing hardwoods
Automobile bodywork Hand washing and waxing a car	Pushing a disabled car
Occupations that require extended periods of walking, pushing or pulling objects weighing less than 75 lbs, standing while lifting objects weighing less than 50 lbs, or carrying objects of less than 25 lbs up a flight of stairs • Tasks frequently requiring moderate effort and considerable use of arms, legs, or occasional total body movements Briskly walking on a level surface while carrying a suitcase or load weighing up to 50 lbs Performing cleaning services	Occupations that require extensive periods of running, rapid movement, pushing or pulling objects weighing 75 lbs or more, standing while lifting heavy objects of 50 lbs or more, walking while carrying heavy objects of 25 lbs or more • Tasks frequently requiring strenuous effort and extensive total body movements Running up a flight of stairs while carrying a suitcase or load weighing 25 lbs or more
Waiting tables or institutional dishwashing Driving or maneuvering heavy vehicles (e.g., semi-truck, school bus, tractor, or harvester, not fully automated, and requiring extensive use of arms and legs	Active and strenuous participation, such as aerobics or physical education instruction • Firefighting • Masonry and heavy construction work
Operating heavy power tools (e.g., drills and jackhammers) Many homebuilding tasks (e.g., electrical work, plumbing, carpentry, dry wall, and painting) Farming, feeding and grooming animals, milking cows, shoveling grain; picking fruit from trees or picking vegetables Packing boxes for shipping or moving Assembly-line work, tasks requiring movement of the entire body, arms, or legs with moderate effort Mail carriers, walking while carrying a mailbag Patient care—bathing, dressing, and moving patients, or providing PT	Coal mining Manually shoveling or digging ditches Using heavy non-powered tools Most forestry work Farming, forking straw, baling hay, cleaning barn, or poultry work Moving items professionally Loading and unloading a truck

+ For an average person, defined here as 70 kg or 154 lbs. The activity intensity levels portrayed in this chart are most applicable to men aged 30 to 50 years and women aged 20 to 40 years. For older individuals, the classification of activity intensity might be higher. For example, what is moderate intensity to a 40-year-old man might be vigorous for a man in his 70s. Intensity is a subjective classification. *The ratio of exercise metabolic rate. One MET is defined as the energy expenditure for sitting quietly, which, for the average adult, approximates 3.5 ml of oxygen uptake per kg of body weight per minute (1.2 kcal/min for a 70-kg individual). For example, a 2-MET activity requires 2 times the metabolic energy expenditure of sitting quietly.

Incorporating an exercise program

It's one thing to intellectually understand why exercise is so beneficial and quite another to be motivated enough to get going on an exercise plan that works—in other words, to undertake a plan that we will incorporate into our daily lives and maintain.

The first thing we have to do is simple: begin! It helps to talk about our plan, perhaps by discussing it with and asking for advice from our doctor, so that when we do start we will keep it safe, realistic, and convenient. Remember, Rome wasn't built in a day. Years of inactivity cannot be shed in one, or even a few sessions, although lots of people feel an immediate improved sense of wellbeing as soon as they begin. Furthermore, because exercise is the one aspect of physical wellbeing that doesn't require any initial investment—other than time and motivation—you can do it at your own pace and in the most comfortable way for you.

Selecting an exercise program

What type of exercising calls to you? Do you enjoy being outside more than inside? Do you enjoy team sports, working out with friends, or would you rather be in a more meditative mode alone? Selecting the appropriate form of exercise will determine how long and how well you continue the program you have selected. Consider your own requirements in terms of time, method, and location, rather than force yourself to comply with someone else's idea of what is fun or acceptable. The preferences and conditions of others may very well not match yours. One of the biggest goals of exercising is to make your program enjoyable and to keep it from becoming too tedious. If you become bored with the program you will likely lose your enthusiasm. When this happens it's a short step to stopping completely.

It is up to you to decide the type of exercise you do, but safety should always be a top priority. This means taking into consideration how to avoid injury and how to deal with any complications that may arise. Always build into your program some quality time to warm up and cool down. This allows your body time to prepare for the activity itself as well as to comfortably wind down when it ends.

Keep the following considerations in mind when you take on a new exercise program: set a plan; set specific and realistic goals; build endurance gradually; listen to your body; and try new programs periodically. Each of these aspects is outlined below.

Plan. Setting a plan is a constructive way of organizing our goals in life, and likely helps in our ongoing growth and development in all aspects. Exercise is no different. Planning your program in a systematic manner in the same way you plan your office work or household chores is the best way to ensure you'll stick with it because it will become part of your everyday routine.

Set realistic goals. Setting goals that are too high, too fast—goals that are perhaps even impossible to achieve—will only make you lose interest in the process itself. Finding something you love to do and doing it in reasonable amounts will keep you much more involved, more directed in the process, and more focused on achieving your goals.

Set specific goals. Goals can be as basic as "I want to walk to work twice a week," or as structured as "I intend to take an aerobics class at the gym." The important thing is to set goals that work with you, your personality, and your life. When you exercise, for how long, with whom, and where are all aspects of scheduling pleasurable routines, and scheduling enjoyable workouts helps us adhere to a regular exercise program.

Be kind to yourself. Build your endurance gradually and increase the time you spend exercising and the amount of effort you expend slowly. Being kind to yourself means not pushing yourself too hard. You are the one who knows your body best; this includes knowing what you are capable of doing and what you are not capable of doing. It means understanding the pluses and minuses we all have and respecting them. If you are a beginner, begin at a beginner's level with exercises that serve your purpose instead of those that may defeat you before you start. Keep your ego in check, too. This is about incorporating something positive into your life for the long run, so it helps to be patient. You can always increase your training over time as you increase your strength.

Listen to your body. Again, you know your own body. While some of us prefer exercising in the morning, others feel better exercising at the end of the day. Give yourself the chance to find out what time is ideal for you, so that you will be less likely to discontinue. It makes sense that only when you are happy and satisfied with what you are doing will you continue doing it. Know that on some days you'll have more energy than on others for any number of reasons. Listen to the messages your body is sending so that you can understand what it is trying to tell you, and then base your decisions on what you learn. I can't tell you how many times I have said to myself, "Tomorrow is another day."

Change it up. To avoid monotony from repeating the same activity or exercise regimen over and over, it helps to introduce workout variations from time to time. If you find yourself dreading your current program, try something new. Typically your body will let you know by resisting the effort it takes to get going! There's no end to the possibilities either, whether you just want to change it for a week or two, or substitute one structured program for another. In the summer, gardening or mowing the lawn can easily substitute for a moderate walking program. If you go to the local gym, try a different piece of exercise equipment or a class. Walking, swimming, bicycling, raking, walking briskly, mopping and scrubbing the floors, golf, tennis doubles, and even rowing are excellent ways to keep up your physical activity. And for those who prefer vigorous exercise, perhaps during the cold of winter instead of swimming laps you might try cross-country skiing or an indoor activity that suits you. Again, the choices are endless, so don't give it up—change it up!

To gain optimum results from the exercises you do, you might try dividing them according to their qualities and functional objectives. For example, some exercises are geared for increasing strength, some for enhancing endurance, others for working on cardio, and still others for increasing flexibility.

Strength and endurance

There are many exercises that increase both strength and endurance, and it's important to know why the combination is so beneficial. When we talk about fitness we normally think of exercise in general, but choosing the right type of exercise to achieve the result you want is just as important.

Endurance, or cardiorespiratory endurance, is the ability of the body's circulatory and respiratory systems to supply oxygen during continuous physical activity. To improve cardiorespiratory endurance we need to undertake activities that will keep our heart rate at a higher beat for an extended period of time, such as brisk walking, jogging, bicycling, or swimming. Endurance increases when we begin slowly and build up our skill, making gradual, steady progress. Even moderate exercise increases the body's oxygen intake by three to six times!

When strength is the primary objective, lifting weights is generally the way to go, as this type of activity gradually builds up muscle fibers and increases strength. Muscular endurance signifies the ability of the muscles to continue to perform lifting without tiring.

It cannot be emphasized enough how important it is to listen to your body's signals. It is not possible to set one standard criterion for how much weight a person should be able to lift, or how steep a hill one should be able to climb, or even how often, how fast, or how long a person should cycle. That's why the simplest thing to do is to listen to what your body is trying to tell you. The level of effort you put forth should agree with you—that is, it should not be too strenuous on the one hand or, on the other, have no effect at all. Begin with the least amount of effort, then build to a moderate effort, and then to a somewhat harder effort to build up your endurance capabilities. As your endurance increases, you can begin to graduate to activities that require much more effort, thereby enhancing your strength capabilities.

Using these guidelines, let's formulate several typical programs for strength *and* endurance.

Exercise Program #1

Warming up. Warm up for five to 10 minutes with a walk or by pedaling on a stationary bicycle. Perform various stretches: for the arms, including biceps and triceps, and for the legs, including quadriceps, hamstrings, and calves. Warming up allows your muscles to do just that—to become ready for the physical exertion to follow, thus reducing your risk of injury.

Weight training. Weight training is advisable on days when you are not doing your aerobic workouts. Giving yourself a day off in between weight training sessions helps the muscles recover properly. Weight training, the most common type of strength training to develop the size and strength of the muscles, uses the force of weight to oppose the force of muscle contraction. The goal of this exercise is to work to build up physical strength. When first starting out with a weight training routine, make sure you choose one that is suitable for your capabilities. In other words, never do more than you are able to do. The lifting of weights, or free weights, includes barbells, dumbbells, and hand weights. Weight machines, incorporating the use of weights in a more standardized format, work the different muscle groups. When getting started, the best approach is to work the whole body. In the beginning, you can generally get away with training each muscle group twice a week with at least one day in between, allowing your muscles time to recover between workouts. The amount of weight you choose is entirely up to you. When starting, however, lighter is always better; as you gain more experience you can gradually increase your weight.

Here is a sample weight training exercise program that incorporates both free weights and weight machines.

*Lat (*latissimus dorsi*) pulls:*	3 sets, 10 to 12 reps each set
Seated cable rows:	2 sets, 10 to12 reps each set
Dumbbell lateral raises:	3 sets, 12 to 15 reps each set
Barbell military presses:	2 sets, 10 to 12 reps each set
Dumbbell chest presses:	3 sets, 8 to 10 reps each set
Barbell biceps curls:	3 sets, 10 to 12 reps each set
Triceps cable pressdowns:	3 sets, 10 to 12 reps each set
Leg press machine:	3 sets, 8 to 10 reps each set
Seated hamstring curls:	3 sets, 10 to 12 reps each set
Seated calf presses:	3 sets, 8 to 10 reps each set

Cool down. Spend at least 5 to 10 minutes cooling down. You can cool down by stretching all the muscle groups you have worked and ending with a full body stretch. Cooling down also helps to bring the heart rate back down to normal levels.

Weight training is advisable on days when you are not doing your aerobic workouts. As explained earlier, taking a day off between weight training sessions helps the muscles recover properly. Doing these exercises twice a week is consistent with the American College of Sports Medicine's guidelines for strength training.

Exercise Program #2

If you are working with weights at least twice a week, doing some cardiovascular exercise at least three times a week is an excellent way to balance your weekly routine. "Cardiovascular exercise is any type of exercise that increases the work of the heart and lungs," says Tommy Boone, Ph.D., a founding member of the American Society of Exercise Physiologists. As suggested earlier, walking, jogging, running, bicycling, step aerobics, and swimming are great ways to get this type of aerobic activity.

Cardiovascular exercises can be done in two ways: slow and steady, or with high intensity. Slow and steady aerobic activities are usually of long duration (45 minutes to an hour), are low impact, great fat burners, and easy on the joints. High intensity aerobic activities are of short duration (20 to 30 minutes), use explosive nonstop movements, burn calories quickly, and have a high impact on the joints. The choice is yours, because either form of exercise will increase your cardiorespiratory endurance. As with weight training, it is important to take a few minutes to warm up prior to exercising and stretch after you are done to cool down in order to relax your muscles and slow your heart rate and breathing to normal levels.

We see from Exercise Programs #1 and #2 that incorporating the aspects of weight training (to gain strength endurance) and aerobics (to work the heart and lungs) with stretching (to gain flexibility) during warming up and cooling down provides the sum total of a well-rounded exercise program. Exercising does not have to stop here, however. There is a myriad of ever evolving and varied methods of exercising to help us achieve our goals. Group activities mentioned in Exercise Program #3, for example, can be a perfect way to get your heart pumping and your body moving.

Exercise Program # 3

Exercise classes are a fantastic way to get in shape and stay in shape while having a great time. These include dancing (such as Zumba®, salsa, ballet, and ballroom dancing), aerobics, and yoga. One class that has found a following is the art of "laughter yoga," as developed by Dr. Madan Kataria. This type of yoga "combines laughter exercises with yoga breathing [to bring] more oxygen to the body and brain, making one feel more energetic and healthy."[45] Currently there are over 6,000 clubs in 60 countries for practicing the art of laughter yoga. Classes and courses dedicated to various meditative practices are also gaining in popularity, such as the Art of Living course, which uses a powerful breathing-based technique called *Sudarshan Kriya*, or healing breath. *Sudarshan Kriya* incorporates specific natural rhythms of breathing to release stress and bring the mind into the present moment. This specific course interweaves a number of breathing techniques with low-impact yoga to productively deal with challenging thoughts and emotions.[46]

So far we have established that exercising is an important component to staying healthy. We also have some ideas about the different routines we might follow. But another aspect of gaining a heightened level of physical fitness is to utilize oxygen as effectively as possible. Doing that depends on *how* we breathe, because good breathing techniques increase the body's oxygen supply both while exercising and at rest. Oxygen is the most vital nutrient of the body. We can do without water for days and food for weeks, but without oxygen we will die in a few short minutes. Thus it is not surprising that a lack of oxygen has been implicated in the deterioration of cellular environments as well. If the cellular environment deteriorates enough, cancer may occur. As early as 1947, scientists in Germany demonstrated this fact through research which showed that the intermittent withholding of oxygen transformed normal body cells into cancer cells. This discovery was later confirmed in 1953 by Drs. Goldblatt and Cameron in the *Journal of Experimental Medicine*,[47] and again in 1955 by Dr. Otto Warburg, the Director of the Max Planck Institute of Cell Physiology in Germany, who stated unequivocally that a lifetime of research had convinced him that cancer was caused by oxygen deprivation to the cells.[48]

In 2001, Höckel, et al. continued to research the relationship between oxygen and cancer. Their research showed that tissue hypoxia, a condition where the entire body, or regions of the body, is deprived of adequate oxygenation (oxygen supply), compromises biologic function. Höckel's study states: "Tumor hypoxia appears to be strongly associated with tumor propagation, malignant progression, and resistance to therapy, and it has thus become a central issue in tumor physiology and cancer treatment."[49] If it is in fact true that inadequate oxygen to cells can create an environment for cancer to grow, then it also appears plausible that the reverse—increased oxygen—may reduce the same risk. The best and easiest way I can think of to increase our intake of oxygen is to improve the way we breathe, something that will inevitably enhance the supply of oxygen to all the cells in the body.

Breathing

By definition, breathing is the act of inhaling and exhaling, bringing oxygen to the body and moving carbon dioxide out of the body. Let's break down the process of breathing so we understand its elements.

When we breathe, gases are exchanged between the cells of an organism and the environment. As we have seen, the main players in this complex physiological process are the lungs and the cardiovascular system. Breathing is achieved by:

- inhalation, whereby the oxygen is brought into the lungs
- circulation, or transport of the oxygen, to the various tissues through dissolution in the bloodstream, and through the exchange of the dissolved oxygen for carbon dioxide
- expiration, a process through which the carbon dioxide is expelled

Breathing is the single paramount activity we undertake in our life span. A normal respiratory rate is somewhere around eight to 14 breaths per minute. Given there are 1,440 minutes in a day, and assuming a resting respiratory rate of, say, 12 breaths per minute, and further assuming that respiratory rate doesn't vary much throughout the day, we normally take in about 12 x 1,440, or 17,280, breaths each day. If our activities increase on any given day, this number will also increase. Most of us have the firm notion that we have no control over our breathing, that our bodies inhale and exhale automatically, and we just go along with it. However, in reality, we can learn to be more aware of our breathing, to breathe more consciously: a technique that can result in an improved state of health. Commonly, on any given day, we actually breathe faster than the average rate of 12 to 14 times a minute because we are unknowingly accustomed to taking quick, short breaths from the top of our chest. Concentrating on our breathing patterns can guide us to breathe more deeply. When we focus on deeper breathing we incorporate not only the diaphragm, but the belly, rib cage, and even the lower back.

Exercise is an activity that naturally increases the heart rate. That is because it is supposed to do just that: escalate the pace of blood supply to the body to meet requirements. When we physically exert ourselves, the need for oxygen to meet our energy demands increases. Breathing, therefore, becomes the mechanism for furnishing the energy that we need. Professional athletes use breathing to their advantage. Most professional athletes breathe consciously *as* they move, rather than making a move ... and then breathing. Bear in mind that gasping for breath after a particularly strenuous bout of exercise is not necessarily an indicator that you have had a good workout, as some may like to believe. Rather, poor breathing practices may lead to harmful changes due to the stress response, which occurs when we feel as if we cannot get enough air. Breathing optimally during exercise, or while we go about our daily routine—in other words, breathing as described in this section—can keep us feeling fit and relaxed.

Many cultures believe that the process of breathing is more than simply a physical function of the body. It has been said that breathing is "the soul of the being," and a tool of communication between the body and mind, and between the conscious and unconscious minds. Indeed, the rhythmic procedure of simple expansion and contraction is in itself an example of consistent, constant movement, similar to the ocean's tide coming in and pulling back, in endless succession. Significantly, breathing is a body function that can be done both voluntarily and involuntarily.

Until recently I myself thought of breathing as little more than the simple act of inhalation and exhalation. With reading and research, however, I have begun to realize how breathing "correctly" can enhance one's feeling of relaxation as it simultaneously boosts the body's oxygen supply.

To start, let's look at an overview of the different types of breathing.

Costal, or chest, breathing. Costal breathing involves the outward and upward movement of the chest wall. The costal diaphragm effects movement of the rib cage in the same way a bellows works. Although we all use our costal diaphragms (described below), we are probably unaware of it. If you put your hands on the rib cage and breathe normally and speak, you will probably feel little or no movement. However, when yawning deeply you may be surprised to see that your hands are pushed up and out as you take in air. This occurs when we take a costal breath. There are three distinct parts of the costal, or in-the-chest, breath cycle:

1. *Inspiration.* As you take a full and fast breath in through the mouth, your ribs expand by moving up and out and your diaphragm contracts downward, creating a vacuum in the thorax and drawing air into the lungs.

2. *Expiration.* As you start to exhale, the ribs begin to move down and in and the diaphragm relaxes upwards, expelling air. The air passes over the vocal cords, enabling speech. When you have finished speaking, any unused air is then comfortably released.

3. *Pause.* When you have released any residual air and the diaphragm is in its fully relaxed or uppermost position, a natural pause occurs. A new cycle begins when you take another breath.

Abdominal breathing. Abdominal breathing is also called diaphragmatic breathing. To understand what that means, we first need to understand what the diaphragm is and what it does. The diaphragm is the large muscle located between the chest and the abdomen, or *thoracic cavity*, which extends across the rib cage. When this muscle contracts during inhalation, it actively flattens, lifting the rib cage up and out and slightly displacing the organs of the abdomen below. This creates suction, or a negative pressure, which draws air into the lungs. This pressure also pulls blood into the chest, improving the return of blood to the heart through the veins. Increased blood flow in turn helps improve energy levels. By virtue of the way abdominal breathing expands the lungs, it not only improves the flow of blood but the flow of lymph as well. Abdominal breathing is an excellent method for improving oxygen-carrying capacity and encouraging relaxation.

Andrew Weil, M.D. is a well-known and respected author, recognized for establishing and popularizing the field of integrative medicine. In his audiobook, *Breathing: The Master Key to Self-Healing*,[50] and on his website (*www.drweil.com*), Dr. Weil expresses the importance of breathing with "mindfulness." According to Dr. Weil, breathing is something we can control to achieve better health and spiritual harmony. He recommends three breathing exercises for stress reduction and relaxation: Stimulating Breath, Relaxing Breath, and Breath Counting.[51]

Stimulating breath is an extension of the breathing techniques of yoga, aimed at increasing vital energy levels and alertness. Following the steps outlined below stimulates a deep sense of invigoration. This type of breathing is felt in the back of the neck, the diaphragm, the chest, and the abdomen. To perform stimulating breaths, follow these simple steps:

1. Inhale and exhale rapidly through the nose, keeping your mouth relaxed and closed. Keep your inhalation and exhalation short and of equal duration, making "breathing noises" as you breathe.
2. Try three in-and-out breath cycles per second. Breathe normally after each cycle.
3. Do this for less than 15 seconds on the first try. Once you get used to doing this, you can gradually increase by 5-second increments to ultimately reach a full minute.

Relaxing breath is a very simple method, takes minimal time, and can be done anywhere. This exercise is a natural "tranquilizer" for the nervous system, in which exhalation takes twice as long as inhalation. Exhaling is done loudly through the mouth, while inhalation is done quietly through the nose. Follow these simple steps to perform relaxing breaths:

1. Exhale through your mouth, making a loud audible sound.
2. Close your mouth and inhale quietly through the nose, counting to 4 in your mind.
3. Hold your breath till you reach a count of 7 in your mind.
4. Exhale completely through your mouth, making a loud sound to a count of 8.

Steps one through four constitute one cycle. Keeping the ratio of 4:7:8 is extremely important. Begin this exercise by doing four breaths at a time for a period of one month; thereafter, increase to eight breaths. It is recommended to practice this type of breathing at least twice a day to get the most beneficial results.

Breath counting, as the name suggests, begins at counting on every exhale, starting with "one" and ending in "five." A Zen practice, breath counting starts with sitting in a comfortable position with your spine straight and your head inclined slightly forward. To begin the exercise, count "one" to yourself as you exhale. The next time you exhale, count "two," and so on, up to "five." Then begin a new cycle, counting "one" on the next exhalation. Never count higher than five, as counts of more than five tend to make the mind wander. For the best results, perform this form of exercise for 10 minutes.

Ancient as well as modern medicine has recognized how our breathing patterns are closely linked to overall wellness. Deep, relaxed breathing has been found to help with asthma, anxiety-related disorders, such as panic attacks, insomnia, and indigestion. Perhaps one of the best known examples of deep-breathing exercise is *pranayama,* the breathing skill (mentioned earlier) which forms a part of the tradition of yoga. In Sanskrit, *prana* means "life force" and *ayama* means "control." *Pranayama* refers to the various methods of inhaling, exhaling, and holding back *prana.* The simplest form of *pranayama* is a breathing technique called *nadi shodhanam* (pronounced naa-di sho-duh-num). *Nadi,* in Sanskrit, means "channel" and *shodhanam* means "purification." In yoga, the practice of *nadi shodhanam* aims to calm, balance, and regulate energy levels through breathing. Primarily this is achieved by alternate nostril breathing.

Practicing *nadi shodhanam*

1. Hold your right hand up with the thumb lightly touching the right nostril. Curl the middle and index fingers toward the palm and close the left nostril with the ring finger pressing gently against it. Take a slow, deep breath through the right nostril.

2. Close the right nostril and release the left nostril at the same time.
3. Let out the breath in a prolonged and slow manner through the left nostril.
4. Repeat this process by inhaling through the left nostril and then exhaling through the right nostril.
5. Steps one through four complete one round of *nadi shodhanam*. Ten to 15 rounds of *nadi shodhanam* performed the right way have a tremendous calming effect, which can be felt almost immediately.

With practice it is possible to shift from the shallow chest breathing we tend to do automatically to deep abdominal, or diaphragmatic, breathing. You can also consider a simple alternative to *nadi shodhanam*, as described below:

1. Choose a quiet environment; loosen any tight clothing and remove any jewelry.
2. Sit comfortably in a chair or lie on your back and close your eyes.
3. Place your hands on your stomach directly above your waistline.
4. Breathe in slowly through your nose, pushing your hands out with your stomach. This helps create the sense of breathing deeply.
5. Hold your breath to a count of 2 to 5: whatever is comfortable for you. Slowly and steadily breathe out through your mouth, feeling your hands move inwards as your abdomen slowly contracts, and until most of the air has been expelled. The process of exhalation is a little longer than that of inhalation.

With experience you will not need to use your hands to check your breathing. Remember that improving your breathing is something that becomes easier and easier if practiced regularly. As with many other things, even breathing requires practice, practice, and more practice.

Health benefits

According to a study by Pal, et al. in 2004, the practice of breathing exercises like *pranayama* are known to improve autonomic function by changing sympathetic or parasympathetic activity. In this study, a total of 60 male undergraduate medical students were randomly divided into a slow-breathing group (practicing slow-breathing exercises) and a fast breathing group (practicing fast-breathing exercises) to practice exercises for a period of three months.

Autonomic function tests were performed before and after each session of breathing exercises. Results of these tests revealed that increased parasympathetic activity and decreased sympathetic activity were observed in the slow-breathing group, while no significant change in autonomic (involuntary) function was observed in the fast-breathing group. The findings of this study show that the regular practice of slow-breathing exercises for as little as three months can improve autonomic function.[52]

In another study involving yoga meditation and breathing, a highly practiced Kundalini yoga meditator was examined. Thoracic and abdominal breathing patterns, heart rate, electroencephalograph (EEG), skin conductance level, and pulse were monitored during pre-baseline, meditation, and post-baseline periods. Analysis of the data collected showed a decrease in respiration rate during the meditative process, from a mean of 11 breaths per minute (pre-baseline) and 13 breaths per minute (post-baseline), to a mean of five breaths per minute during meditation using predominately abdominal/diaphragmatic breathing. The increase in alpha brain waves during meditation suggested to researchers that changes in breathing patterns may contribute to the development of *alpha EEG*.[53] Benefits of Alpha EEG brain waves include: relaxation; creativity; enhanced problem-solving; emotional centering; fear, tension, and anxiety reduction; a more positive outlook; and an overall unfolding and flowing of inner awareness.

A paper published by Ohnishi and Ohnishi in 2006 also reports health benefits through the use of "Ki-energy." Broadly defined, Ki- (or "chi" or "qi") energy is the vital force that underlies functioning of the body, mind, and spirit. Ki-energy is considered to have a specific wavelength that not only exists in each of us, but can also be purposefully generated and transmitted through air to be received by another individual. This energy may be enhanced through the practice of what is called the Nishino Breathing Method. This research has shown that practice of Nishino's Ki-energy can inhibit division of cancer cells, protect isolated mitochondria from heat deterioration, and reduce lipid peroxidation in heat-treated mitochondria.[54,55]

The Nishino Breathing Method was developed by Kozo Nishino, a Japanese qi expert who studied medicine prior to applying himself to the art of ballet at the Metropolitan Opera's School of Ballet in New York City. Upon his return to Japan after his studies, Nishino founded the Nishino Ballet Company. It was at this point he embarked on a study of the mystics and of the Japanese martial art Aikido. The Nishino Breathing Method was born of his knowledge of Western medicine techniques, dance, and the Japanese martial arts. Nishino has been teaching this method for over 20 years and has worked with more than 10,000 students.

The Nishino Breathing Method is a process of energy creation that is similar to the way a plant draws water from the earth. Three elements make up this type of breathing, starting with *sokushin*, in which inhalation occurs through the soles of the feet. Upon inhalation through the nose, one first becomes aware of the soles of the feet and then feels the energy rising upward from the feet to the knees, to the thighs, and to the *tanden*, the second element, found in the area of the umbilical. From the tanden, the energy is then steadily propelled upward along the spine, eventually reaching the *hyakue*, the third element, at the top of the head. At this point, if one lightly holds one's breath, and then slowly exhales through the mouth, the energy from the hyakue flows back to the tanden, in the front of the body, and down the midline. Finally, upon full exhalation, the energy is directed downward through the soles of the feet into the earth. Over time, a natural energy exchange, or *taiki*, is said to occur within the body. This energetic communication is felt not only inside the practitioner's own body, but between the practitioner and the bodies of others. In taiki practice sessions, anybody can be a recipient of this kind of strong life energy.

In a study that followed both beginning and advanced students of the Nishino Breathing Method (NBM), for example, it was found that not only did NBM improve microcirculatory response, increase immune activity, and lower stress levels in all participants, but that results were significantly higher in the NBM method experts compared to those who were beginners of the practice.[56] A study by Kimura, et al. in 2005 has further demonstrated that practice of the Nishino Breathing Method has been seen to decrease stress levels and increase the immune response of the practitioner after only one class.[57]

Constructive breathing techniques have a beneficial impact on all the various systems of the body, as indicated below.

Respiratory system. Breathing correctly relaxes tight chest and back muscles and increases diaphragmatic movement, improving overall air flow.

Lymphatic system. Breathing serves as a pump for the lymphatic system. The deep rhythmic movement of breathing helps circulate the lymph, which aids in the detoxification of the body.

Circulatory system. The circulatory system benefits from correct breathing by way of improved blood circulation and increased oxygen-carrying capacity. Increased oxygen to the cells of the body facilitates better organ functioning.

Nervous system. Proper breathing is a quick way to stimulate the parasympathetic nervous system. This response calms the minds and facilitates a sense of relaxation.

Digestive system. Diaphragmatic breathing massages the organs involved in the digestive system, enhancing the digestive process.

Endocrine system. Breathing correctly balances hormone levels, having a positive impact on the endocrine system's cells, tissues, and organs.

It is really quite extraordinary how simple methods of correct breathing can have such profound physiological benefits.

Stress

I recently overheard a group of high-school students complaining how "stressed" they were from studying for their mid-term examinations. As I listened to their complaints with amazement, it was then that I realized that stress really can affect anyone, regardless of age or experience.

Stress is defined as a physical, mental, or emotional factor that causes the body to experience physical and/or mental tension. What exactly are "stress factors"? According to Dr. Hans Selye, an Austrian physician who spent 50 years studying the causes and consequences of stress, stress factors are any outside forces which create challenges in our daily lives: "No one can live without experiencing some degree of stress all the time," said Selye. "You may think that only serious disease or intensive physical or mental injury can cause stress. This is false. Crossing a busy intersection, exposure to a draft, or even sheer joy are enough to activate the body's stress-mechanism to some extent. Stress is not even necessarily bad for you; it is also the spice of life, for any emotion, any activity causes stress."[58] Dr. Selye's research uncovered that a stress-induced hormonal system could lead to physiological breakdowns and ultimately contribute to what he called "diseases of adaptation." Based on Selye's research and conclusions, many would have to agree that stress is that which both challenges and tests us.

Another popularly cited definition of stress originated with Dr. Richard S. Lazarus, a pioneer in the field of emotion and stress. Dr. Lazarus said that stress is a condition or feeling experienced when a person perceives that "demands exceed the personal and social resources the individual is able to mobilize."[59] One of the appropriate responses to stress is the release of powerful neurochemicals and hormones that prepare us to respond to that stress, whether actual or imagined. However, prolonged exposure to these chemical compounds long after the stress has passed can lead to health problems of all kinds. It is a known fact that prolonged, unmanageable stress has detrimental effects on both our physical health and emotional wellbeing. Consequently, the most important thing about stress is how we handle it. Since living in today's world provides an abundance of stress, which few of us can avoid altogether, it is up to each of us to stay as balanced as possible. This means adopting the best strategies for coping in order to best adapt and maintain our equilibrium, or what the great neurologist Walter Cannon called *homeostasis*.

Cornell University's Gannett Health Services has designed a graph to explain mental and physical performance in relation to stress (see Figure 4-15). According to the Cornell model, positive stress can drive us to action and move us into our "peak performance zone," bringing a sense of passion and stimulation into our lives. On the other hand, negative stress can result in fatigue, anxiety, and feelings of helplessness. If this response persists over time, we are sure to experience ramifications in terms of our health.

FIGURE 4-15. The Stress Continuum. Cornell Slope Stress Continuum: *What's healthy? What's not?* 2009. (Source: reprinted with permission from Cornell University. (*http://www.gannet.cornell. edu/images/_slope_JEA.gif.* Modified slightly for reproduction purposes)

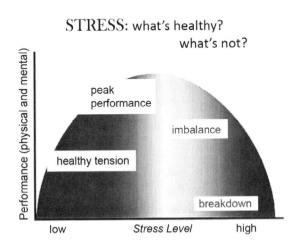

- **Healthy tension.** Healthy tension comes from stimulating challenges and demands that motivate us to improve our performance and efficiency. This kind of tension has the added benefit of increasing joy and excitement in our lives.

- **Peak performance.** In order to reach our personal best, whether it's taking an examination, running a race, giving a presentation at work, parenting, or managing any other personal challenge, we need to be well prepared physically, mentally, and emotionally. This foundation of preparedness allows us to access what we need to achieve our peak performance.

- **Imbalance.** When stress builds up, the protective functions of our body and mind can become compromised. We may feel irritable or overwhelmed, have problems sleeping and/or eating, or experience aches or pains.

- **Breakdown.** If stress is left unchecked, symptoms will worsen, causing forgetfulness, severe physical complaints, illness, and feelings of anxiety, panic, and/or depression. Seeking help at this stage is critical.

"I'm so stressed." We hear this said often, but what does it really mean? Stress is our internal response to the external "events" of our daily living. In other words, stress is what our bodies and minds perceive as we adapt to our ever-changing world. When most of us think of the word "stress," we tend to think of the term as a negative byproduct of some of our experiences. However, as explained earlier, stress is not all bad.

There are actually two sides to the stress coin: *distress* and *eustress*. While both are equally challenging, their long-term impact on the body yields very different results. And although both stresses are cumulative in nature, distress has a negative connotation, while eustress refers to the type of stress connected to positive or happy events in one's life.

Eustress comes from a Greek word, *eu*, meaning "good." When attached to "stress" it signifies the "good" kind of stress—the kind of stimulation that prepares us both mentally and physically for an impending challenge. For example, an athlete gains strength during competition, a painter experiences a stroke of inspiration while painting, or a student feels challenged trying to solve a math problem. When we are engaged in these types of activities, or in other activities that stimulate and motivate us, we find that complacency and boredom tend to disappear. Eustress is what we experience when we have been promoted at a job, get married, have a baby, or go on vacation. These types of "in spirit" activities energize us to grow and develop.

Distress, on the other hand, occurs when an individual cannot adapt to the stress that occurs. As a result, the normal physiological equilibrium of any number of bodily organisms becomes disturbed. It is when the body is unable to process this stress response appropriately that an imbalance ensues, and the individual's health and wellbeing becomes compromised.

Distress is broken down into two types: *acute* and *chronic*.

Acute stress. We experience acute stress in response to immediate, perceived physical, emotional, or psychological threat. This threat can be real or imagined, because it is the perception of that threat that triggers our response. During an acute stress response, the autonomic nervous system becomes activated. Acute stress feels intense, especially since it often occurs as a result of some unexpected, sudden change in our routine. When the threat passes, our body becomes aware of the actual nature of the change. With that awareness comes the capacity for the body to then return to its original, non-threatened state.

Chronic stress. Chronic stress is stress of a different kind. It can affect our body for a long period of time—even indefinitely. In this state of ongoing physiological stimulation, the body experiences so many stressors that the autonomic nervous system rarely has a chance to activate a relaxation response. People who are plagued by too many changes or upsets in their personal lives, employment, and/or environment often experience ongoing chronic stress—and the conditions which develop in response to the ongoing bombardment. Chronic stress has three components:

1. the precipitating event or condition, and our assumptions and belief systems relative to that event or condition
2. our ongoing perception of the event or condition
3. our responses (physiological, behavioral, and emotional) to that event or condition

Psychologists Suzanne Segerstrom, Ph.D., and Gregory Miller, Ph.D. have researched and analyzed the results of nearly 300 studies on the causes of stress by sorting them into different categories and then statistically evaluating their relationships. Their investigation found five different "stressor" categories, as follows:

1. *Acute time-limited stressors*: challenges, such as public speaking or mental math
2. *Brief naturalistic stressors*: real-world challenges, such as academic tests
3. *Stressful-event sequences*: focal events, such as loss of a spouse or major natural disaster, which give rise to a series of related challenges
4. *Chronic stressors*: persistent demands that force people into restructuring their roles and identities without any clear purpose, such as caregiving for an ill spouse, permanent disability, or having to relocate from your native country due to an act of war
5. *Distant stressors*: traumatic experiences from the distant past which impact the immune system due to their long-lasting emotional and cognitive consequences, such as combat trauma or child abuse[60]

Acute time-limited stressors and brief naturalistic stressors are those responsible for our aforementioned fight or flight response. This is purely an adaptive response. These stressors are also called "brief stressors" because they enhance the physiology by helping the body meet the existing challenge. Stressful-event sequences are longer in duration and intensity than brief stressors. As a result, they can have detrimental effects on the immune response over the long term. In other words, the studies conducted showed that the longer the duration of the stress, the more participants' immune systems seemed to shift from potentially positive adaptive changes to potentially negative ones. This shift was shown to have a huge psychological and physiological impact. For example, chronic stressors are events that are beyond our control; therefore, in their intensity, they become responsible for transforming our identities and social roles. Distant stressors, such as memory events, can also have long-term stress-related physiological consequences, as they tend to be relived and replayed over and over again in our mind's eye. Since we know that a weakened immune function naturally allows further susceptibility to disease, Segerstrom and Miller's research revealing that chronic stress affects physiology and causes a decline in immune function is significant.

Events such as a spouse's death, divorce, marriage, separation, a jail term, the death of a close relative, injury or illness, being fired from a job, and retirement are the most commonly cited reasons for stress. Of course, stress doesn't knock on the door before it comes in, so we are often unprepared for its impact. Plus, stress can affect anyone, at any time, for any reason. Furthermore, there's no telling what people will find stressful. Our individual outlooks, personalities, support systems, and responses all contribute in determining what each of us might consider stressful.

Understanding what has caused our stress will make a difference to whether we feel capable or incapable of handling it. If we are reacting negatively, the first step in processing the nature of the stress is to identify exactly why and how the event or events occurred and why we feel so uncomfortable. How we react to this stress—how our stress is manifested in signs and symptoms—varies from person to person. Some of us will experience distress in the form of physical aches and pains, such as lower-back aches, headaches, stomach upsets, and skin outbreaks. Many experience bouts of depression, hypersensitivity, anxiety, and crying. Whatever the cause of our stress, however, it is clear that the earlier we take measures to alleviate our reactions to the stressful circumstances, the better we may be able to control their effects. Some of the common warning signs and symptoms of stress are listed in Table 4-2.

TABLE 4-2. Warning signs and symptoms of stress. (Source: *www.helpguide.org/stresssigns.htm*)

Cognitive symptoms	Emotional symptoms
Memory problems	Moodiness
Indecisiveness	Agitation
Inability to concentrate	Restlessness
Trouble thinking clearly	Short temper
Poor judgment	Irritability, impatience
Seeing only the negative	Inability to relax
Anxious or racing thoughts	Feeling tense and "on edge"
Constant worrying	Feeling overwhelmed
Loss of objectivity	Sense of loneliness and isolation
Fearful anticipation	Depression or general unhappiness

(continued on next page)

Physical symptoms	Behavioral symptoms
Headaches or backaches	Eating more or less
Muscle tension and stiffness	Sleeping too much or too little
Diarrhea or constipation	Isolating oneself from others
Nausea, dizziness	Procrastination, neglecting responsibilities
Insomnia	Use of alcohol, cigarettes, or drugs to relax
Chest pain, rapid heartbeat	Nervous habits (e.g., nail biting, pacing)
Weight gain or loss	Teeth-grinding or jaw-clenching
Skin breakouts (hives, eczema)	Overdoing activities (e.g., exercising, shopping)
Loss of sex drive	Overreacting to unexpected problems
Frequent colds	Picking fights with others

Unfortunately, we cannot possibly shut out all stress from all aspects of our lives. Stressors of one kind or another penetrate our lives daily; the news coverage alone accounts for an overabundance of scenes of death, accidents, war, earthquakes, floods, violence, and terrorist attacks—broadcast around the clock—on television, on the Internet, and in newspapers and magazines. Watching the news can easily make our stress levels soar. Our physical reactions (as listed in Table 4-2) to these events serve as defense mechanisms, meant to help the human body deal with perceived threats and dangers. They are not meant to be triggered regularly, by news coverage and media; if they are, we may see a detrimental effect on our health.

The fight or flight response. Originally, the phrase "fight or flight" was coined to describe the physiological response or ability that enables us to physically stay and fight, or to run away (take flight) when faced with danger. However, this response can also be activated in situations where neither fighting nor running is necessary. When this happens, we tend to perceive everything in our environment as a possible threat to our survival. Within seconds, sequences of nerves fire. Chemicals such as adrenaline, noradrenaline, and cortisol are released into the bloodstream. Blood is shunted away from our digestive tract and directed into the muscles and limbs, which require extra energy for running and/or fighting. Our respiratory rate increases, our pupils dilate, our sight sharpens, and our impulses quicken. As a result, our body receives a burst of energy and strength that helps get us through the situation at hand.

Cortisol is also responsible for curbing functions that are fight or flight influenced, such as the suppression of the immune response and altering of the growth process and digestive and reproductive systems. This response can also alter mood to cause depression and affect memory and motivation.

Clinical studies indicate that stress, chronic depression, social interaction, and other psychological factors may influence both the onset and progression of cancer. In one such study by Antoni, et al. in 2006, researchers revealed that clinical and experimental stress can significantly influence the underlying cellular and molecular processes that facilitate malignant cell growth. Antoni explains: "As cancer treatment evolves toward a more patient-specific approach, consideration of the influence of bio-behavioral factors provides a novel perspective for mechanistic studies and new therapeutic targets."[61]

Reactions to stress. Our response to stress is amazingly self-regulatory. This means that the body is enabled to return to normal when the crisis has passed. Specifically, as hormone levels in the bloodstream decline, our heart rate, blood pressure, and respiration, as well as other systems of the body, return to average levels. Physiological factors are not the only components that help us return to normalcy. Psychological factors, such as relaxation, happiness, and optimism also begin to re-emerge when the threat is over. Yet, as the American Psychological Association reports, stress continues to be a growing problem in the United States. In the APA's 2009 Stress in America survey, 75% of all U.S. adults reported experiencing moderate to high levels of stress in the past month (24% to an extreme level; 51% to a moderate level) and nearly half (42%) reported that their stress had increased in the past year. Nearly half (43%) of all adults say they eat too much or eat unhealthy foods as a result of stress, and 37% report skipping a meal because they are under stress. Sixty-six percent of all adults living in the U.S. have been told by a healthcare provider that they have one or more chronic conditions, most commonly high blood pressure or high cholesterol.[62]

Katherine C. Nordal, Ph.D., the APA's executive director for professional practice, states, "The prevalence with which Americans continue to report increasing and extreme stress levels is a real concern. Also, people say that their levels of stress and lack of willpower are preventing them from making lifestyle and behavior changes that are necessary for improving and maintaining good health. It's clear that people need tools and support to better manage extreme stress in order to prevent serious health consequences. Unfortunately, our current healthcare system does not do a very good job in this regard. And insurance companies often don't cover preventive services or the kinds of services people need in order to better manage chronic illness."[62]

An estimated 1 million employees do not report for work on any given workday because of purported problems due to stress. Job-related stress is estimated to cost U.S. industry $300 billion annually due to absent workers, diminished productivity, and employee turnover, as well as medical, legal, and insurance fees. Stress has been shown to cause 60 to 80% of industrial accidents and lawsuits demanding compensation for workers involved in job-related stress claims. These types of claims average more than four times those for physical injury claims. Furthermore, stress is a leading factor contributing to the lack of response to treatments in cases of heart disease, cancer, lung ailments, and quite possibly many other diseases.

As we have seen, the stress response consists of a series of biochemical and physiological changes. Elevated levels of adrenaline, noradrenaline, and cortisol over long periods of time suppress the immune system, making us susceptible to infectious disease from microorganisms as well as chronic diseases such as cancer. It is also a well-known fact that people under stress have a greater tendency to use or abuse cigarettes, alcohol, and other drugs excessively, further affecting the central nervous system, cardiovascular system, digestive system, musculoskeletal system, immune system, respiratory system, reproductive system, and endocrine system. Working to make a conscious effort in reversing this process is critical to staying healthy and disease-free.

Anger. On the APA's website, in the article "Controlling Anger—Before It Controls You," Jerry Deffenbacher, Ph.D., a psychologist who specializes in anger management, states, "Some people really are more 'hotheaded' than others are; they get angry more easily and more intensely than the average person does. There are also those who don't show their anger in loud, spectacular ways, but are chronically irritable and grumpy. Easily angered people don't always curse and throw things; sometimes they withdraw socially, sulk, or get physically ill."[63] This statement shows us how differently people react when they are angry. The next question is how an individual's reaction to anger will affect his or her health.

In a study from the Department of Psychology at Ohio State University the effects of certain types of expressed anger on wound-healing was examined, where the 98 participants involved received blister wounds on their non-dominant forearms. After blistering, the wounds were monitored daily for eight days to assess the speed at which the wounds would heal. Researchers found that individuals who exhibited less anger control were more likely to heal more slowly. These participants had also shown a higher level of cortisol reactivity during the blistering procedure, and it was this enhanced cortisol secretion that was shown to relate to the longer healing time.[64] In another study which examined the different effects of expressed and suppressed anger, it was found that both types of anger were predictive indicators for the development of ischemic heart disease.[65]

Anger *can* be managed. Start by identifying and being aware of the particular factors in your life that are causing the reaction you feel. Some schools of thought suggest that the ideal way to combat anger is to identify and discuss the events that precipitate the anger. The Department of Health and Human Services is one government entity that has addressed concerns related to anger by providing tools for effective anger management. HHS's 12-week cognitive behavioral anger management group treatment program has been shown to be successful in helping participants learn the skills to control their anger.[66]

Relaxation

By dictionary definition, relaxation is "the act of relaxing or the state of being relaxed, the refreshment of body or mind, or a reduction in strictness or severity." This broad interpretation includes virtually any method or activity that helps us attain a state of relaxation, of being calm, thereby decreasing stress and tension. When we achieve a relaxed state of mind we let go of worry and the mind's constant "noise," or chatter that normally inhabits our thought processes. Because the mind cannot be separated from the body, any tension in our mind is always reflected in the workings of our body and vice versa.

An offshoot of relaxation is the absence of tension in the muscle of the body. In a physically relaxed state, tension seems to disappear effortlessly from our muscle groups in such a way that we may not even be aware of the shift. In the same way that stress causes a lengthy chain of events, relaxation also causes a significant series of physiological changes.

Relaxation has been shown to:

- slow the heart rate
- slow the breathing rate
- lower blood pressure
- reduce the need for oxygen
- increase the blood flow to major muscles
- reduce muscle tension

As a result you may:

- have more energy
- experience fewer physical symptoms

- be less reactive under emotional responses, such as anger or frustration
- experience improved concentration
- have a greater ability to handle daily problems
- experience increased efficiency in the activities of daily life

Relaxation techniques are tools for bringing us back to feeling calm and peaceful. On its website, the University of Maryland Medical Center classifies relaxation techniques into three main types.[67]

Autogenic Training/Therapy (AT). *AT* is a relaxation-inducing process that combines visual imagery with body awareness and focuses on easy, natural breathing and on slowing the heart rate. Autogenic training also focuses on a feeling of warmth and comfort in the limbs, a state that further induces the body to relax. During Autogenic Therapy, the participant enters a place of passive concentration, a state of mind that occurs when we intentionally relinquish willpower or any active, concentrated effort. In essence, the more passive we are, the greater the relaxation we will experience. Developed by psychiatrist Dr. Johannes Schulz, AT is known to help balance the parasympathetic and sympathetic nervous systems; it is this balance that contributes to a greater sense of wellbeing.

AT has been compared to meditation and self-hypnosis. The technique revolves around autosuggestion, where individuals learn simple mental exercises that allow them to enter deep states of relaxation and experience relief from the negative effects of stress. Exercises consist of silently repeating simple phrases while focusing on different organs of the body. These "autosuggestions" are designed to focus attention on the bodily sensations associated with the feeling of relaxation. Physical suggestions of a warmth and heaviness in the limbs, warmth in the solar plexus, calm and regular breathing and heartbeat, and a cool forehead are some of the suggestions used to elicit the relaxation response.[68]

One example of performing autogenic relaxation is as follows: Begin to breathe deeply, passively releasing muscle tension with each exhale. Beginning with your right hand, say to yourself: "My right hand is relaxed, heavy, and warm; my right hand is completely limp and relaxed." Allow this to happen. Repeat as the relaxation fills your hand. When you feel relaxed in your right hand, move on to your arm and repeat the same relaxation process. Take some time with the process, repeating the relaxation phrases a few times before moving on to your left hand and arm. When you feel ready, move to another area of the body with a different set of muscles.

Progressive muscle relaxation. Another effective method of relaxation is called Progressive Muscle Relaxation, or PMR. This technique was developed in the early 1920s by American physician Edmund Jacobson, who suggested that since muscular tension accompanies anxiety, the reduction of anxiety can be achieved by relaxing muscular tension.[69] Jacobson's work showed how the voluntary relaxation of certain muscles reduced symptoms of anxiety in his patients. Throughout the course of his research, Jacobsen observed that practicing relaxation techniques was found to be effective against illnesses such as ulcers, insomnia, and hypertension. Practicing the technique of Progressive Muscle Relaxation on a regular basis by slowly tensing and releasing the muscles of the body has been shown to bring about significant levels of relaxation in many individuals.

An example of performing PMR is as follows.

The first step is to sit or lie down comfortably. Check for tension in each of the muscle groups in your body; the major areas where tension is likely are the shoulders, jaw, forehead, neck, and back. When you focus on a group of muscles and begin the relaxation process, start by tensing the muscle group, hold the tension for 10 seconds, and then relax the muscles slowly for 10 to 15 seconds so that the feeling of draining the tension from the body sets in. It helps to repeat the process to reinforce the feeling of letting the tension drain from the muscles. Repeat the tensing of each muscle group, followed by the relaxation, 10 to 15 times before you move on to the next set of muscles. If you would like to try this technique, here is one step-by-step procedure you can follow:

- Sit in a comfortable chair or lie on the bed in a comfortable position. Try to find the highest degree of comfort you can. Take off your shoes, avoid tight clothes, and do not cross your legs.
- Take a deep breath and exhale slowly. Breathing techniques can be incorporated when working with the muscles or independently. Repeat.
- Concentrate on the muscles and feel them tensing and relaxing alternately.
- Tense each muscle group for 10 seconds and hold each relaxation period for 10 to 15 seconds.
- Do not tense all your muscles simultaneously; concentrate on one specific muscle group at a time.

Here are some recommendations for relaxing the different muscle groups, as follows:

- *Hands.* Clench/tense the fists, then relax the fingers to full extension (straightening and back) in a relaxed position.
- *Biceps and triceps.* Tense and then relax the biceps, and then the triceps.
- *Shoulders.* Pull the shoulders back and then relax. Push them forward in a hunched position, and relax.
- *Lateral neck.* With your shoulders straight and relaxed, bend your head slowly to the right side as far as you can. Hold, and then relax. Bend to the left. Hold tension, then relax again.
- *Forward neck.* Bend your chin into your chest. Hold, and then relax.
- *Mouth.* Open your mouth as far as possible. Bring the lips together or purse as tightly as possible. Hold, and then relax.
- *Tongue (roof and floor).* Push your tongue into the roof of your mouth. Hold, and relax. Push it into the bottom of your mouth. Hold, then relax.
- *Eyes.* Open your eyes wide. Hold, and then relax. Close your eyes tight. Hold, and relax again. Make sure that your eyes, forehead, and nose are fully relaxed after each tensing.
- *Breathing.* Breathe in as deeply as possible. Then take another deep breath. Let it out and breathe normally for 15 seconds. Do this process in two steps: breathe in, breathe in some more; breathe out, and then breathe out normally for 15 seconds.
- *Back.* With your shoulders resting on the back of a chair, push your body forward so that your back is arched. Hold, then relax.
- *Buttocks.* Tense your buttocks and raise your pelvis off the chair. Hold, then relax. Tense your buttocks and raise your pelvis off the chair again. Hold; relax again.
- *Thighs.* Extend legs and raise them about six inches off the floor (or the footrest). Hold, then relax. Next dig your heels into the floor or your footrest. Hold; relax again.
- *Stomach.* Pull in your stomach as much as possible. Tense, then relax. Push out the stomach and tense it again. Hold, then relax.
- *Calves and feet.* Point your toes with your legs on the floor/foot rest. Hold, then relax. Bend the toes up as far as possible. Tense again, then relax.
- *Toes.* Keeping your legs relaxed, dig your toes into the floor. Hold, then relax. Bend the toes up as far as possible. Tense again, and then relax.

When you have completed this full-body exercise, give yourself a few minutes to stay in the totally relaxed state you have achieved in order to experience how your body felt before and after the exercise. Do you feel less tense? Does your body feel calmer, rejuvenated? It's a good idea to integrate this routine regularly and to keep a record of your "progress"—any changes or feelings you experience. Over time you can eliminate steps for body parts which do not appear to be causing you particular tension, but doing them all will ensure you spend enough time to get the full benefit of the session. These exercises are not designed to keep all tension away, but rather to help you to be aware of certain elements, such as how you are feeling at any given time, how you are reacting to stress, and where your tension may be focused. When you start performing tensing-and-relaxing exercises on a regular basis you will likely begin to see the benefits on your overall level of tension. The entire process of this muscle relaxation sequence takes about 30 minutes the first few times, but with practice that time may decrease to 15 or 20 minutes.

Meditation practice. In the U.S., the two most popular forms of meditation include Transcendental Meditation®, or TM®, and mindfulness mediation. TM®, a practice established by Maharishi Mahesh Yogi, is derived from Hindu traditions which use a *mantra*, a repeated word, sound, or phrase, to help the mind settle inward to a quiet, peaceful state of consciousness. The goal of TM® is to achieve a state of relaxed awareness. Mindfulness meditation instead has its roots in Buddhism. In one common form of mindfulness meditation, the individual focuses on the flow of breath in and out of the body. The individual meditating learns to focus attention on what is being experienced, without reacting to or judging that experience. This practice helps the individual experience thoughts and emotions that come up in normal daily life with a greater sense of peace and balance.

The therapeutic benefits of relaxation techniques have been well documented, notably in reference to their effects on cancer patients. In 2008, for example, Kwekkeboom, et al. published a study that validated progressive muscle relaxation and guided imagery as a complementary therapy for cancer patients with pain. Post-study interviews were conducted with 26 hospitalized patients with cancer pain who had completed trials of guided imagery and PMR. Researchers in this study found that despite the fact that pain results varied from patient to patient, the majority of participants perceived that the complementary interventions worked for their pain and many reported a clinically significant change in their overall pain levels.[70]

The National Center for Complimentary and Alternative Medicine references several published studies regarding the highly beneficial effects of meditation on physical and emotional wellbeing,[71] and the overwhelming common finding is irrefutable: meditating provides an opportunity to tap into a power that already resides within us, a power we can then draw out and draw on for healing and self-improvement. The process of meditation has revealed undeniable evidence of the interconnectedness between the mind and body. For example, there are encouraging studies citing the influence of mediation on breast and prostate tumors, and a preliminary study has found an association between meditation practice and levels of melatonin produced by the pineal gland.[72] In another study of a mindfulness-based stress reduction meditation program for early-stage breast and prostate cancer patients, researchers revealed a significant improvement in the participants' quality of life, stress symptoms, sleep patterns, and positive changes in behavior patterns, such as exercise levels and caffeine consumption. Further noted was the fact that while T-cell production of interleukin 4 (IL-4) increased during this period, interferon-gamma and NK-cell production of interleukin-10 decreased. The authors of the study state, "These changes in the immune profiles of these patients are consistent with a shift in the balance from a Th1 (proinflammatory) to a Th2 (anti-inflammatory) environment, and are behaviorally associated with a shift away from a depressive pattern to one more consistent with healthy immune function."[73]

Sleep

Sleep is vital for the survival of all living things. Sleep is a natural state of rest, an instinctive periodic state of inactivity adopted by the body under conditions of fatigue. Over the years, we have begun to reconsider the meaning of sleep, where "sleep scientists" are now addressing the various factors involved in either inducing or repressing the common state of what we call "sleep." Consequently, a behavioral definition has evolved by observing the common traits of a majority of sleeping individuals to include a typical posture of lying down, little movement, and a reduced response to external stimulation. The hallmark of sleep is a behavioral disengagement, during which we do not normally respond to low-intensity sounds or touches, and which is reversed when a person returns to the state of wakefulness. Sleep is considered "reversible," in that it is a temporary state that occurs in order to allow the body to rest.

Sleep is also considered to be the ultimate form of relaxation and is vital for normal motor and cognitive function. During deep sleep, muscles fully relax, breathing and the heart rate slow down, and the body temperature drops. We may appear physically inactive during sleep; however the brain is far from dormant, and this is evidenced by measurements shown on an electroencephalogram, or EEG. In electroencephalography, electrodes connecting the instrument to the individual's scalp transmit the brain's activity to a computer, which translates the electrical activity into wavy lines drawn on a moving piece of paper, or as an image on a computer screen. By recording brain waves in this manner, scientists have been able to document differences in the various patterns of brain waves produced between the stages of sleep and wakefulness.

We now know that there are two main stages of sleep: non–rapid eye movement, or NREM sleep (also known as "quiet sleep"), and rapid eye movement, or REM sleep (also known as "active" or "paradoxical sleep").

Stage 1. NREM sleep is a period of lighter sleep that includes four phases. In phase one, we are half awake and half asleep. Muscle activity slows down and is accompanied by slight, occasional twitching. During this period we are sleeping lightly enough that we can be awakened very easily. When we awaken someone in this stage of sleep, we often hear them say, "I'm awake," or "I wasn't really asleep."

Within 10 minutes of entering the light sleep of NREM, we enter phase two, which lasts for about 20 minutes. In this stage, breathing becomes shallower, body temperature decreases, and the heart rate begins to slow down. In phase three of NREM sleep, we enter a phase when slow *delta waves*, the waves of high amplitude but low frequency, begin to emerge. This is the transitioning phase between light sleep and a very deep sleep. Phase four is considered the actual delta wave phase. Our breathing and heart rates are at their lowest levels during this period of very deep sleep. If we are awakened from this deep state of sleep, we often have difficulty adjusting and may feel groggy and disoriented for a few moments.

Stage 2. REM sleep is the stage of sleep we enter approximately 70 to 90 minutes after we fall asleep. We generally have three to five REM sleep cycles each night, and it is during this period when most dreaming occurs. The brain is extremely active during this stage and is characterized by eye movement and irregular heart and breathing rates. Increased brain activity also takes place during this period. REM sleep is referred to as "paradoxical sleep," because as our brain and other body systems become more active, our muscles become more relaxed. We dream due to our increased brain activity, but we sleep due to the inert quality of our voluntary muscles.

Babies divide their sleep time equally between the two stages of sleep. As we grow older, however, our NREM period increases and time spent in REM sleep decreases. Middle-aged adults spend 20% of their time in REM, while the elderly generally spend less than 15% of their sleep time in that stage. An average adult is required to sleep eight hours every day. That means that if we sleep eight hours per day, over a year we will spend the equivalent of 122 days asleep. At this rate, a 75-year-old will have spent a total of 25 years, or one third of his or her life, sleeping. Taken from that perspective, it seems like an awful lot, doesn't it?

Do we really need that much sleep? Why do we sleep at all? The answers to these kinds of questions continue to inspire much debate. Regardless of the many open questions, we do know—and there is widespread consensus—that sleep is something we cannot do without.

Lack of sleep

It is an unfortunate truth that many of us do not get enough sleep. Currently, lack of sleep has actually become an indentifiable, and commonly encountered, disorder. According to a report published in the *Journal of the American Medical Association*, insufficient sleep continues to be a growing health concern. Based on the data compiled, sleep insufficiency has been associated with numerous physical and mental health problems, injury, loss of productivity, and mortality. It was reported that approximately 29% of all U.S. adults report sleeping less than seven hours a night and 50 to 70 million adults have chronic sleep and wakefulness disorders. A CDC analysis of 2006 data from the Behavioral Risk Factor Surveillance System (BRFSS) in four states has shown that an estimated 10% of adults report receiving insufficient rest or sleep on all days during the 30 days preceding the data collection, with females being almost 3% more likely than males to experience this condition.[74]

Sleep and a healthy immune system

Sleep has two main benefits. First, it enhances the restorative ability of the body, allowing our organs and muscles to recuperate from the strenuous work of our daily lives, and second, it helps the body adapt to ever-changing conditions. In addition, sleep contributes to our capacity for learning and memory.

In children we find that the immune system and hormones responsible for growth and development function at their optimal capacity during sleep. In fact, it is through sleep deprivation studies that we have come to understand the tremendous importance of sleep for overall functioning at all ages.

Several independent study groups have conducted sleep deprivation studies. In one study by the Department of Psychiatry at the University of California and the San Diego Veterans Affairs Healthcare System, the effects of nocturnal sleep, partial-night sleep deprivation, and sleep stages were examined on circulating concentrations of interleukin-6 (IL-6) in relation to the secretory profiles of growth hormone, cortisol, and melatonin in 31 healthy male volunteers. Researchers of this study found that loss of sleep decreased the participants' nocturnal interleukin-6 levels, and that lower interleukin-6 levels affected the integrity of their immune system functioning.[75]

In another study, investigators examined the relationship between sleep and the recuperation from sickness caused by infectious disease. To evaluate this relationship, sleep patterns were classified in rabbits inoculated with *E. coli*, *S. aureus*, or *C. albicans* on the basis of the duration of the period of enhanced sleep. In this case, patterns characterized by long periods of enhanced sleep were associated with a more favorable prognosis and less severe clinical signs than the patterns which were characterized by relatively short periods of enhanced sleep and followed by prolonged sleep suppression. The authors of the study concluded that getting adequate amounts of sleep over the course of an infectious disease aids in the recuperative process.[76]

And that's just the beginning.

The overwhelming contribution of sleep toward the maintenance of a healthy immune system has also been illustrated in other scientific research. In one study, participants were denied sleep in order to examine the effect of sleep deprivation on levels of circulating lymphocytes, the white blood cells of the immune system. In this study, the marked decrease of lymphocytes and DNA synthesis in those participants who were deprived of sleep for 48 hours was shown to contribute to the decreased ability to fight off sickness and disease.[77] Furthermore, natural killer (NK) cells revealed a significant decrease in destructive activity after only one night of sleep deprivation.[78]

Sleep and mental alertness

Innumerable studies support the fact that sleep is necessary for mental alertness, the learning process, and our "declarative memory," or the ability to recall and recognize complex facts. Regular intervals of sleep are also essential for learning basic visual discrimination tasks and developing motor skills. One such study has demonstrated that human memory consolidation is strongly dependent on REM sleep,[79] while another has revealed that REM sleep significantly enhances anagram problem solving.[80] Sleep has also been shown to have an effect on blood sugar, where studies have found that six hours (or less) or nine hours (or more) of sleep is associated with both an increased prevalence of diabetes mellitus and impaired glucose tolerance. The authors of this study further cited that because this effect was present in subjects without insomnia, voluntary sleep restriction may contribute to the large public health burden of diabetes mellitus.[81]

Another interesting study examined the effect of sleep on the development of "insight," where insight is defined as a "sudden gain of explicit knowledge allowing qualitatively changed behavior."[82] Subjects in this study were asked to transform strings of digits into new strings by following two explicit rules for eight hours. What researchers found was that the more times the participants performed the task, the more rapidly they were able to execute it. This outcome supported the idea that repeated performance exposed subjects to a "hidden rule" which, when recognized, made the task much simpler. In this particular case, more than twice as many subjects gained insight into the "hidden rule" after a period of sleep than when they had not recently slept, regardless of the time of day.

Insomnia and managing sleeplessness

Do you or does someone you know suffer from the inability to fall asleep or stay asleep? Although most of us suffer at least occasionally from this problem for one reason or another, it can become a significant detriment to our health when our lack of sufficient sleep persists and becomes true insomnia. Physicians regard insomnia, or the trouble falling asleep, as more of a symptom than a disease. It appears insomnia is generally due to some underlying cause, which can be associated with a psychological or medical condition or due to the accompanying use of certain pharmacological agents.

Intervention to deal with insomnia includes *stimulus* and *temporal control,* which together comprise a set of changes designed to do two things: first, to re-associate the bed/bedroom with sleep and second, to re-establish a consistent sleep schedule. For example, using the bed/bedroom primarily for sleep means avoiding certain activities, such as reading and television-watching, going to bed only when sleepy, getting out of bed when unable to sleep, arising at the same time every morning, and avoiding naps.[83] The effective management of insomnia begins with recognition and adequate assessment, because knowing where changes have to be made and implementing those changes is the first step toward getting a sound night's sleep. For example, although it is not uncommon to fall asleep with the television on when we're tired enough, it has been found that the constant bright light and the effect of recently watched programs that may include natural disaster or violence can make it more difficult to fall asleep—and sleep well. Corrective action, particularly in terms of controlling stimulus and restricting sleep patterns, helps many people to find non-pharmacological alternatives to insomnia, and thereby create durable long-term improvements in sleep habits.[84]

One way to ensure a good night's sleep is to incorporate physical activity into one's daily routine. The benefits of physical activity in improving the quality and duration of sleep have been well studied, to the degree that exercise is now popularly regarded as the most cost-effective technique for health management in people with insomnia. Other effective behavioral modifications include avoiding temperature extremes, large meals, tobacco, alcohol, and caffeine (which notably impairs sleep)[85] just before bedtime. Making the effort to limit fluid intake in the evening and restrict the use of the bedroom to sleep and for sleep-related activities also sets a pre-sleep pattern for more conducive, productive sleep.

Sleep and good health

Sleep is a necessity that literally empowers. To quote an Irish proverb, "The beginning of good health is sleep." Adequate and proper sleep revitalizes the body and brain, and enhances our mental alertness, perceptive ability, thought processes, reflexes, and communication skills. It enables us to follow safety procedures and promotes general good health.

Some tried and true practical techniques that help millions of people fall asleep include listening to the soothing sounds of nature, such as a gentle rain, a soft wind, or ocean waves, regulating the temperature and light in the bedroom, and avoiding loud alarm clocks and electronic gadgets. Physicians specifically advise avoiding heavy, carbohydrate- and fat-rich foods just before bedtime, as they create an increase in blood glucose levels and often cause one to wake up during the night with strong feelings of hunger due to the resultant plunge in glucose levels. Taking a hot shower or a warm bath before bedtime or light reading that is not suspense-filled, fear-producing, or anxiety-ridden are also ways to be lulled into a deep, relaxed, rewarding sleep.

Sleep and hormones

Melatonin is a hormone that has been widely studied due to its involvement in the regulation of sleep patterns. You may have heard of melatonin in the form of a supplement, promoted to regulate sleep problems related to travel and jet lag. Inside the body, melatonin is secreted mainly by the pineal gland in the brain, but small levels of synthesis also occur in other areas of the body, such as the eye, gastrointestinal tract, skin, bone marrow, and lymphocytes. Melatonin is secreted primarily at night, since the trigger for melatonin secretion is decreased light exposure. During the day, light induces the retina of the eye to continuously send impulses to the pineal gland, thereby shutting down the production of melatonin. Darkness, on the other hand, decreases the impulses sent to the brain, and the pineal gland secretes melatonin to induce sleep.

Apart from controlling the sleep-wake cycle, melatonin acts as an antioxidant, regulating several antioxidant enzymes (such as glutathione peroxidase, glutathione reductase, and glucose 6-phosphate dehydrogenase).[86,87] In studies involving cancer, melatonin has been shown to have a direct, marked inhibitory effect on MCF-7, or human breast cancer cell growth in culture, where melatonin completely blocks the stimulation of MCF-7 cell proliferation.[88] Melatonin has also been shown to significantly improve the quality of wound healing and scar formation,[89] and to have growth inhibitory effects on ovarian carcinoma,[90] endometrial carcinoma,[91] human uveal melanoma,[92] prostate tumor cells,[93] and intestinal tumors.[94]

Melatonin has been found not only to inhibit tumor growth, but to modify the immune response with regard to infection, inflammation, and autoimmunity:[95] data supported by the discovery of the existence of both nuclear and membrane receptors for melatonin in the immune system.[96] Physiologically, it has been widely assumed that the pineal gland is the major source of melatonin; however, studies have now revealed that human lymphocytes synthesize and release large amounts of melatonin elsewhere in the body. Melatonin's versatility includes many proven factors: it has been linked to antioxidant, oncostatic, anti-aging, and immunomodulatory (capable of modifying or regulating one or more immune functions) properties;[97] shown to prevent some chemotherapy-induced side-effects, particularly myelosuppression (a condition in which bone marrow activity is decreased, resulting in fewer red blood cells, white blood cells, and platelets) and neuropathy (a nerve problem that causes pain, numbness, tingling, swelling, or muscle weakness); and found to increase the efficiency of the immune system by stimulating the release of cytokines (small proteins).[98]

In another study, when laboratory rats were administered doses of melatonin, T-helper cells, considered important for cellular immunity, were observed to increase in number.[99] It is clear, therefore, that melatonin's immune-enhancing potential, in addition to its antioxidant potential, contributes greatly to its anti-tumorogenic properties.

Knowing that melatonin can significantly influence our sleep patterns and that it can be found in plant form, we can immediately and easily begin boosting our melatonin level by following a plant-rich diet. Oats, sweet corn, and rice are the most abundant sources, but melatonin also occurs naturally in vegetables like cabbage and radish sprouts, and in ginger, tomatoes, bananas, and barley in small amounts. That is why melatonin's potential antitumor and protective qualities can be attributed in part to its dietary intake through the consumption of vegetables, fruits, and whole grains.

Tryptophan and sleep

Tryptophan is an amino acid with a sleep-inducing effect as well. Tryptophan converts into serotonin, a promoter of REM sleep; increased levels of tryptophan, therefore, increase our ability to achieve deep sleep. Tryptophan is present in milk and milk products, honey, egg whites, soy products, lentils, hazelnuts, peanuts, sesame seeds, sunflower seeds, whole grains, rice, and tuna. While turkey also contains high amounts of tryptophan, it is comparable to amounts contained in other meats, so it may well be that the Thanksgiving drowsiness many of us suffer has more to do with what goes along with the turkey, such as carbohydrates and alcohol, than consumption of the turkey itself.

Diet

It may surprise you to learn that the word *diet* is derived from the Greek word *diatia*, meaning "way of life"—not "way to lose weight." Although human beings consume foods of both plant and animal origin, our dietary habits are largely molded by the society and culture in which we live. Various cultures have different accepted dietary preferences as well as taboos based on beliefs and religion. For instance, Judaism advocates the consumption of "kosher" (from the Hebrew, *kasrut*) foods which are considered to be fit, proper, or correct based on Kashrut, the body of Jewish law dealing with what foods can and cannot be eaten and how these foods must be prepared. Similar laws exist according to the Islamic faith, which recommends the use of *halaal* (Arabic for "permitted") foods. Americans are known to consume more red meat than people in other countries, and the Japanese consume more rice and fish. Latin American diets include more rice and beans, while lentils and pita bread (flat bread made out of wheat and yeast) is a typical staple food in Middle Eastern countries.

With all the varied diets to choose from, some are known to be healthier than others. The Mediterranean diet, for example, which includes a variety of cuisines from southern Italy, France, certain regions of Spain, and other countries bordering the Mediterranean Sea, is popularly considered one of the healthiest diets. This diet consists of a variety of fruits, vegetables, bread and cereals, potatoes, beans, nuts, and seeds. Most food preparation is done with olive oil, the oil of choice, and eggs, dairy products, fish, poultry, and wine are consumed in low to moderate quantities. Because the type of food we consume is largely related to what foods are indigenous to our environment, our culture, and our beliefs, our "diet"—and our way of life—is a reflection of the sum total of the foods we choose to eat.

Whole foods

By definition, *whole foods* are foods that have remained as close to their natural state as possible in that they have had little to no processing and have retained most, if not all, of their original nutrients and fiber. Whole foods provide our bodies with just the right amount of ingredients to be and stay well. Our store shelves are filled with tempting, easy-to-prepare products, but eating these foods as a regular diet often comes at a significant negative health cost. As Dr. Loren Cordain, member of the faculty of the Department of Health and Exercise Science at Colorado State University and considered by many as the world's leading expert on Paleolithic diets, states in his research, "In the United States and most Western countries, diet related chronic diseases represent the single largest cause of morbidity and mortality. These diseases are epidemic in contemporary Western society and typically afflict 50 to 65% of the adult population." Cordain contends that it is the excessive consumption of dairy products, cereals, refined cereals, refined sugars, refined vegetable oils, fatty meats, salt, and combinations of these foods that contributes to virtually all chronic diseases of the modern era.[100]

What exactly is "processed food"? If it's boxed, bagged, canned, or jarred, and has a list of ingredients on the label, it's *processed*. Processed foods have been purposely altered from their natural state for "safety" and convenience reasons. Processed foods include canned, frozen, dehydrated, heat-treated, sun-dried, and convenience foods, and can contain color, stabilizers, emulsifiers, bleach, flavor, softeners, preservatives, and sweeteners. Many people are unaware that processed foods are those which have undergone refining, a method that literally strips the vitamins, fiber, protein, and fat content—in essence, everything nutritious—out of the food. It is only at the last phase of the product's processing that manufacturers make any attempt to restore what has been lost.

When it comes to health and disease prevention, it is therefore important to eat the *whole* food. In other words, to derive the maximum benefit from the grain, fruit, or vegetable you eat, do not throw away the pulp, peel, and seeds, as you may have been taught. These parts are filled with health-enhancing nutrients! Whole foods are generally rich, not only in vitamins and minerals, but in phytochemicals, fiber, protein, complex carbohydrates, and fats.

Do you remember as a kid learning about the "four basic food groups"? Do you remember the meat group, the dairy group, the grain group, and the group consisting of fruits and vegetables? These general guidelines were the ones widely accepted in the 1950s and were designed to ensure we met our "daily requirements." Since then, however, food groups and their constituents have been revised to adhere to the U.S. Department of Agriculture's new guidelines, in the form of a program called "MyPyramid." The USDA's website, *www.mypyramid. gov*, tells us that, "One size doesn't fit all. MyPyramid offers personalized eating plans and interactive tools to help you plan and assess your food choices." This program was in part created to advance and promote dietary guidance for all Americans based on the epidemic increases in type 2 diabetes and obesity afflicting a large and rapidly growing number of children and adults.[101]

In the past, many so-called "food pyramids," formulated by a number of different groups, including the USDA, provoked considerable controversy because they did not differentiate between protein groups, refined grains and whole grains, and saturated and unsaturated fats. These pyramids not only failed to emphasize exercise, weight control, and the possible importance of taking a daily multivitamin, but actually advocated for the ingestion of "discretionary calories" in the form of wine, beer, candy, soda, and caloric sweeteners. The most recently updated and recognized pyramid, established in 2008 by the Harvard School of Public Health, is called the "Healthy Eating Pyramid." The Healthy Eating Pyramid, in my opinion, is the most well rounded and thoroughly researched pyramid to date and is said to be "based on the latest science, unaffected by businesses and organizations with a stake in its messages, [and] a simple, trustworthy guide to choosing a healthy diet (see Figure 4-16).[102]

FIGURE 4-16. Harvard University's "Healthy Food Pyramid." (Sources: Food Pyramid©2008 Harvard University, The Healthy Eating Pyramid, The Nutrition Source, Department of Nutrition, Harvard School of Public Health. Reprinted with permission: *http://www.thenutritionsource.org*, and Eat, Drink, and Be Healthy, by Walter C. Willett, M.D., and Patrick J. Skerrett. Free Press/Simon & Schuster, Inc. 2005.)

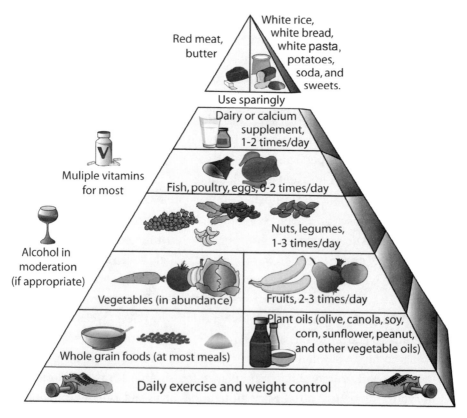

Noted at the top of this pyramid are foods are to be eaten sparingly due to the inherent health risks which far outweigh any benefits. These include: red meat, butter, white rice, white bread, white pasta, potatoes, soda, and sweets.

Based on the different food groups expressed in the Harvard food pyramid, we can begin to determine our caloric requirements according to age, gender, and lifestyle. *Calories* are simply measurements of energy. A "small" calorie, or *gram calorie*, is approximately the amount of energy required to raise the temperature of 1 g of water 1° centigrade. A "large" calorie, or *kilogram calorie* (kcal), refers to the amount of energy required to raise the temperature of 1 kg of water, or 2.2 lb of water, the same amount: that is, 1°. In essence, 1 kcal equals 1,000 calories.

The caloric value of a food, or the calories contained in a food product, is the amount of energy released when the food is completely digested. Most caloric values, as set forth by the USDA and in food industry tables, are based on "indirect calorie estimation," an estimate determined by use of the Atwater system. The Atwater system was created to calculate total caloric value by adding up the average values of the calories provided by a food's energy-containing nutrients, such as carbohydrates, proteins, fats, and alcohol.

What determines an individual's specific caloric requirement? An individual's caloric requirement depends, in general, on two things: size and activity level. Men and women who are sedentary will maintain their body weight by consuming about 13 calories per pound of body weight each day. Moderate physical activity increases this requirement to 16 calories, and intense activity to 18 calories per pound. In general, to maintain a current body weight, a 125-lb woman who undertakes a moderate activity level needs 2,000 calories a day and a 175-lb man needs about 2,800 calories a day.[103]

Fats and alcohol generate more energy than carbohydrates and proteins. When we consume more fats—that is, more calories or energy units than our body has the capacity to expend in energy—our bodies simply react by storing the excess, depositing it in various places on our bodies, as if to say, "We'll stay around to see if you need us later." Unfortunately, fatty deposits stick around longer than we might like if we continue to expend less energy than we take in. This is what leads to being overweight, and sometimes to chronic obesity—both conditions that have been shown to increase the risk for cancer. What's the best way to address this issue? By being aware and always trying to balance the body's energy intake with the body's energy output.

According to this new pyramid, a typical diet should include the following:

Whole-grain foods. Our bodies need carbohydrates for energy. Whole-grain foods and flours include 100% whole wheat, brown rice, bulgur, corn, buckwheat, oatmeal, spelt, and wild rice. Whole grains are nutrient-rich and take longer to digest than highly processed carbohydrates, such as white flour products, so they help control blood sugar and insulin levels. That is why calories from whole grains have further health benefits in that they help reduce the risk of diabetes and heart disease.

Plant oils. The average American receives one third or more of his or her daily calories from fats. As we mentioned, trans fats in particular have negative repercussions on the body's ability to stay healthy, so it's important to reassign our fat intake from healthier plant oils instead. Good sources of healthy unsaturated fats include olive, canola, soy, corn, sunflower, peanut, flaxseed, and other vegetable oils. Healthy fats actually improve cholesterol levels when they replace highly processed trans-fat foods.

Vegetables and fruits. A diet rich in fruits and vegetables can help lower blood pressure and protect us from heart attack, stroke, and any number of different cancers. Abundant amounts of vegetables and fruits contribute to overall maintenance and good health.

Fish and poultry. Fish is an ideal source of omega-3 oil, shown to reduce the risk of heart disease. Chicken and turkey are low in saturated fat, something that is essential for maintaining a healthy heart. Eggs have been maligned in recent years for containing high levels of cholesterol, but they have their positive attributes too, including high levels of protein, essential vitamins, and minerals.

Nuts and legumes. Nuts and legumes are excellent sources of protein, fiber, vitamins, and minerals. Almonds, walnuts, pecans, peanuts, hazelnuts, and pistachios are all tasty sources for adding to a daily requirement of proteins and vitamins. There are literally dozens of types of legumes, ranging from black beans, garbanzos, and kidney beans, to those that can be sprouted, such as mung and alfalfa. Legumes are available in dried, fresh, frozen, and tinned forms.

Dairy or calcium. Healthy, strong bones need calcium, vitamin D, and exercise. Dairy products, traditionally Americans' primary source of calcium by way of milk and cheese, are not the only way to ensure we get what we need, however, especially since many individuals have an intolerance to dairy. Calcium can also be found in nondairy products, such as dark green, leafy vegetables (kale and collard greens, for example), as well as in dried beans and legumes. Furthermore, with homogenization, pasteurization, and the addition of hormones and antibiotics to milk-related products, serious questions are being raised about the potential health risks of some dairy products. Milk products also naturally contain a high level of saturated fat. If you do drink milk, it is advisable to consume low-fat, organic products.

Balancing work and home

In the constant struggle to balance life at work and home, buying the ingredients to cook a meal often takes a back seat to more convenient, prepared meals. To confuse issues even more, the food products we buy are labeled with complex, if not misleading, information. For example, some products promote a reduction in fat content—but compared to what? Sometimes this advertised "lower fat" has been compensated by an increase in sugar content. Because foods claim to be everything from "reduced-fat," "low-fat," "calorie-free," "low-calorie," "fat-free," and "all natural," often misnomers at the very least, it behooves us to learn more about the labels on the products we purchase and the system behind those labels.

United States food labeling regulations

Through the years, food labeling regulations in the United States have been revised in a number of ways in order to reflect the goal of enhancing health awareness.[104] But do we really read food labels? Though many of us may not take the time to actually read the tiny print on product labels, I highly recommend it. In a few seconds, we not only get complete information on the nutrient, calorie, fat, and carbohydrate content of the product, but can instantly begin to assess what kinds of potentially unhealthy substances we are about to ingest. Recently the FDA has begun to regulate the use of certain misleading words or phrases on food packaging. For example, in the past any food product could claim to be "light" regardless of whether that designation was assigned to color, texture, or even taste. Today, for a food product to earn the label of "light," it must contain half the fat, one third the calories, or half the salt of its regular, "not light" counterpart, as indicated below in this table of nutrient claims and descriptors provided by Colorado State University.[104]

TABLE 4-3. Glossary of nutrient claims and descriptors. (Source: *http://www.ext.colostate.edu/pubs/food-nut09365.html*, 2010).

Term	Description
Calorie free	Fewer than 5 calories per serving
Cholesterol free	Fewer than 2 mg cholesterol and 2 g or fewer of saturated fat per serving
Enriched or fortified	Has been nutritionally altered so that one serving provides at least 10% more of the Daily Value of a nutrient than the comparison food
Extra lean	Fewer than 5 g fat, 2 g saturated fat, and 95 mg of cholesterol per serving and per 100 g
Fat free	Less than 0.5 g of fat per serving
Free	"Without," "no," or "zero" can all be used in place of "free"
Fresh	Generally used on food in its raw state; cannot be used on food that has been frozen or cooked, or on food that contains preservatives
Fresh frozen	Foods that have been quickly frozen while still fresh
Good source	One serving provides 10 to 19% of the Daily Value for a particular nutrient
Good source of fiber	Contains 10 to 19% of the Daily Value for fiber (2.5 to 4.75 g) per serving. If a food is not "low fat," it must declare the level of total fat per serving and refer to the nutrition panel when a fiber claim is mentioned
High	One serving provides at least 20% or more of the Daily Value for a particular nutrient

(continued on next page)

High fiber	Contains 20% or more of the Daily Value for fiber (at least 5 g) per serving. If a food is not "low fat," it must declare the level of total fat per serving and refer to the nutrition panel when a fiber claim is made
Lean	Fewer than 10 g of fat, 4 g saturated fat, and 95 mg cholesterol per serving and per 100 g in meat, poultry, or seafood
Light	1. At least one third fewer calories per serving than a comparison food; or 2. Contains no more than half the fat per serving of a comparison food. If a food derives 50% or more of its calories from fat, the reduction must be at least 50% of the fat; or 3. Contains at least 50% less sodium per serving than a comparison food; or 4. Can refer to texture and/or color, if clearly explained; for example, "light brown sugar"
Low	"Little," "few," or "low source of" may be used in place of "low"
Low calorie	40 calories or fewer per serving
Low cholesterol	20 mg or fewer of cholesterol and 2 g or fewer of saturated fat per serving
Low fat	3 g or fewer per serving
Low saturated fat	1 g or less saturated fat per serving and 15% or less calories from fat
Low sodium	140 mg or fewer per serving
More	One serving contains at least 10% more of the Daily Value of a nutrient than the comparison food
Percent fat free	A claim made on a "low fat" or "fat free" product which accurately reflects the amount of fat present in 100 g of food; a food with 3 g of fat per 100 g would be "97% fat free"
Reduced	A nutritionally altered product which must contain 25% less of a nutrient or of calories than the regular or reference product
Salt or sodium free	Less than 0.5 g of sugars per serving
Sugar free	Less than 0.5 g of sugars per serving
Unsalted	Has no salt added during processing. To use this term, the product it resembles must normally be processed with salt and the label must note that the food is not a sodium-free food if it does not meet the requirements for "sodium free"
Very low sodium	Fewer than 35 mg or less sodium per serving

Although the claim descriptions listed above are helpful, it is important to keep in mind a few significant points. First of all, although "fat-free" and "sugar-free" tell the consumer that there is no fat or sugar in the food product, the food may still be considered "fat-free" if it contains 0.5 or fewer gm per serving. And, while a food may be considered "sugar-free," it may not be carbohydrate-free. The descriptor "healthy," though not included in this table, is a word commonly used on many products we see on our grocery shelves. This term means that the food may contain no more than 3 gm of fat, including 1 gm of saturated fat, and 60 mg of cholesterol per serving.

Flavorings also play an important role in the products we eat. Under the Code of Federal Regulations, the definition of "natural flavor" or "natural flavoring" is: "the essential oil, oleoresin, essence or extractive, protein hydrolysate, distillate; any product of roasting, heating, or enzymolysis, which contains the flavoring constituents derived from a spice, fruit or fruit juice, vegetable or vegetable juice, edible yeast, herb, bark, bud, root, leaf or similar plant material; [and] meat, seafood, poultry, eggs, dairy products, or fermentation products thereof, whose significant function in food is flavoring rather than nutritional." *Whew!* In contrast, "artificial flavor" is defined by the FDA as any substance that does not fit the definition of a "natural flavor." The term "artificial flavor" or "artificial flavoring" means "any substance [whose] function … is to impart flavor [and] is not derived from a spice, fruit or fruit juice, vegetable or vegetable juice, edible yeast, herb, bark, bud, root, leaf or similar plant material, meat, fish, poultry, eggs, dairy products, or fermentation products thereof."[105]

Diet redesign

It is true that it takes a little more thought and planning to design a healthy diet, but I can tell you firsthand what a difference it makes in the way you'll feel. I try to plan my weekly menu, including all my regular meals and snacks, in advance. It's always a good idea to spend some time drawing up a comprehensive list of what you'll need during the week so that when you get to the store you're not tempted to buy all sorts of things that you can do without. Shopping when you're hungry is never a good idea either, because it makes you vulnerable to impulse buying. I like to make the following day's lunch the previous night so I do not feel compelled to purchase unhealthy food on the run. Overall, the idea is to train ourselves to be more organized. That means planning ahead with regard to every stage of our dietary habits: making lists, buying items, preparing foods, eating meals, and freezing when and if necessary.

The healthy diet. What constitutes a healthy diet? A healthy diet is comprised of all the nutrients required to support our bodies in leading a healthy lifestyle. Healthy foods increase energy levels, improve the way the body functions, and enhance the strength of the immune system. When we eat healthfully, not only are we satisfying our requirements for essential nutrients and fiber, but we are in a firm position to be able to adapt to life's challenges. In essence, we just feel better all around.

New diet guidelines. In 2010, the *Dietary Guidelines for Americans* continues to reflect our ever-changing lifestyles and evolution.[106] Published jointly every five years since 1980 by the Department of Health and Human Services and the Department of Agriculture, these guidelines provide reliable, basic information about how good dietary habits can promote health and reduce risk for major chronic diseases. This research also forms the basis for all federal food and nutrition education programs. New guidelines emphasize the importance of dietary choices and physical activity for optimum health and focus on the need for weight control, a trend that has gained considerable momentum in the last decade.

Organizations such as the American Cancer Society and the American Heart Society have joined forces to study the dietary patterns of Americans. Their research has led them to propose that for the maintenance of overall health an adult diet should be rich in vegetables, fruits, and whole-grain products, and should include at least 20 to 30 gm of fiber.[107,108] According to the Dietary Reference Intakes published by the USDA, 45 to 65% of our calories should come from carbohydrates, 10 to 35% from protein, and 20 to 35% from fat.[109]

Nutritional overview

The nutrients that we derive from the food we eat can be broadly divided into two components: *macronutrients and micronutrients*. The first group, macronutrients, is comprised of carbohydrates, proteins, and fats. The second group of micronutrients consists of all the other nutrients we consume in smaller amounts, such as vitamins and minerals. Vitamins and minerals, though relatively small in quantity compared to the macronutrients we consume, are the critical catalysts that keep our body functioning smoothly by supporting the metabolism. The metabolism is made up of the total physical and chemical processes by which our material substance is produced, maintained, and destroyed, and by which energy is made available. In other words, we all have an intrinsic metabolic capacity to generate some of the nutrients we need, discard what we do not, and generate energy in the process.

For example, every time we exercise we have the ability to synthesize glucose from stored fat and carbohydrates to generate energy. These "stored" organic compounds are considered *non-essential* nutrients because we are able to manufacture them on our own to meet the body's requirements. However, there are also nutrients that we are either unable to synthesize in the body or unable to synthesize in acceptable amounts suitable for good health. These are called *essential nutrients*, meaning that we must consume them through our intake of foods to meet daily requirements. The six basic nutrients required for healthy bodies are: carbohydrates, proteins, fats, vitamins, minerals, and water.

The Recommended Dietary Allowance (RDA) system was developed during World War II by Lydia J. Roberts, Hazel K. Stiebeling, and Helen S. Mitchell, members of a committee established by the U.S. National Academy of Sciences in order to investigate issues of nutrition that might "affect national defense."[110] These devised standards were to be used for our armed forces and for civilians in the general population who required food relief. Roberts, Stiebeling, and Mitchell researched and compiled available current information and submitted their findings for review. Their final set of guidelines, called RDAs, or Recommended Dietary

Allowances, were accepted in 1941. These allowances were meant to provide superior nutrition for civilians and military personnel in order to ensure a "margin of safety" for basic nutritional requirements. Today the RDA system provides nutritional facts to help guide the general public and health professionals. Under this system, recommendations are utilized in the United States and Canada for the dietary composition of foods in schools, prisons, and hospitals, for industries developing new food products, and with regard to healthcare policy and public health matters. Today, guidelines for the Recommended Dietary Allowance have a more expanded role, as outlined in the Dietary Reference Intake system.[111] Currently, the Dietary Reference Intake is a composition of the following:

- **Estimated Average Requirements** (EAR). The EAR is the median intake value that is estimated to satisfy the requirement of 50% of the people in a particular age or gender group.
- **Recommended Dietary Allowances** (RDA). The daily dietary intake levels of a nutrient considered sufficient to meet the requirements of nearly all (97 to 98%) healthy individuals in each life-stage and gender group. According to the Food and Nutrition Board, "The RDA is intended for use primarily as a goal for the usual intake of individuals."
- **Adequate Intake** (AI). If there is not enough evidence to establish an EAR, then by definition, no RDA can be established. In this case there is inadequate scientific evidence to indicate requirements; therefore, observed levels of intake have to be greater than the estimated requirements. In these cases, AI is established instead of RDA. The AI represents the observed or calculated mean intake level in healthy people.
- **Tolerable Upper Intake Levels** (UL). This is the highest level of continued daily nutrient intake that is likely to pose no health risk in an age or gender group. UL, by definition, is considered a safe level of intake for a particular group.

Macronutrients

As we talked about earlier, macronutrients are nutrients that our body needs in significant amounts. Proteins, carbohydrates, and fats are the macronutrients we consume that provide the bulk of our energy, and are three of the six basic nutrients required by the body to stay healthy.

Proteins make up the antibodies of the immune system, the hormones of the endocrine system, the enzymes in the digestive system, and the blood-coagulating factors of the circulatory system. The name *protein* is derived from the Greek word *prota*, meaning "of primary importance." Proteins are composed of small units called amino acids, basic structural building blocks that are connected together by peptide bonding, the primary linkage for all protein structures.

Nearly all the enzymes in the body are proteins. Hemoglobin, for example, the oxygen-carrying component of our blood, is a protein. Proteins are important in maintaining the structure of the cells and in "cell signaling," the ability of cells to perceive and correctly respond to their microenvironment. When errors in cellular communication occur, they are responsible for diseases such as diabetes, autoimmune disease, and cancer. Twenty different amino acids are necessary for the body's continued health. Amino acids are classified into two groups: *essential amino acids* and *non-essential amino acids*. An essential amino acid is a necessary and indispensable amino acid that cannot be made by the body; therefore, it must be supplied through food. Some essential amino acids are isoleucine, leucine, lysine, methionine, phenylalanine, tryptophan, threonine, and valine. Histidine is an unusual amino acid because it is considered "semi-essential." This means that histidine starts out as essential when we are infants, but becomes non-essential when we reach several years of age, due to the fact that we begin to synthesize it on our own. Non-essential amino acids are made by the body from the essential amino acids, or during the normal breakdown of proteins. Some non-essential amino acids are arginine, alanine, asparagine, aspartic acid, cysteine, glutamic acid, glutamine, glycine, proline, serine, and tyrosine.

Meat, fish, eggs, and dairy products are very good sources of essential amino acids. Others can be found in whole grains, corn, and wheat. Lentils and legumes, nuts, soy milk, cheese, yogurt, peanut butter, poultry, beans, and tofu are rich sources of protein. It is recommended we ingest more than the average requirement of high-protein foods each day to provide enough foundation for the body to have the ability to repair tissues, facilitate muscle growth, and create blood cells and disease-fighting antibodies. Protein foods are also sources of vitamin B, iron, and zinc.

"Average" daily requirements for protein increase when other considerations arise, such as injury, pregnancy, breast-feeding, strenuous exercise, and/or bodybuilding activities. Unlike carbohydrates and fats, dietary proteins do not remain stored in the body. Whatever is left over is converted into either fat or carbohydrate, and then either utilized or stored in this new form.

The average requirement for dietary protein for an adult is calculated based on 0.8 gm of protein per kg of body weight, or .37 per lb of body weight. This amount should be the daily minimum. Therefore, a 165-lb (75 kg) man needs about 60 gm, equivalent to slightly over 2 oz of protein per day. A woman who weighs 130 lbs (59 kg) requires about

47 gm of protein daily. During pregnancy and during lactation (breast-feeding), these requirements increase, as do requirements for athletic individuals.

Carbohydrates. The best way to a healthy body is through a balanced approach. When it comes to diet, however, this does not mean we should consume equal amounts of fats, proteins, and carbohydrates. In fact, in a healthy diet the body needs slightly more carbohydrates than it does fats and protein. This is because carbohydrates are the body's most preferred source of energy. Carbohydrates ordinarily comprise about 60% of daily food intake and play a vital role in digestion and metabolism and in providing energy. Most carbohydrates are of plant origin, organic compounds made of hydrogen, oxygen, and carbon. Simple carbohydrates, or simple sugars, are composed of monosaccharide or disaccharide units. Common monosaccharides, carbohydrates composed of single-sugar units, include:

- *glucose*, the immediate source of energy in the body
- *galactose*, a milk sugar
- *fructose*, a sugar found in fruits and honey

Those carbohydrates composed of two sugars are specifically referred to as disaccharides, or double sugars. They contain two monosaccharides linked together and include:
- *sucrose*: common table sugar (glucose + fructose)
- *lactose*: major sugar in milk (glucose + galactose)
- *maltose*: product of starch digestion (glucose + glucose)

Both monosaccharides and disaccharides are considered simple carbohydrates—organic compounds made of one or two sugars. A simple sugar is just what the name implies: simple, such as the sugar in your sugar bowl. Candy, cake, syrups, and soda are examples of simple carbohydrates. Simple sugars are absorbed quickly, the way gum loses its sugary flavor when chewed or the way candy melts in your mouth. Complex carbohydrates, on the other hand, are made of three or more linked sugars. These carbohydrates take longer to digest and are usually packed with fiber, vitamins, and minerals. Examples of complex carbohydrates are vegetables, legumes, and fruits.

Complex carbohydrates, or *polysaccharides*, are composed of simple sugar units in long chains, called *polymers*. The polysaccharides of particular importance in the study of human nutrition are *starch, oligosaccharides, glycogen,* and *fiber*.

Starches. Starches are chains of glucose banded together and derived from plants. Starch represents the main type of digestible complex carbohydrate. In Canada, most of the United States, and Europe, our staple grain is wheat. Rice is the staple grain in Asia and corn is the most commonly consumed grain in most parts of South America and the southern United States. The U.S. is the largest producer of corn in the world. The second highest source of starch is the bean and pea family. Foods in this family contain about 40% starch by weight and contain substantial amounts of protein as well. Our third major source of starch is—you guessed it—tubers, or potatoes, yams, and cassavas.

Oligosaccharides. Oligosaccharides are carbohydrates found naturally in many plants in small amounts. They are made up of only a few simple sugars (generally three to 10) linked together. Plants with large quantities of oligosaccharides include chicory root, from which most commercial inulin is extracted, Jerusalem artichokes, onions, leeks, legumes, and asparagus. Oligosaccharides are typically low-glycemic-index carbs, which means they help maintain stable blood glucose levels when eaten as part of a meal.

Glycogen is a polysaccharide made up of glucose molecules used to store energy in the body. Glycogen is a highly branched structure that allows the bonds between glucose molecules to be quickly broken down by enzymes for immediate energy use. The primary storage sites for glycogen in the human body are the liver and the muscles.

Fiber. The recommended daily amount of fiber is 25 gm for women and 38 gm for men. Fiber-rich food allows us to stay feeling fuller longer; this helps us control our weight by lessening our urge to eat more often. Increasing our intake of complex carbohydrates and decreasing our cravings for refined foods creates a foundation for improved health in many ways.

Complex carbs like fruits and vegetables have a number of nutritional benefits other than weight control. They contain vitamins, minerals, phytochemicals (non-nutritive plant chemicals with protective or disease-preventive properties), and other nutrients that are rarely present in simple-sugar food items. Ninety percent of foods higher in complex carbohydrates are also lower in calories. Plus, it generally takes more time and energy to eat a 100-calorie peach than it does to consume 100 calories of soda! Calorie for calorie, complex carbohydrates are more nutritious and useful to the body.

The National Academy of Sciences Institute of Medicine Food and Nutrition Board has determined that the Dietary Reference Intake for carbohydrate consumption is 130 gm per day for both children and adults.[111] If you are considering losing weight through a "low carbohydrate diet," you may want to know that these diets are designed to restrict consumption of carbs to less than the percentage of daily caloric intake recommended. The increased consumption of protein and fat is encouraged to compensate for part of the calories that formerly were coming from carbohydrates.

Fats. Fats are a group of compounds that contain glycerol and fatty acids. In humans, *adipose*, or fatty tissue is the body's means of storing energy over extended periods of time. Fat has gotten a bad name over the past few years, and most of us suffer from the misguided impression that all fat is bad. Not so; fats are a necessary part of our diets because they supply the body with some beneficial essential fatty acids and help in the following ways:

- Fat is a source of energy. One gram of fat provides about nine calories.
- Fat aids the body in absorbing vitamins.
- Fats are an important source of calories and nutrients for infants and toddlers, forming the basic building blocks for cell membranes.
- Fat gives taste to foods and a feeling of fullness.
- Fat provides insulation and padding for our internal organs.
- Dietary fat plays a major role in the body's cholesterol levels.

Dietary fat is broken into these major categories: *saturated*, *trans fats*, *unsaturated* (*monounsaturated* and *polyunsaturated*), and *dietary cholesterol*. These categories can be further broken down into healthy fats and unhealthy fats.

Harmful fats. Saturated and trans fats (trans-fatty acids) are less healthy fats. They have been shown to increase the incidence to coronary heart disease, LDL ("bad" cholesterol), and cancer.

Saturated. Saturated fats are typically solid at room temperature. Saturated fats are derived mainly from animal sources, including meat and dairy products. Cottonseed and tropical oils, such as palm and coconut oil, also contain some saturated fats. Because saturated fats have no double bonds between the carbon atoms they are considered fully saturated. These fats may or may not contain cholesterol, which is only found in animal products.

Trans fats. Trans fats result from the hydrogenation of vegetable oil. Hydrogenation is the process of adding hydrogen to make the oil more saturated. When the oil is saturated it changes the configuration of the food, producing a straighter structure. Complete hydrogenation converts unsaturated fatty acids to saturated ones; as a result, the liquid vegetable oil becomes a solid fat like margarine. This process increases the shelf life and flavor stability of foods. Trans fats can be found in vegetable shortenings, crackers, cookies, snack foods, and other foods made with hydrogenated oils. They can also be heated and reheated without degradation, which is why they have become a mainstay for fast food frying. As of January 2006, the amount of trans fats in food products must be listed on all food labels.

Other fats are listed below:

Cholesterol. Cholesterol is the principal *sterol*, any of a group of solid, mostly unsaturated, polycyclic alcohols found in humans, and is an essential component of cell membranes. Cholesterol has been identified in cell signaling and is an important precursor molecule for the synthesis of Vitamin D, sex hormones, and steroid hormones. Cholesterol can be synthesized by the body as well as consumed through the diet. Major dietary sources of cholesterol include egg yolks, beef, cheese, pork, poultry, and shrimp. Typically, the body makes all the cholesterol it needs, so increasing its consumption is not necessary. Saturated fatty acids are the main culprits in raising blood cholesterol, and increased blood cholesterol increases the risk of various diseases.

Healthy fats. Healthy fats raise your HDL ("good" cholesterol), reduce inflammation, improve circulation, and play a number of other beneficial roles. Unsaturated fats are considered the "healthy fats." They are predominantly found in foods from plants, such as vegetable oils, nuts, and seeds, and are liquid at room temperature.

There are two types of unsaturated fats:

Monounsaturated. Monounsaturated fats are typically liquid at room temperature, but change to solid when cold. Structurally they have a single double bond in the fatty-acid chain, while the remainder of the carbon atoms in the chain are single-bonded. Monounsaturated fats are found in high concentrations in olive oil, nuts, avocados, and sesame seeds.

Polyunsaturated. Polyunsaturated fats are typically liquid at room temperature and when chilled. Structurally these fats have more than one double bond in the fatty-acid chain. Having more than one double bond contributes to the fat's fluidity at both room and chilled temperatures. The two main types of polyunsaturated fats are omega-6 fatty acids and omega-3 fatty acids, neither of which can be produced by the body. Foods high in polyunsaturated fats are grain products, fish (such as salmon, herring, mackerel, and halibut), fish oil, and shellfish. Two polyunsaturated fatty acids that cannot be made in the body are linoleic acid (an omega-6 fatty-acid) and alpha-linolenic acid (an omega-3 fatty-acid). These must be provided by diet and are therefore known as essential fatty acids. Within the body both can be converted to other polyunsaturated fatty acids, such as arachidonic acid, eicosapentaenoic acid (EPA), and docosahexaenoic acid (DHA). Good sources of omega-6 fatty acids include grains, seeds, nuts, safflower oil, sunflower oil, corn, and soybean oil. Good sources of omega-3 fatty acids include flaxseeds, hemp seeds, mustard seeds, walnuts, linseed oil, and canola oil.

Consuming *both* omega-6 and omega-3 fatty acids is important for continued good health, but we also need to consume them in the right amounts. A healthy diet should consist of a 1:1 ratio of omega-6 fatty acids to omega-3 fatty acids. It has been estimated that the present Western diet is noticeably "deficient" in omega-3 fatty acids, with a ratio of omega-6 to omega-3 of 15–20:1.[112] Why? Because many diets now include large quantities of oils used for cooking and in prepared foods, and these are the oils (such as corn oil, safflower oil, cottonseed oil, peanut oil, and soybean oil) that primarily contain omega-6s. In addition, while our omega-6 intake has been increasing, our intake of omega-3 foods has been steadily on the decline.

Consuming too much omega-6 and too little omega-3 is known to cause blood clots, constrict arteries (leading to increased risk of heart attack), and increase inflammation and the symptoms of arthritis. This imbalance may block an individual's ability to respond to insulin, and thus contribute to high blood-sugar levels, and the potential for obesity as well. Increased hormonal levels may also occur on this type of diet, again leading to the onset of certain types of cancers.

Cod liver oil is a good example of one of the most effectual sources of omega-3 fatty acids, as well as vitamins A and D. Children were once given cod liver oil to build strong bones and prevent colds; now adults are advised to take cod liver oil to promote better cognitive function and a healthy heart. Cod liver oil is derived from cod livers, and can be purchased as a ready-prepared nutritional supplement. Cod livers are steamed and pressed to extract the oil, resulting in a pale yellow liquid that is thin and oily with a mild to very strong odor. Cod liver oil has been shown to help prevent heart disease, cancer, and arthritis; to improve memory and brain function; to reduce inflammation; and to be a complementary measure for the treatment of multiple sclerosis.

The Mediterranean diet. The Mediterranean diet is inspired by cultural dietary choices followed by some of the countries where olive trees grow—in the Mediterranean basin. A Mediterranean meal plan incorporates the traditionally healthy living habits of people from this region and includes an abundance of vegetables, legumes, beans, whole grains, fruits, nuts, seeds, and olive oil, as well as the moderate consumption of fish, occasional poultry, and minimal amounts of red meat and sweets (see Table 4-4). The food of this diet is fresh, unprocessed, and unrefined; it is also low in saturated and trans fats. If you feel so inclined, including a glass of wine with your dinner is considered a healthy part of this type of diet. People following a Mediterranean-style diet show a reduced risk of cardiovascular and cancer mortality as well as a reduced risk of diabetes and obesity. The focus of the Mediterranean diet is not necessarily to limit total fat consumption, but to make better choices in the fats you eat.

TABLE 4-4. The healthy Mediterranean diet.

Eating a Mediterranean diet
Include a high consumption of fruits, vegetables, breads, cereals, potatoes, beans, nuts, and seeds
Consume olive oil, an important source of monounsaturated fat
Consume dairy products, fish, and poultry in low to moderate amounts and little red meat
Consume no more than 4 eggs per week
Consume wine in low to moderate amounts
Consume sweets sparingly, if at all

Benefits of healthy fats

High blood pressure. As the heart pumps out blood it pushes against the walls of the arteries. This force is called *blood pressure*. If maintained at acceptable levels, this pressure poses no health risk; however, if this pressure rises and stays high over time, serious health consequences may be experienced. Clinical studies suggest that diets or supplements rich in omega-3 fatty acids lower blood pressure significantly in individuals whose pressure is elevated and that supplementing one's diet with oils, fish, seeds, and nuts can assist in keeping blood pressure at safe, acceptable levels.

Heart disease. The heart is the driving force of the cardiovascular system. Through the body's blood vessels, the heart pumps blood and nutrients to every cell of the body. If the pumping action of the heart becomes insufficient, the brain and vital organs can suffer. Some associated consequences of heart disease are arteriosclerosis, atherosclerosis, angina, heart attack, and stroke. Clinical evidence suggests that the EPA and DHA found in fish oil help reduce risk factors for heart disease, including high cholesterol and high blood pressure. There is also strong evidence that these substances can help prevent and treat atherosclerosis by inhibiting the development of plaque and blood clots, which tend to clog arteries. One of the best ways to help prevent and treat heart disease is to eat a low-fat diet consisting of monounsaturated and polyunsaturated fats (including omega-3 fatty acids) and to replace foods rich in saturated and trans-fat.

Diabetes. Diabetes is a disease caused when the body does not produce or properly use insulin. There are four different types of diabetes. Type 1 results from the body's inability to produce insulin; type 2 results when the body becomes insulin-resistant or fails to use the insulin properly; gestational diabetes occurs in women who are pregnant; and pre-diabetes is a state which occurs when a individual's blood glucose levels are higher than normal, but not high enough for a diagnosis of type 2 diabetes. Individuals with diabetes have been shown to have high triglyceride and low HDL levels. Omega-3 fatty acids from fish oil can help lower triglycerides and raise HDL levels.

Weight loss. Those of us who struggle with weight often find ourselves embroiled in other health-related issues as well: poor blood-sugar control, for example, and/or diabetes and high cholesterol. Weight-loss programs that include exercise and diets rich in foods with high omega-3 fatty-acid content (such as salmon, mackerel, and herring) help control blood sugar and cholesterol levels.

Arthritis. Arthritis is a joint disorder featuring chronic inflammation of the joints. Joints are the points where two different bones come together and function to move the body parts connected by the bones. Arthritis literally means "inflammation of one or more joints." The use of omega-3 fatty acid supplements has been shown to decrease morning stiffness and joint tenderness and to reduce drug usage.

Osteoporosis. Osteoporosis is a disease that causes bones to become thin and weak and thus break easily. Throughout our growing years and into adult years, the body utilizes the mineral calcium to ensure normal bone production and formation. If calcium intake is not sufficient, or if the body does not absorb enough calcium from the diet, bone production and bone tissues may suffer, potentially contributing to the development of osteoporosis. Omega-3 essential fatty acids have been shown to increase calcium levels, deposit calcium in the bones, and improve bone strength. In addition, studies suggest that people who are deficient in certain essential fatty acids (particularly EPA, the omega-3 fatty acid found in fish) are more likely to suffer from bone loss than those with normal levels of these fatty acids.

Depression. Depression is comprised of a group of symptoms that reflect a sad and/or irritable mood and exceed normal situational feelings of sadness or grief. In the case of depression, this sadness is characterized by a greater intensity and duration and by more severe symptoms and functional disabilities than might normally be experienced. It has been found that low levels of omega-3 fatty acids (or an unhealthy balance of omega-3 to omega-6 fatty acids) can increase the risk for depression. Since omega-3 fatty acids are important components of nerve cell membranes, helping nerve cells communicate with each other is an essential step in maintaining good mental health.

Bipolar disorder. When electrical and chemical elements in the brain fail to function properly, one of the results is bipolar disorder, an illness that affects thoughts, feelings, perceptions, and behavior. In one four-month, double-blind, placebo-controlled study of 30 patients undergoing usual treatment for bipolar disorder, omega-3 fatty acids were added to some of the participants' diets, while placebos containing olive oil were added to others'. Significantly, researchers found that the patient group receiving omega-3 fatty acids had a considerably longer period of remission than the group receiving the olive oil placebo.[113]

Skin disorders. The skin is one of the most vulnerable organs of the body. There are many disorders of the skin which, if left untreated, require clinical care by a physician or other healthcare professional. Along with clinical care, studies have shown that omega-3 fatty acids protect against photocarcinogens (substances which generate free radicals) in animals and show promise as photoprotective agents.[114,115]

Asthma. Asthma is a chronic disease that inflames and narrows the *airways*, tubes that carry air in and out of the lungs. When reactive airways narrow, the flow of air is reduced. If this reaction response continues, swelling and inflammation will occur; this narrows air passages even further and reduces air flow even more. Asthma is associated with the body's production of pro-inflammatory fatty compounds called leukotrienes, secreted by the immune system's white blood cells (leukocytes) as a reaction to common environmental allergens and pollutants. One way to counter the body's excess production of leukotrienes is to enhance intake of omega-3 fatty acids. In one clinical research study, for example, when 14 subjects with bronchial asthma were given supplements of perilla seed oil (omega-3 fatty acids) and corn oil (omega-6 fatty acids), a significant improvement in pulmonary function and the generation of leukotrienes in the omega-3 group as compared to the omega-6 group was observed.[116]

The following general dietary recommendations are for daily dietary fat from the USDA and the USHSS Dietary Guidelines for Americans 2010.[117]

- Consume fewer than 7% of calories from saturated fatty acids
- Limit dietary cholesterol to less than 300 mg per day
- Avoid trans fatty acids from commercial sources, while consuming small amounts of trans fatty acids from natural sources
- Redefine cholesterol-raising fats as saturated fats and trans fatty acids, to make up less than 5% of caloric intake.
- Consume two servings of seafood per week to provide an average of 250 mg per day of n-3 fatty acids.

In addition, specific recommendations were made to reduce the intake of foods high in solid fat (fats that are solid at room temperature) and added sugars, suggesting that most Americans consume no more than 5 to 15% of their total calories from these sources.

Vitamins

Vitamins, organic substances found in plants and animals, are essential for the proper growth and functioning of the body. Vitamins have diverse functions, such as behaving as hormones and antioxidants, regulating cell growth and differentiation, and acting as metabolic catalysts for many biological processes. In 1912, Polish biochemist Kazmierz Funk (1884–1967) of the Lister Institute in London coined the term *vitamine*. The word originates from the contraction of two words: "vital" and "amine," from "vita," meaning life, and "amine," from compounds found in the thiamine Funk isolated from rice husks. "Vitamine" was later shortened to "vitamin," since it was discovered that not all vitamins have a nitrogen-containing "amine" group.

Not all vitamins are derived from the diet. For example, vitamin D is produced by the skin and only by exposure to the sun. History traces knowledge of the effects of vitamins back almost 3,500 years, when the ancient Egyptians discovered that night blindness, which we now know is caused by a vitamin A deficiency, could be treated with the ingestion of liver.

In 1747, a Scottish surgeon named James Lind discovered that scurvy, a disease common among sailors whose vessels stored no fresh produce and marked by swollen and bleeding gums, bruising, and joint pain, could be prevented by eating citrus fruits. Today we know that scurvy is a disease caused by vitamin C deficiency, and that vitamin C is found in large amounts in citrus fruits. It was Hungarian researcher Dr. Albert Szent-Gyorgyi who earned the Nobel Prize in Medicine in 1937 for the definitive discovery of vitamin C. From the early 1900s, when vitamins were initially "discovered," all the way through the 1950s, most physicians worldwide have based their studies and diagnoses on vitamin deficiencies, laying the foundation for a new era in vitamin research.

Measuring vitamin intake

The International System of Units, or the metric system, provides a decimalized universal system of measurement. The basic elements of this system are as follows: *meter* is the standard unit for length, *liter* for volume, *gram* for weight, and *Celsius* for temperature. Metric units are used around the world for personal, scientific, and commercial purposes. When it comes to vitamins, abbreviations for units of weight are a common sight on food and supplementation labels. For example, you might see a product that has 250 mg of vitamin C, 6 mg of B12, and so on. The abbreviations mcg, mg and gm stand for metric measurements of weight. The mcg, or microgram, is the smallest unit of weight. A milligram, or mg, is the middle measurement, and the gm, or gram, is the largest of these measurements. There are 1,000 micrograms to each milligram, and 1,000 milligrams to each gram. Gram units are the most widely used and recognized measurements in vitamin labeling, food preparation, and shopping around the world.

To provide some scale relative to how much a gram weighs, let's look at some examples of products we see in our daily lives. A paper clip or a U.S. bank note (irrespective of denomination) weighs approximately 1 gm. A U.S. penny weighs about 2.5 gm, and a packet of sugar at the local diner about 4 gm. One can of Coca Cola contains approximately 39 gm of sugar, roughly equivalent to almost 10 packets of sugar! On a much smaller scale, the weight of a single grain of sand is 1 mg, or 1/1,000th of a gram. Even smaller is a microgram (mcg, or *ug*), equivalent to 1/1,000,000th, or 1 millionth, of a gram.

Besides the gram unit on a label, it is also quite common to see the abbreviation *IU*, which stands for International Units, and is a measurement of the potency of the vitamin. IU applies to fat-soluble vitamins, such as A, D, and E. There is no fixed definition for IU, as there is for grams, milligrams, or micrograms. This is because the IU measurement is based on the potency of the nutrient, so the actual IU value will depend upon the specific substance being measured. Despite this difference, it is possible to determine the relationship of weight to International Units, as illustrated below:*

Vitamin E

> 1 IU = 0.735 mg d-alpha tocopheryl acetate
>
> 1 IU = 0.671 mg d-alpha tocopherol
>
> 1 IU = 0.861 mg d-alpha tocopheryl succinate

Vitamin A (acetate)

> 1 IU = 0.344 mcg (or µg)

Vitamin D

> 1 IU = 0.025 mcg
>
> 40 IU = 1 mcg (or µg)

Vitamin content conversion. Vitamin content in food can also be measured in International Units. International Units can be defined as units of measurement that evaluate the potency of a substance. Because International Units measure potency instead of quantity, there is a different international unit-to-milligram conversion ratio for each particular substance. (Source: http://www. apinchofhealth.com/forum/vbb/ showthread.php?t=2326.)

Again, vitamins are substances that are essential for normal cell function, growth, and development. There are 13 "essential" vitamins, which are required for the body to function. They are: vitamins A, C, D, E, K, B1 (thiamine), B2 (riboflavin), B3 (niacin), B5 (pantothenic acid), B6, B12, biotin, and folate (folic acid).

Vitamins are grouped into two categories: *fat-soluble* and *water-soluble*. Fat-soluble vitamins are stored in the body's fatty tissue for use at a later time. Water-soluble vitamins must be used by the body right away; any that are not used immediately are excreted through the urine. Vitamin B12 is the only water-soluble vitamin that can be stored in the liver for many years.

The Dietary Reference Intakes for vitamins are listed in Table 4-5.

TABLE 4-5. Dietary Reference Intakes (DRIs): Recommended vitamin intakes for males and females, ages 19 to 70. (Source: Food and Nutrition Board, Institute of Medicine, National Academies, 2009)

Males	Age 19–30	Age 31–50	Age 51–70	Females	Age 19–30	Age 31–50	Age 51–70
Vitamin A	900 µg	900 µg	900 µg	Vitamin A	700 µg	700 µg	700 µg
Vitamin C	90 mg	90 mg	90 mg	Vitamin C	75 mg	75 mg	75 mg

(continued on next page)

Vitamin D	5 µg	5 µg	10 µg
Vitamin E	15 mg	15 mg	15 mg
Vitamin K	120 µg	120 µg	120 µg
Thiamin	1.2 mg	1.2 mg	1.2 mg
Riboflavin	1.3 mg	1.3 mg	1.3 mg
Niacin	16 mg	16 mg	16 mg
Vitamin B6	1.3 mg	1.3 mg	1.7 mg
Vitamin B12	2.4 µg	2.4 µg	2.4 µg
Folate	400 µg	400 µg	400 µg
Pantothenic acid	5 mg	5 mg	5 mg
Biotin	30 µg	30 µg	30 µg
Choline	550 mg	550 mg	550 mg

Vitamin D	5 µg	5 µg	10 µg
Vitamin E	15 mg	15 mg	15 mg
Vitamin K	90 µg	90 µg	90 µg
Thiamin	1.1 mg	1.1 mg	1.1 mg
Riboflavin	1.1 mg	1.1 mg	1.1 mg
Niacin	14 mg	14 mg	14 mg
Vitamin B6	1.3 mg	1.3 mg	1.5 mg
Vitamin B12	2.4 µg	2.4 µg	2.4 µg
Folate	400 µg	400 µg	400 µg
Pantothenic acid	5 mg	5 mg	5 mg
Biotin	30 µg	30 µg	30 µg
Choline	425 mg	425 mg	425 mg

Vitamin function

Vitamins perform specific functions. That means that our bodies need to receive enough of all the vitamins to avoid deficiencies and potential health problems down the road.

- Vitamin A helps form and maintain healthy teeth, bones, soft tissue, mucous membranes, and skin.
- All the B vitamins are important for the function of the metabolism. Vitamin B6, also known as pyridoxine, helps the body use the protein we consume, helps form red blood cells, and helps maintain brain function, among other attributes.
- Vitamin B12 specifically helps form red blood cells and maintain the central nervous system.
- Vitamin C, or ascorbic acid, is an antioxidant. Vitamin C promotes healthy teeth and gums, helps the body absorb iron and maintain healthy tissue, and promotes wound healing.
- Vitamin D, known as the "sunshine vitamin," is produced by the body in response to being in the sun. Ten to 15 minutes of sunshine three times per week is enough to produce the body's requirement of vitamin D, which promotes absorption of calcium, essential for the normal development and maintenance of healthy teeth and bones. Vitamin D also helps maintain proper blood levels of calcium and phosphorus.
- Vitamin E, an antioxidant known as tocopherol, plays a role in the formation of red blood cells and helps the body utilize vitamin K.

- Vitamin K is not considered an "essential" vitamin as such, but without it our blood would not coagulate. Some studies suggest vitamin K promotes strong bones in the elderly.
- Biotin metabolizes proteins and carbohydrates and is essential in the production of hormones and cholesterol.
- Niacin is another B vitamin. It helps to maintain healthy skin and nerves and to lower cholesterol.
- Folate works with vitamin B12 to help form red blood cells. Folate contributes to the production of DNA, which controls tissue growth and cell function. Low levels of folate are linked to birth defects, such as spina bifida. Many foods are now fortified with folic acid.
- Pantothenic acid is necessary for metabolizing the food we eat. It also plays a role in the production of hormones and cholesterol.
- Riboflavin (B2) works with the other B vitamins to ensure the body's growth and red blood cell production.
- Thiamine (B1) helps the body change carbohydrates into energy, ensures heart functioning, and contributes to nerve cell health.

Vitamins are widely available from the natural foods we eat, so before you reach for a vitamin supplement, try getting your vitamins from natural food sources. Here are some of the best sources for each:

Fat-soluble vitamins

- *Vitamin A:* eggs, meat, milk, cheese, sweet potatoes, carrots, liver, kidney, and cod
- *Vitamin D:* cheese, butter, margarine, cream, fortified milk, fish, oysters, and cereals
- *Vitamin E:* wheat germ, corn, nuts, seeds, olives, spinach and other green, leafy vegetables, asparagus, and vegetable oils
- *Vitamin K:* cabbage, cauliflower, spinach, soybeans, and cereals

Water-soluble vitamins

- *Folate:* green, leafy vegetables and fortified foods
- *Niacin (B3):* dairy products, poultry, fish, lean meats, nuts, eggs, legumes, and enriched breads and cereals

- *Pantothenic acid (B5) and biotin:* eggs, fish, dairy products, whole-grain cereals, legumes, yeast, broccoli and other vegetables in the cabbage family, white and sweet potatoes, and lean beef
- *Thiamine (B1):* fortified breads, cereals, and pasta, whole grains, lean meats, fish, dried beans, peas, soybeans, dairy products, and fruits and vegetables
- *Vitamin B2 (riboflavin):* spinach, broccoli, mushrooms, eggs, milk, liver, oysters, and clams
- *Vitamin B6 (pyridoxine):* bananas, watermelon, tomato juice, broccoli, spinach, acorn squash, potatoes, white rice, and chicken breast
- *Vitamin B12:* meat, eggs, poultry, shellfish, and milk and milk products
- *Vitamin C (ascorbic acid):* citrus fruits and juices, strawberries, tomatoes, broccoli, turnip and other greens, sweet and white potatoes, and cantaloupe; most other fruits and vegetables contain vitamin C as well

If vitamins are "good," are more vitamins "better"?

The question of vitamin supplementation is not a simple one to answer. If we all realize that a diet rich in appropriate vitamins and minerals keeps us strong, energetic, and healthy, it might be natural to think that supplementing our diet would continue to allow us to feel this way. In fact, there are several reasons why people make the decision to supplement. For anyone who has recovered from cancer, for example, supplementation becomes an insurance policy, a first line of defense to make sure that our body gets what it needs. Many of us in this situation may feel that one of the reasons we got sick in the first place was because we were lacking "something," and the lack of vitamin intake is generally the first thing that comes to mind—especially with all the reports about the multiple benefits of ingesting adequate amounts.

The first question is whether current RDA requirements for vitamins and minerals are sufficient. With that said, many of us are learning that heavily processed foods, such as those that come in cans, plastic wrappers, boxes, and bags, on store shelves and in freezer sections, offer unquestionably insufficient essential vitamins. Some of us have trouble taking in adequate amounts of vitamins due to allergies to certain vitamin-rich foods or have taste preferences that reduce overall vitamin intake. Still others may require medications that cause an unavoidable loss of essential nutrients.

In essence, there is a myriad of reasons why we might choose to supplement our diets. The important thing to recognize, however, is that more does not necessarily mean better. In the case of vitamins, for example, taking too much of a good thing can have a detrimental effect in the form of toxicity or overdose symptoms.

In terms of vitamin supplementation, there are a few factors that warrant mentioning. The first is that there are two types of supplements: synthetic vitamin supplements and natural vitamin supplements. A synthetic vitamin is a laboratory simulation of its real counterpart substance found in nature that is made to mimic the way natural vitamins function in the body. These synthetic, or "isolated," nutrients do not exist on their own in a natural form. They lack the enzymes, coenzymes, trace elements, activators, and many other still unknown factors that work together to do what nature naturally does in the body. Generally speaking, synthetic vitamins cannot be used or recognized by the body in the same way as their natural versions because they have been highly processed and contain artificial ingredients, dyes, preservatives, sugars, starch, and other additives. Natural vitamin supplements, on the other hand, contain a complex array of enzymes, coenzymes, minerals, and nutrients—the precise "cofactors" the body needs to absorb and utilize. If you do choose to complement your body's intake with vitamin supplementation, taking whole food supplements is the best choice to ensure your body gets what it requires.

Research supports the fact that those who have had cancer are increasingly motivated to supplementation. For example, when researchers led by Cornelia Ulrich at the Fred Hutchinson Cancer Research Center in Seattle reviewed 32 studies conducted between 1999 and 2006, they found that 64 to 81% of cancer survivors reported taking extra vitamins or minerals (excluding multivitamins) compared to the general adult American population, of which only 50% reported taking supplements.[118] It is good to know that cancer survivors are taking a more active approach and including complementary options for their health; however, those who are still undergoing treatment need to be cautious. In fact, the American Cancer Society indicates that the use of vitamins and supplements during cancer treatment should be avoided. For instance, it has been shown that the taking of antioxidant supplements during treatment may interfere with the outcome of chemotherapy and radiation. Oncologists have suggested that this may be because treatment is more effective when the body is temporarily kept in a state of cellular vulnerability rather than a state of high defensive alert. This is one reason why it is always advisable to confer with a physician prior to beginning any supplementation program.

It is also important to understand that the best way to ensure our bodies receive their daily requirement of essential vitamins is for us to have balanced diets, and that balanced diets are those that contain a variety of foods from the food pyramid guide (see page 188). Because there is so much research showing that consuming higher amounts of fresh fruits and vegetables can be linked to a reduced risk for most types of cancer,[119] results from the research have become the basis for dietary guidelines endorsed by the U.S. Department of Agriculture and the National Cancer Institute. Currently, these organizations both recommend at least five servings of fruits and vegetables per day.

Vitamins and cancer

Ongoing research in the field of vitamins and their effects on cancer suggests a strong correlation between dietary intake and the reduction of various types of cancer. Below are some of the direct links that have been made between vitamins and a decreased risk for cancer.

Vitamin A and beta-carotene. Beta-carotene, and vitamin A in particular, has been linked to a lower risk of many types of cancer.[120] A higher intake of fresh fruits and vegetables, or other food sources of these vitamins, has been shown to reduce the risk of most types of cancers.[121-123]

Vitamin D. A wealth of research (laboratory, animal, and epidemiologic) suggests that vitamin D may be protective against some cancers, including epidemiologic studies suggesting that a higher dietary intake of calcium and vitamin D specifically correlates with a lower incidence of cancer in general.[124-30] For over 50 years researchers have observed an inverse association between sun exposure and cancer mortality[131] and between lower levels of vitamin D in the blood and increased colon and colorectal cancer risk.[132-140]

Vitamin E. Antioxidants have the ability to help protect cell membranes against the damaging effects of free radicals (which may contribute to the development of chronic diseases such as cancer),[141] and include vitamin E. Studies reveal that vitamin E has potent anti-tumor properties,[142] and that one specific form of vitamin E possesses unique biological properties which prevent and combat cancer by inducing programmed cell death (*apoptosis*) of human prostate, breast, leukemia, gastric, and other human cancer cells.[143]

Vitamin C. Many studies investigating the role of vitamin C in cancer prevention have shown that higher intakes of vitamin C are associated with the decreased incidence of cancers of the mouth, throat and vocal chords, esophagus, stomach, colon-rectum, and lungs. Researchers from the Linus Pauling Institute have studied biochemical, clinical, and epidemiologic evidence of vitamin C in chronic disease prevention, for example, and it was found that consuming no more than 86 mg of vitamin C daily showed no difference in cancer risk, while consuming at least 90 to 110 mg of vitamin C daily showed significant cancer risk reduction.[144]

Vitamin C amounts have also been shown to have an effect on lung cancer prevention. In one study involving 870 men over a period of 25 years, the men who consumed less than 60 mg of vitamin C daily showed a significant 2.8-fold increase of lung cancer incidence as compared to men who consumed more than 100 mg per day.[145]

In another research study, called the Nurses' Health Study, 82,324 women between the ages of 33 and 60 were studied to evaluate vitamin C in relation to breast cancer risk. Findings in this study showed that premenopausal women with a family history of breast cancer who consumed an average of 205 mg per day of vitamin C from foods had a 63% lower risk of breast cancer than those who consumed an average of 70 mg per day.[146] The Swedish Mammography Cohort Study in 2001 also revealed that a high intake of vitamin C was inversely related to breast cancer incidence among overweight women.[147]

A number of observational studies have further found dietary vitamin C intake to be associated with a decreased risk of stomach cancer,[148] that vitamin C inhibits the formation of carcinogenic compounds, specifically nitrosamines in the stomach, and that vitamin C supplementation may be useful in reducing the risk of developing gastric cancer.[149]

Vitamin B. B vitamin deficiency has been shown to increase cancer risk. According to a study led by Dr. Zhenhua Liu in 2007, for example, "population-based studies reported that 18 to 25% of adults have low vitamin B-6 status and 10 to 20% of healthy elders are thought to have marginal vitamin B-12 status." The author goes on to state that depletion of B vitamins has a substantial impact on gene expression and, as a result, "is of considerable potential importance in defining the dietary risk factors for colorectal cancer."[150]

It has also been found that a diet rich in B vitamins may decrease the risk of pancreatic cancer. A 2007 study by Dr. Eva Schernhammer, et al., for example, concluded that "among participants who achieve their intake of these factors exclusively through dietary sources, there may be an inverse relation between circulating folate, B6, and B12 and risk, particularly among subjects who maintained a normal BMI [Body Mass Index]."[151]

"A person who has reason to be concerned about their risk of developing this cancer, which is relatively rare but quite deadly, should maintain a normal weight and eat their fruit and vegetables," advises Dr. Schernhammer, the study's lead investigator and assistant professor at Harvard Medical School. In this study, however, nutrients from dietary supplements were found *not* to reduce the risk for contracting cancer. Dr. Schernhammer states, therefore, that although this study, along with a previous study in Finland and two other large American studies, had similar findings, it is still uncertain why the ingredients of the vitamin pills act differently from vitamins obtained directly from food. Once again, since food is our best source for dietary needs, whole-grain cereals and green vegetables, all good sources of vitamin B, are important to include in any regular dietary regime.

Folic acid. Folic acid, or folate, is a type of B vitamin that plays an important role in the production and maintenance of new cells and tissues. Since folate is involved in the synthesis, repair, and function of DNA, a deficiency of folate may allow for abnormal DNA replication and, as a result, provide an opening for the progression to cancer.

Some evidence associates low blood levels of folate with a greater risk of breast, pancreatic, and colon cancer. Researchers in the Nurses' Health Study, for example, who followed 88,756 women for 14 years who were free of cancer, found that the women who had been taking multivitamins containing folic acid for more than 15 years had a markedly lower risk of developing colon cancer.[152] Other evidence has revealed that alcohol consumption has an antagonist effect on folate, a result which increases the potential risk for colon cancer.[153]

Folic acid and methotrexate. *Methotrexate* is a drug that has been found to inhibit the action of folic acid.[154,155] In doing so, methotrexate can have a toxic effect on the rapidly dividing cells of bone marrow and gastric mucosa, while primarily working to inhibit cancer growth. *Leucovorin*, or *folinic acid*, is a folic acid-based drug used in conjunction with this type of chemotherapy to protect the bone marrow and mucosa from the effects of methotrexate. Research continues to determine the ways in which folinic acid can be used in cancer treatment regimens.[156]

Minerals

Minerals, like vitamins, are also natural substances, and comprise the group of inorganic elements essential for normal body function in human and animal life. Minerals can be found in water as well as in foods. Minerals are derived from plants that extract the elements from the earth's soil. Humans and animals then consume the plant matter, fulfilling their need for the nutrients. Minerals serve to aid in a variety of biological processes, such as building skeletal and soft tissue, regulating blood pressure, clotting blood, balancing fluid levels, and activating enzymes, cell membranes, and oxygen transport. Several minerals, in diverse combinations, are constantly required to support our metabolism. Minerals required for our physiological functions can be classified into two groups: *macrominerals* and *microminerals*. Macrominerals are those minerals we need in amounts of milligrams; microminerals, or *trace elements*, are the minerals we need in amounts of micrograms.

Macrominerals required for the human body's proper functioning are calcium, chloride, magnesium, phosphorus, potassium, and sodium. Required, but in smaller amounts, are the microminerals boron, chromium, cobalt, copper, iodine, iron, manganese, molybdenum, nickel, selenium, sulfur, and zinc.

The Dietary Reference Intakes for minerals are listed in Table 4-6.

TABLE 4-6. Dietary Reference Intakes (DRIs): Recommended mineral intakes for males and females, age 19 through 70. (Source: Food and Nutrition Board, Institute of Medicine, National Academies, 2009)

Males	Age 19–30	Age 31–50	Age 51–70	Females	Age 19–30	Age 31–50	Age 51–70
Boron	not determinable	not determinable	not determinable	Boron	not determinable	not determinable	not determinable
Calcium	1,000 mg	1,000 mg	1,200 mg	Calcium	1,000 mg	1,000 mg	1,200 mg
Chromium	35 µg	35 µg	30 µg	Chromium	25 µg	25 µg	20 µg
Copper	900 µg	900 µg	900 µg	Copper	900 µg	900 µg	900 µg
Fluoride	4 mg	4 mg	4 mg	Fluoride	3 mg	3 mg	3 mg
Iodine	150 µg	150 µg	150 µg	Iodine	150 µg	150 µg	150 µg
Iron	8 mg	8 mg	8 mg	Iron	18 mg	18 mg	8 mg
Magnesium	400 mg	420 mg	420 mg	Magnesium	310 mg	320 mg	320 mg
Manganese	2.3 mg	2.3 mg	2.3 mg	Manganese	1.8 mg	1.8 mg	1.8 mg
Molybdenum	45 µg	45 µg	45 µg	Molybdenum	45 µg	45 µg	45 µg
Phosphorus	700 mg	700 mg	700 mg	Phosphorus	700 mg	700 mg	700 mg
Selenium	55 µg	55 µg	55 µg	Selenium	55 µg	55 µg	55 µg
Zinc	11 mg	11 mg	11 mg	Zinc	8 mg	8 mg	8 mg

Specific macrominerals and microminerals aid the body's functioning in the following ways:

- *boron:* metabolizes calcium
- *calcium:* forms bone and teeth, clots blood, aids in normal muscle function, releases enzymes, contributes to normal heart rhythm
- *chloride:* balances electrolytes
- *chromium:* contributes to insulin action, metabolic processing, and storage of carbohydrates, protein, and fat
- *cobalt:* forms B12
- *copper:* contributes to the enzymes necessary for energy production and antioxidant action; forms the hormone epinephrine, red blood cells, bone, and connective tissue
- *fluoride:* forms bone and teeth
- *iodine:* forms thyroid hormones
- *iron:* forms many enzymes and is an important component of muscle cells, hemoglobin, and cytochrome pigment

- *manganese:* contributes to bone formation and the formation and activation of certain enzymes
- *magnesium:* forms bone and teeth; contributes to normal nerve and muscle function, and activates enzymes
- *molybdenum:* metabolizes nitrogen, activates certain enzymes, and helps break down sulfites
- *nickel:* aids in enzyme function
- *phosphorus:* forms bone, teeth, and the nucleic acids RNA and DNA and produces energy
- *potassium:* aids in normal nerve and muscle function and electrolyte balance
- *sodium:* aids in normal nerve and muscle function and helps the body maintain a normal electrolyte and fluid balance
- *selenium:* acts as an antioxidant and aids in thyroid gland function
- *sulfur:* aids in protein synthesis
- *zinc:* forms many enzymes and insulin, and is required for healthy skin, the healing of wounds, and growth

The following shows a list of foods that contain significant amounts of particular minerals:

- *boron:* fruit, vegetables, and nuts
- *calcium:* dairy products, calcium-fortified foods, canned fish with bones (salmon, sardines), and green, leafy vegetables
- *chromium:* liver, processed meats, whole-grain cereals, and nuts
- *chloride:* salt, meat, sardines, cheese, green olives, and sauerkraut
- *cobalt:* green, leafy vegetables, meat, and organ meats
- *copper:* organ meats, shellfish, cocoa, mushrooms, dried legumes, dried fruits, peas, tomato products, and whole-grain cereals
- *fluoride:* seafood, tea, and fluoridated water
- *iodine:* seafood, iodized salt, eggs, and cheese
- *iron:* red meat, leafy green vegetables, fish (such as tuna and salmon), eggs, dried fruits, beans, whole grains, and enriched grains
- *phosphorus:* dairy products, meat, poultry, fish, cereals, nuts, and legumes
- *potassium:* legumes, potato skins, tomatoes, and bananas

- *manganese:* whole-grain cereals, pineapple, nuts, tea, beans, and tomato paste
- *magnesium:* nuts, soybeans, and cocoa
- *molybdenum:* legumes, whole-grain breads and cereals, and dark green vegetables
- *nickel:* meat, liver, seafood, peanuts, fortified cereals, and whole grains (depending on the nickel content of soil where grains were grown)
- *selenium:* meats, seafood, nuts, and cereals (depending on the selenium content of soil where grains were grown)
- *sodium:* salt, sea vegetables, green olives, milk, meat, sardines, cheese, green olives, and sauerkraut
- *sulfur:* meat, eggs, and legumes
- *zinc:* meat, liver, seafood, peanuts, fortified cereals, and whole grains (depending on the zinc content of soil where grains were grown)

Minerals and cancer

Selenium and cancer. Selenium is a mineral with a well-evidenced anticancer effect. Once thought to be useful only in the treatment of dandruff, selenium has more recently been found to function as a cofactor for the metabolic reduction of antioxidant enzymes and to play a role in the functioning of the thyroid gland. Hence, selenium has begun to take a place in the spotlight, based on continued research showing a positive correlation between selenium and cancer prevention and a possible link between cancer and selenium deficiency.[157-161]

Research suggests that selenium affects cancer risk in two ways: as an antioxidant, protecting the body from damaging effects of free radicals, and possibly by preventing or slowing tumor growth. Certain breakdown products of selenium are believed to prevent tumor growth by enhancing immune cell activity and suppressing the development of blood vessels to the tumor.

In one such study, taking a daily supplement containing 200 µg of selenium did not affect recurrence of skin cancer, but significantly reduced the occurrence and death from total cancers, where the incidence of prostate cancer, colorectal cancer, and lung cancer was notably lower in the group given the supplements.[162] Other studies have shown evidence that selenium may protect normal tissues from chemotherapy toxicity,[163] that methyl selenium may improve the chemotherapeutic action of prostate cancer,[164] and that selenite concentrations may strongly inhibit the growth of the sarcomatoid mesothelioma cells.[165]

Further research has indicated that cancer incidence, including that of the lung, colorectum, breast, pancreas, and prostate, is lower among people who have higher blood levels or higher intakes of selenium;[166-171] that adequate amounts of selenium can improve immune response through the increased production of interferon and other cytokines, T-cell proliferation, and T-helper cells;[172] and that selenium influences both the innate, nonadaptive, and the acquired, adaptive, immune systems.[173]

Calcium and cancer. Some studies suggest a strong relationship between calcium intake and colorectal cancer risk, such as the Nurses' Health Study, where more than 135,000 men and women were observed relative to calcium intake. Overall, those participants who supplemented with more than 700 mg of calcium per day were found to have a 35 to 45% reduced risk of cancer of the lower part of the colon, compared to those who had a calcium intake of 500 mg or less per day.[174] Furthermore, the National Institutes of Health–American Association of Retired Persons (NIH–AARP) Diet and Health Study, which analyzed results from following more than 293,000 men and 198,000 women, also revealed that high intakes of total calcium, dietary calcium, and supplemental calcium were associated with an approximate 20% lower risk of colorectal cancer among men and an approximate 30% lower risk of colorectal cancer among women.[175]

Magnesium. This trend is the same for a number of other minerals, including magnesium, where studies show that an adequate consumption of magnesium may correlate to a reduced risk of cancer. For example, in one large prospective study covering more than 14 years, a high magnesium intake was seen to reduce the occurrence of colorectal cancer in women.[176] In another study, when 35,196 Iowa women (age 55 to 69) were studied over a 17-year period, results showed that those women with diets high in magnesium had a reduced occurrence of colon cancer.[177] Further studies have also revealed statistically significant inverse trends in risk for both colon and proximal colon cancer in overweight subjects who consume higher amounts of magnesium.[178]

Given these findings, we can see that magnesium plays an important role in offsetting the risk for cancer, especially as a low magnesium level is known to be a common side effect of certain anticancer drugs, specifically cisplatin and cyclosporine, and anti-EGFR (epidermal growth factor receptor) agents, including cetuximab and panitumumab.[179] Magnesium is also a cofactor for more than 300 enzymes and is involved in numerous transport mechanisms; therefore it is not surprising that hypomagnesemia (low magnesium levels) has been associated with considerable morbidity. This is why a proactive approach is recommended in managing hypomagnesemia in cancer patients receiving this type of chemotherapy.[179]

Still other studies have revealed that: magnesium hydroxide has been shown to have anti-carcinogenic effects on colon epithelium, or tissue, in animal studies;[180] magnesium plays a role in gene stability and DNA;[181] and that magnesium improves insulin response[182,183] and action,[184,185] due to the fact that hyperinsulinemia is a risk factor for colorectal cancer.[186,187] In the case of insulin, resistance occurs when the body's cells do not respond properly to the insulin produced and when glucose does not get absorbed by the body's cells for use as energy. When this happens, the body needs to produce extra insulin to maintain normal blood sugar levels. Eventually, if the pancreas is unable to keep up with this extra demand, one of the results can be long-term high blood sugar levels and type 2 diabetes.

Zinc. Zinc is a good example of a mineral that is found in small amounts, but packs a significant punch in terms of our health. It is generally scientifically accepted that zinc deficiency can negatively affect the immune system because of zinc's essential role in gene regulation of lymphocytes and in the normal development and function of cells involved in the immune response, such as neutrophils and natural killer cells.[188] High zinc concentration in bodily tissue has also been strongly associated with a reduced risk of developing esophageal squamous cell carcinoma,[189] and zinc supplementation in conjunction with chemotherapy and radiotherapy has been shown to improve overall survival in patients with advanced *nasopharyngeal carcinoma* (cancer of the part of the pharynx behind and above the soft palate, directly continuous with the nasal passages).[190]

Because the taking of manufactured nutrients and supplements in relation to cancer will always be shrouded in controversy, and because Mother Nature does always seem to know best, until more research is done, the best approach remains to receive one's daily intake from dietary sources.

Fiber

Fiber is simply the part of any fruit, vegetable, whole grain, or legume that cannot be digested or absorbed. As a result, fiber passes through the stomach and intestine and into the colon virtually unchanged. Whole-grain breads, bran flakes, whole-wheat-based foods, and barley are among the foods that contain high fiber, as are nuts, seeds, and legumes. Dried fruits, such as apricots, dates, prunes, and raisins are high in fiber as well. Oranges, apples (eaten with the skin), kiwi, mangos, bananas, and pears are also excellent fiber sources. Among vegetables significant for their fiber are broccoli, spinach, carrots, green peas, and celery. Again, the best route is to obtain our dietary fiber naturally from high-fiber foods instead of trying to add them in by eating extra bran or through supplementation. According to the Harvard School of Public Health, the average American only consumes 15 gm of dietary fiber a day, considerably less than the recommended intake. In 2002, the Food and Nutrition Board of the National Academy of Sciences Research Council issued DRIs for fiber (see Table 4-7). In the past, no national standardized recommendation for fiber existed. The new DRIs represent desirable intake levels established using the most current scientific methodology.

TABLE 4-7. Dietary Reference Intakes (DRIs) for fiber for males and females, age 9-50. (Source: Food and Nutrition Board, Institute of Medicine, National Academies, 2009)

Males	grams of fiber per day	Females	grams of fiber per day
Age 9–13	31 gm	Age 9–13	26 gm
Age 14-18	38 gm	Age 14-18	26 gm
Age 19–50	38 gm	Age 19–50	25 gm
Age 51+	30 gm	Age 51+	21 gm

The Nutrition Facts panel on food labels provides us with the amount of dietary fiber provided in a single serving of food. We can also refer to the front of a food's package to see if it lists any of the following nutrient content claims:

- "High fiber food": 5 gm or more of fiber per serving
- "Good source of fiber": 2.5 to 4.9 gm of fiber per serving
- "More, or added, fiber": at least 2.5 gm of fiber per serving

Dietary fiber is either *soluble*, because it dissolves in water, like oats, oat bran, psyllium husk, barley, legumes, and pectin, or *insoluble*, because it does not dissolve in water, like wheat bran, nuts, seeds, or vegetables. Soluble fiber, like all fiber, cannot be digested, but does change through bacterial fermentation. Insoluble fiber passes through the digestive tract relatively unchanged.

A high-fiber diet has many benefits in that it:

- **Lowers the risk of digestive conditions,** such as hemorrhoids, irritable bowel, and diverticular disease

- **Prevents constipation.** Fiber increases weight and size of stool and softens stool, reducing the chances for constipation
- **Lowers blood cholesterol.** Soluble fiber helps reduce low-density lipoprotein levels, or bad cholesterol
- **Assists in weight loss.** High-fiber foods are less energy-dense, which translates into a reduction of calories for the same amount of food
- **Improves blood-sugar levels.** Soluble fiber can slow the absorption of sugar, something that can help those with diabetes improve blood-sugar levels
- **Reduces the risk of cancer.** There is strong evidence that dietary fiber aids in reducing the risk of breast, colorectal, and esophageal cancer

"Nutrition facts" labels

The American Institute for Cancer Research has published a booklet entitled *The AICR Guide to the Nutrition Facts Label*.[191] The purpose of this booklet is to educate the general public about the meanings behind all the numbers on our current food labels. It teaches us to compare numbers on a single label and then compare corresponding numbers between labels on different food products. These comparisons enable us to be better informed about the choices available for our health.

The "Nutrition Facts Label" appears on the packaging of a product, usually on the back. The numbers and percentages it lists give us a good indication of whether the product is an appropriate food choice. Utilizing the information we find on the labels, we can make determinations to consume what is "good" and avoid what is not.

Let's look at a label as it appears on a typical box of macaroni and cheese in more detail so we can understand how to use these labels most beneficially (see Table 4-8).

TABLE 4-8. Nutrition facts for a sample label of macaroni and cheese product.

Nutrition facts: Serving size 1 cup (228 gm) Servings per container 2 (Amounts as they appear on actual food labels are indicated.)	
Amount per serving	
Calories 250	Calories from fat 110
Total fat 12 gm	**% Daily value*** 18%
Saturated fat 3 gm	15%
Trans fat 1.5 gm	-

(continued on next page)

Cholesterol 30 mg	-
Sodium 470 mg	20%
Total carbohydrate 31 gm	10%
Dietary fiber 0 gm	0%
Sugars 5 gm	-
Protein 5 gm	-
Vitamin A	4%
Vitamin C	2%
Calcium	20%
Iron	4%

*% Daily Values are based on a 2,000-calorie diet. Your Daily Values may be higher or lower depending on your calorie need:

	Calories	2,000	2,500
Total fat	Less than…	65 gm	80 gm
Saturated fat	Less than…	20 gm	25 gm
Cholesterol	Less than…	300 mg	300 mg
Sodium	Less than…	2,400 mg	2,400 mg
Total carbohydrates	-	300 gm	375 gm
Dietary fiber	-	25 gm	30 gm

In Table 4-9 the first thing we see is the size of each individual serving and then the number of servings available in the container.

TABLE 4-9. Serving sizes per container as indicated on label of macaroni and cheese product.

Serving Size	1 Cup (288 gm)	Servings per container 2

Based on each serving size, we then read the accompanying number of calories all the way through to the percentage of iron listed. If we were to consume two servings contained in this package, we would simply multiply the numbers related to each nutrient listed in the food product by 2. For example, if we consume the entire packet in our sample of two servings, we would multiply everything from calories to iron by 2 to get an accurate idea of how much we are ingesting. In this case, one serving provides 12 gm of fat, so two servings would equal 24 gm of total fat.

Calories. The caloric count on the label tells us two things: first, how many calories there are in one serving, and second, how these calories contribute to a total day's caloric content (see Table 4-10). There are 250 calories in a serving, which is equivalent to one eighth of a total daily intake of 2,000 calories. This means that there is plenty of room left for consuming other foods and beverages. If most of us consume three meals per day as well as a couple of snacks, each meal should not constitute more than approximately 500 calories (based on a 2,000-calorie-per-day consumption). "Calories from fat 110" on the label signifies that 44%—or close to half—of the calories in that serving are from fat. Since it is generally recommended that fewer than 30% of our daily intake of calories should come from fat, this is one of the important considerations we need to look at before we think of buying and consuming a particular type of food. This does not mean that every item we eat during the day needs to have fewer than 30% of its calories from fat. However, it helps to be aware of meals and foods with a higher caloric content from fat, so we can then balance it out by making a decision to consume other foods with lower fat content on that same day.

TABLE 4-10. Calories per container as indicated on label of macaroni and cheese product.

Calories 250		Calories from fat 110	
	Calories	2,000	2,500

Total fat. The "Total Fat" is the sum of all the different fats included in the food product in one serving (see Table 4-11). This total fat is then compared to the recommended limit of fat consumption in a day based on an average person's total food consumption. For example, for an individual with a 2,000-calorie-per-day diet, the recommended total fat consumption should be fewer than 65 gm of fat. In this case, our label says that this product contains 12 gm of fat, or about 18% of the recommended 65 gm. Again, in general, anything over 20% on the Nutrition Fact Label is considered a high amount, and 5% or less is considered low.

TABLE 4-11. Fats per container as indicated on label of macaroni and cheese product.

Total Fat 12 gm		18%
Total Fat	less than 65 gm	

Saturated fat. This particular line on the label tells us how much saturated fat is present in this product: in this case, 3 gm (see Table 4-12). An individual on a 2,000-calorie-per-day diet is generally recommended to consume fewer than 20 gm of saturated fat per day. Three grams, therefore, is about 15% of the daily recommended requirement. In this case, 3 gm does not by itself appear to be too high, considering fewer than 20 gm are recommended; however, if we bear in mind that 20% is our high-water mark, 15% is pretty close to that level. Since saturated fats contribute to raising cholesterol levels, it is advisable to choose products with the lowest levels of saturated fat.

TABLE 4-12. Saturated fats per container as indicated on label of macaroni and cheese product.

Saturated Fat 3 gm		15%
Sat Fat	less than 20 gm	

Trans fat. While "Trans Fat" is listed on the label, at this time recommended levels of trans fat have not been set and so are not indicated on food labels (see Table 4-13). Trans fats, just like saturated fats, have been shown to raise cholesterol levels. If we add the amount of trans fat to the amount of saturated fat on this label, we arrive at a total of 4.5 gm, which is 22% of the recommended limit of fewer than 20 gm. Together, that means the fat content raises the levels of this undesirable fat in the product to a high degree.

TABLE 4-13. Trans fats per container as indicated on label of macaroni and cheese product.

Trans Fat	1.5 gm

Cholesterol. The amount of cholesterol present in a food product is shown on this line (see Table 4-14). In this package of macaroni and cheese, the amount of cholesterol is 30 mg, or 10%. An individual on a 2,000-calorie-per-day diet is recommended to consume fewer than 300 mg of cholesterol. This product contains 30 mg, or 10%, of the total recommended allowance. Again, we are advised by health professionals and research that we are best served by choosing foods with the lowest amounts of all three: saturated fat, trans fat, and cholesterol.

TABLE 4-14. Cholesterol per container as indicated on label of macaroni and cheese product.

Cholesterol 30 mg		10%
Cholesterol	less than 65 gm	300 mg

Sodium. This line on the food label tells us how much sodium is present in one serving of the food product (see Table 4-15). In a 2,000-calorie-per-day diet, the recommended amount of sodium is less than 2,400 mg. This product contains 470 mg, which is 20% of the recommended amount. While 20% may not seem like a lot relative to the total recommended daily amount, this one serving of food contains a high level of sodium content in relation to the rest of the day's food consumption.

TABLE 4-15. Sodium per container as indicated on label of macaroni and cheese product.

Sodium 470 mg		20%
Sodium	less than	2,400 mg

Carbohydrates. The total carbohydrate content in a single serving of this product from both naturally occurring and additive sources is revealed here (see Table 4-16). Again, as part of a 2,000-calorie-per-day diet, our recommended total carbohydrate intake based on daily values is 300 gm, or about 45 to 65%, of the total 2,000 calories. Since our recommended total carbohydrate consumption is listed here, there is no guideline for "less than" on the label.

TABLE 4-16. Carbohydrates per container as indicated on label of macaroni and cheese product.

Total Carbohydrate 31 gm		10%
Total Carbohydrate	300 gm	

Dietary fiber. This line records the amount of dietary fiber in one serving of the food product (see Table 4-17). In a 2,000-calorie-per-day diet, 25 gm is the recommended total amount for consumption. Again, we find there are no "less than" amounts of fiber listed because 25 gm of dietary fiber is the goal for maintaining good health. In this particular product, there is no dietary fiber at all, so consuming this product would not help us in reaching our daily allotment of 25 gm of dietary fiber.

TABLE 4-17. Dietary fiber per container as indicated on label of macaroni and cheese product.

Dietary Fiber 0 gm		0%
Dietary Fiber	25 gm	

Sugar. Food labels do not incorporate any recommended limits or goals for sugar intake (see Table 4-18). This is because sugar is not a substance required to stay healthy. Sugar is purely a superfluous substance; in other words, it adds calories without adding nutrition. However, sugar amounts listed on a label *do* provide information about the product's sugar content and are an important consideration in making our dietary decisions. Because 1 teaspoon contains approximately 4 gm of sugar, in this case we can conclude that the amount of sugar in this product is fairly low. We can also assess sugar levels by looking for other types of sugars that may be included in the product but do not appear under the name of "sugar," such as honey, corn syrup, fructose, high-fructose corn syrup, maltose, or dextrose. All of these sugars enhance flavor and add calories, but have no nutritional value.

TABLE 4-18. Sugar per container as indicated on label of macaroni and cheese product.

Sugar 5 gm	

Protein. Again, as with sugar and carbohydrates, food labels do not express recommended limits for protein (see Table 4-19). Americans normally consume high-protein foods in their intake of meats, poultry, and dairy products. Vegetables are relatively low sources of protein, so those who choose a vegetarian diet need to pay particular attention to this line to help ensure they are consuming somewhere in the vicinity of 50 gm of protein per day.

TABLE 4-19. Protein per container as indicated on label of macaroni and cheese product.

Protein 5 gm	

Vitamins. Near the end of our food product label we will find a listing of vitamins and minerals that *may* be present in the product (see Table 4-20). Manufacturers are required to list the amounts of vitamin A and C, minerals, calcium, and iron content in all products. In our example, one serving of macaroni and cheese contains 4% of vitamin A, signifying that one serving contains 4% of the recommended daily value. The product provides 20% of the recommended calcium, 2% vitamin C, and 4% iron. This product lacks adequate amounts of vitamin A, C, and iron.

TABLE 4-20. Vitamins per container as indicated on label of macaroni and cheese product.

Vitamin A		4%
Vitamin C		2%
Calcium		20%
Iron		4%

Choosing products using food labels

Reading our food label line by line helps us choose food products for their overall benefits—or reject them for their drawbacks—in meeting our nutritional needs. In this case, one box of macaroni and cheese is shown to contain a high percentage of calories from fats, both saturated and trans fats. It also contains high amounts of sodium. This product is also noticeably low in vitamins and contains no fiber at all. So, while it may taste good, it contains high amounts of substances we don't need and few of the ones we do. Only the 20% amount of calcium has any measure of benefit. Naturally, we're not expected to completely discontinue buying products like these, but limiting how much we eat of them and how often we eat them is the best approach.

Phytochemicals

How often did we all hear, "You can't have dessert until you finish your vegetables" when we were growing up? Well, it turns out this was good advice because we now know just how important it is to include large amounts of fruits and vegetables in our diet, not only for good general nutrition, but also for fighting cancer. Fruits and vegetables of all kinds are rich in plant chemicals called *phytochemicals*. For our purposes, all we need to know is that in whatever form they take, phytochemicals help us stay healthy.

The phytochemical equation

Plants are like humans in the sense that they also produce disease-preventing, non-nutritive chemical compounds, or phytochemicals, to protect themselves against bacteria, viruses, and fungi. Though phytochemicals are not essential for sustaining life, they play a major role in a healthy diet, and doctors and researchers believe that phytochemicals help prevent various human diseases, such as diabetes, hypertension, and cancer. There are thousands of phytochemicals: some of the well-known ones are lycopene (found in tomatoes), isoflavones (found in soy), and flavonoids (found in fruits). All brightly colored fruits and vegetables, as well as whole grains and beans, are good sources of phytochemicals. Phytochemicals act as antioxidants, protect the body's nutrients, and prevent against carcinogens, depending on their source—in other words, in which color and type of fruit or vegetable they appear.

Color-coded phytochemicals

There's nothing more beautiful than a selection of multicolored fruits and vegetables. In fact, including a wide variety of colored foods in our diet in the form of fruits and vegetables from each color group is one way to balance our approach and ensure the most benefit from what we consume. By eating all the colors—red, orange, green, blue, and so on—we know we're getting a full range of phytochemicals that help prevent various forms of cancer. Below are some of the major food families that can be identified by their specific color and contain particular phytochemicals.

> **The red food family:** All variations of tomatoes (such as whole, paste, juice, and soup), watermelon, pink grapefruit, pink guavas, and apricots are good sources of the phytochemical lycopene. Including these foods in your daily diet may reduce the risk of prostate cancer.

The purple/red family: The phytochemical anthocyanin is found in red raspberries, strawberries, cranberries, red cabbage, kidney beans, sweet cherries, beets, red apples, red onions, red beans, plums, red grapes, pomegranates, eggplant, prunes, black currants, elderberries, and other plant foods, giving them their distinguishable purple/red color. This phytochemical can help protect against cancer, and is also good for vision and cardiovascular health.

The green family: The fruits and vegetables included in this family are marked by various shades of green. Cabbage and other cruciferous vegetables, such as broccoli, Brussels sprouts, kale, cauliflower, bok choy, watercress, rutabaga, arugula, and turnips, are rich in the phytochemicals sulforaphane, isothiocyanate, and indoles, and help protect against breast cancer.

The deep orange/yellow family: The fruits and vegetables in this group are rich in *beta-carotene* and need to be included in the diet. This powerful antioxidant supplies fruits and vegetables with these characteristic colors, and contributes to reducing the risk of cancer and heart disease and bolstering the eyesight and the body's immune system. Carrots, pumpkins, mangoes, apricots, cantaloupe, sweet potatoes, peaches, butternut squash, and others in the orange/yellow family are all rich in beta-carotene.

The other family included in this group is the yellow/orange variety, which includes oranges, grapefruit, lemon, papaya, pears, pineapple, yellow pepper, and yellow raisins, all good sources of the phytochemical bioflavonoid. Along with vitamin C, these foods may also reduce the risk of cancer.

The white/allium family: In this case, white really is a color! Foods in this group include garlic, leeks, shallots, chives, and onions. Beneficial in terms of their antibacterial, antiviral, and antifungal effects, they contain the phytochemical allicin, which also helps protect against cancer and heart disease.

Not all fruits and vegetables can be strictly branded by color and grouped into families, though most of them are rich in phytochemicals. Some of these that also contribute to a daily healthy diet include nuts, seeds, grains, beans (legumes), tea, and chocolate. Note that raw or steamed vegetables hold onto more of their phytochemical properties, and so maintain a higher nutrient value or content than overheated and boiled vegetables.

Garlic, onions, leeks, and chives are known for their notable anticancer effects. The sulfur-containing compounds in these vegetables can inhibit enzymes involved in carcinogen activation, as well as suppress proliferation of cancer cells. Cruciferous vegetables are those in the cabbage family, such as broccoli, Brussels sprouts, cauliflower, kale, and turnips. Cruciferous vegetables manage to block carcinogens from damaging the body's cells and the genetic material in those cells, while citrus fruits, grapes, and other fruits help to excrete carcinogens from the body. Soybeans and dried beans specifically help prevent the development of tumors, and whole grains, also abundant in phytochemicals, have been proven to prevent cellular damage.

As of this writing, the National Cancer Institute has identified 35 plant foods that possess cancer-protective properties.[192] The foods and herbs with the highest anticancer activity include garlic, soybeans, cabbage, ginger, licorice root, and the umbelliferous vegetables, including carrots, celery, coriander, parsley, and parsnips. Additional foods with cancer-protective properties include onions, flax, citrus, turmeric, cruciferous vegetables, tomatoes, sweet peppers, brown rice, whole wheat, oats, barley, various herbs (such as mint, rosemary, thyme, oregano, sage, and basil), cucumber, cantaloupe, and berries.

While most of us are aware that certain foods we eat can hurt us, there are many foods that can help us as well; not surprisingly, fruits and vegetables are number one in this category. Due to their importance, the Centers for Disease Control and Prevention, in conjunction with 11 other organizations, including the American Cancer Society and the National Cancer Institute, has started an aggressive campaign called The National Fruit and Vegetable Program. The goal of this program is to increase public awareness about the significance of fruits and vegetables in the daily diet.[193] According to David Heber, M.D., Ph.D., director of the UCLA Center for Human Nutrition, "Virtually every disease of aging—including heart disease, diabetes, and many common forms of cancer, such as breast cancer and prostate cancer—results from damage to DNA, which can be prevented by the substances found in fruits and vegetables." Heber goes onto state that "80 to 90% of cancers are not inherited, but result from the defects in DNA during your lifetime from accumulated damage that could be prevented by increasing fruit and vegetable intake."[194] Dr. Hai Liu Rui of the Department of Food Science at Cornell University agrees. "Epidemiological studies have consistently shown that regular consumption of fruits and vegetables is strongly associated with reduced risk of developing chronic diseases, such as cancer and cardiovascular disease." Rui goes on to explain, "The additive and synergistic effects of phytochemicals in fruits and vegetables are responsible for their potent antioxidant and anticancer activities. The benefit of a diet rich in fruits, vegetables, and whole grains is attributed to the complex mixture of phytochemicals present in these and other whole foods."[195]

Phytochemicals exist in more than 150,000 edible plants on earth. It is well known that plants produce these chemicals to protect themselves, but even more startling is the research demonstrating that these same phytochemicals protect humans against many diseases as well. Incredibly, humans today eat only 150 to 200 of the 150,000 plants worldwide! Though the average American eats only three servings of plant foods on a daily basis, for years the National Cancer Institute has encouraged Americans to eat five to nine servings of fruits and vegetables per day, based on their prolific health benefits. Below is a list of naturally occurring plant compounds and the phytochemicals in their composition (see Table 4-21).

TABLE 4-21. Essential phytochemicals.

Naturally occurring plant compounds	Essential phytochemicals present
Alkaloids	caffeine
	theobromine
	theophylline
Anthocyanins	cyanidin
Carotenes	lycopene
Coumestans	flavan-3-ols
Flavonoids	epicatechin
	hesperidin
	kaempferol
	naringin
	nobiletin
	proanthocyanidins
	quercetin
	resveratrol
	rutin
	tangeretin
Hydroxycinnamic acids	chicoric acid
	coumarin
	ferulic acid
	scopoletin
Isoflavones	daidzein
	genistein
Lignans	silymarin
Monophenols	hydroxytyrosol
Monoterpenes	geraniol
	limonene
Organosulfides	allicin
	glutathione
	indole-3-carbinol
	isothiocyanate
	sulforaphane
Phenolic acids	capsaicin
	ellagic acid
	gallic acid
	rosmarinic acid
	tannic acid

(continued on next page)

Phytosterols	beta-sitosterol
Xanthophylls	astaxanthin
	beta-cryptoxanthin
Other phytochemicals	damnacanthal
	digoxin
	phytic acid

The wide range of phytochemicals offers many different mechanisms of action. Here are a few ways in which phytochemicals can work:

As antioxidants. Most phytochemicals have "antioxidant activity." This means they protect our cells against oxidative damage caused by free radicals generated by things like air pollution, exposure to sunlight, radiation, pesticides, drugs, and cigarette smoke, and in doing so, reduce the risk of developing certain types of cancer and heart disease. Phytochemicals with this capability include: allyl sulfides (onions, leeks, garlic), carotenoids (fruits, carrots), flavonoids (fruits, vegetables), and polyphenols (tea, grapes).

As hormonal regulators. Some phytochemicals, called *isoflavones,* which are found in soy, can faintly mimic the estrogen hormone. Estrogen provides benefits like lowering cholesterol levels, building strong bones, supporting a healthy heart, relieving hot flashes associated with menopause, and so on. Isoflavones may also reduce the risk for reproductive cancers (such as breast and ovarian cancer) and osteoporosis, as well as enhance intercellular communication. Because they are considered "weak" phytoestrogens, isoflavones may act as "anti-estrogens" in that they compete with the more potent, naturally occurring internal estrogens (e.g., 17b-estradiol) for the ability to bind to estrogen receptors. This may explain why populations that consume significant amounts of soy (for example, in Southeast Asia) have reduced risk of estrogen-dependent cancer. Although some studies about the benefits of soy remain controversial, others appear much more conclusive in their findings.[196,197]

As enzyme stimulators. Indoles, found in cabbage, stimulate enzymes that remove and/or neutralize carcinogens. Other phytochemicals that interfere with enzymatic function in this way are protease inhibitors (e.g., soy and other beans) and terpenes (e.g., citrus fruits and cherries). Proteases belong to the class of enzymes known as hydrolases, the enzymes that are responsible for breaking down proteins into smaller units and have been identified in promoting cancer progression.

Preventing potentially harmful DNA replication. Saponins are phytochemicals found in chickpeas, sprouts, and beans. They have been found to have a cytostatic effect on cancer cells. This means they interfere with DNA replication to prevent the multiplication of cancer cells.

Antibacterial effect. Garlic is one example of a phytochemical called *allicin*. Allicin's antibacterial properties may inhibit the growth of some types of bacteria.

Physical action. Some phytochemicals physically bind to cell walls, thereby preventing pathogens from adhering as well. Proanthocyanidins are responsible for the anti-adhesion properties of cranberry, which is known to reduce the risk of urinary tract infection and improve dental health.

Another example of phytochemicals in action is red wine. You may have heard about the potentially favorable effects of red wine consumption. Apparently, this is due to the phytochemical resveratrol, a substance that shows a dramatic tendency to decrease the risk of many types of cancer. However, the question of whether the best source of resveratrol is red wine is still being debated, considering its high caloric content and alcohol's possible role in certain types of cancer. Other potentially healthier sources of resveratrol include grapes, berries, and peanuts. Although resveratrol is a natural antibiotic produced when plants are under attack by pathogens such as bacteria or fungi, it can also be produced through chemical synthesis and sold as a nutritional supplement.[198] In this case, it is primarily derived from an herb called Japanese knotweed. Resveratrol has been found in mouse and rat experiments to protect against cancer by acting as an antioxidant, anti-mutagen, and anti-inflammatory.[199]

Dozens of studies have reported on resveratrol's anticancer activity on the cells of breast, skin, gastric, colon, esophageal, prostate, and pancreatic cancer and leukemia.[200] For example, Garvin, et al. have revealed that resveratrol inhibited angiogenesis and induced apoptosis in human breast cancer,[201] and Zhou, et al. have shown that resveratrol induces apoptosis in human esophageal carcinoma cells.[202]

Soybeans are in a class of their own. They contain several forms of anticarcinogens, including protease inhibitors, phytosterols, saponins, phenolic acids, phytic acid, and isoflavones.[203] Of these isoflavones, genistein and daidzein are particularly noteworthy because soybeans are their only significant dietary source. Among the major seed oils, flaxseed oil is a rich source of the omega-3 fatty acid, alpha-linolenic acid, and it has been demonstrated that dietary flaxseed inhibits human breast cancer growth and metastasis.[204] In another study involving plant compounds, it was found that frequent tomato, or lycopene, intake was associated with a reduced risk of prostate cancer.[205]

Phytochemicals have actually been used as drugs for thousands of years. For example, Hippocrates is thought to have prescribed willow tree leaves to abate fever; salicin was originally extracted from the white willow tree and later synthetically produced to become the staple, over-the-counter drug called aspirin; and Taxol (paclitaxel), an important cancer drug, is a phytochemical initially extracted and purified from the Pacific yew tree. It is estimated that 5,000 individual phytochemicals have been identified in fruits, vegetables, and grains.[206]

Vegetables, fruits, and whole grains contain a wide variety of phytochemicals with the potential to modulate cancer development based on their dietary fiber, antioxidant content, stimulation of enzyme systems, and anti-inflammatory response. These processes in turn help prevent the formation of potential carcinogens, block the action of carcinogens on tissue, or act on cells to suppress cancer development. At this time, specific phytochemicals are allowed only limited healthcare claims on food packaging by the FDA because qualified health claims on conventional food must be supported by credible scientific evidence, something that requires both extensive testing and funding.

More information on garlic. Garlic (Allium sativum) is an amazing herb, probably the herb most widely quoted in scientific literature for its medicinal properties. Garlic's purported health benefits are numerous, including its cancer/tumor preventive properties, and its antibiotic, anti-hypertensive, and cholesterol-lowering properties. One study undertaken in China has shown a strong inverse relationship between stomach cancer risk and increased consumption of allium vegetables,[207] and in a study that examined results from human studies and 22 animal epidemiologic studies, allium vegetables were shown to have a strong protective effect against different types of cancer.[208] Studies have also confirmed an inverse relationship between garlic consumption and the reduced risk of colorectal cancer,[209] allium vegetables (including garlic) and the reduced risk of prostate cancer,[210] and the moderately protective role of onion and garlic intake against developing endometrial cancer.[211]

Tea and phytochemicals. Tea is second only to water as the most widely consumed beverage in the world. Tea is packed with phytochemicals, notably polyphenols, which comprise up to 30% of the total dry weight of fresh tea leaves. Catechins are the predominant and most significant of all tea polyphenols; green tea alone has four major catechins. Scientific studies have shown that consuming five or more cups of green tea per day has been associated with the decreased recurrence and the improved prognosis of stages I and II breast cancer in Japanese women.[212]

In Table 4-22 (on the next page) you will find a list of phytochemical-rich foods for easy shopping.

TABLE 4-22. Phytochemicals and their food sources.

Phytochemical	Food source
Allium	Garlic, leeks, chives, and onions
Allyl sulfide	Allium vegetables—onions, garlic, chives, and leeks
Apigenin	Chinese cabbage, bell pepper, garlic, French peas, guava, and celery
Carotenoids	Yellow-orange vegetables and fruits, green, leafy vegetables, and red fruits
Catechins	Green tea, black tea, wine, coffee, and apples
Coumestans	Clover and alfalfa sprouts
Curcumins	Turmeric
Flavonoids	Most fruit, vegetables, grains, and nuts
Gingerols	Ginger
Indoles and isothiocyanates	Cruciferous vegetables—broccoli, cabbage, cauliflower, Brussels sprouts, cabbage, kohlrabi, rutabaga, Chinese cabbage, bok choy, horseradish, radish, and watercress
Isoflavones	Tofu, soybeans, tempeh, soy milk, and textured vegetable protein
Lignans	Soybeans and flaxseed
Liminoids	Citrus
Lycopene	Solanaceous vegetables—tomatoes and peppers
Phenolic acids	Berries, grapes, nuts, and whole grains
Phthalides and polyacetylenes	Carrots, parsnips, parsley, coriander, and cilantro
Phytic acid	Wheat bran
Phytates	Grains and legumes
Quercetin	Apples, onions, tea, berries, cruciferous vegetables (broccoli, cauliflower, Brussels sprouts, bok choy), various seeds and nuts, some medicinal botanicals, including ginkgo biloba, and St. John's wort
Saponins	Beans and herbs
Terpenes	Cherries, citrus, and herbs

Consider the following tips for increasing phytochemical-rich foods in your diet:

- Use fresh or steamed vegetables instead of dried or canned.
- Keep cooking to a minimum.
- Eat a variety of the many delicious fruits available.
- Add fresh garlic (not garlic powder) to almost any meal—or simply add to the amounts called for in any recipe.

- Eat whole, not refined, grains. Phytochemicals are found in the highest concentrations in the nutrient-rich fiber that coats the starchy center of the grain. It is this fiber that is usually lost during processing.
- Eat the largest variety of vegetables you can. Try new vegetables as often as you can by incorporating them into your meals on a regular basis. You never know what you're going to like!
- Ethnic cuisines are great sources for discovering new kinds of foods, including vegetables. Local Asian or Latin American grocery stores are just two places where you can find interesting, inviting vegetables to add to your diet.

Probiotics

The term *probiotic* means "for life." Probiotics are foods or dietary supplements containing potentially beneficial bacteria and certain yeasts. According to the World Health Organization, probiotics are defined as "live microorganisms, which, when administered in adequate amounts, confer a health benefit on the host."[213] Probiotics have been recognized for years as an important functional requirement for human health, traditionally used to restore imbalances due to aging, stress, illness, traveling, and/or the use of medication (such as antibiotics). Probiotics have been shown to assist, encourage, and even restore the body's naturally occurring gut "microflora," the microorganisms that normally live in the digestive tract and perform a number of useful functions. It is estimated that 100 trillion microorganisms representing more than 500 different species inhabit every normal, healthy bowel. These microorganisms are involved in carbohydrate fermentation and absorption, systemic immune function support, the reduction of allergic reactions, as well as metabolic function and the repression of pathological microbial growth. Therefore, it is not uncommon for doctors to recommend a course of probiotics after a course of antibiotic therapy to help restore what has been depleted.

It is believed that the earliest use of the word "probiotic" was by Dr. Werner Kollath (1892–1970), one of the pioneers of the health food movement in Germany. Kollath established hygiene as science, using the word "probiotic" to describe inorganic and organic supplements that could help restore health to patients suffering from malnutrition and the aftereffects of eating high amounts of refined food. The term was also loosely used in 1965 by Lilly and Stillwell in *in vitro* studies relative to the growth of protozoa when they defined probiotics as "growth promoting factors produced by microorganisms."[214]

The true, original concept behind probiotics, however, evolved from the work of Russian scientist and Nobel Laureate Eli Metchnikoff at the beginning of the 20th century. It was Metchnikoff's thesis that Bulgarian peasants lived longer because they consumed large quantities of sour, or fermented, milk, which contains the bacteria *Lactobacillus bulgaricus*. Metchnikoff believed that the growth of *Lactobacillus* in the gastrointestinal tract replaced other putrefactive bacteria, thereby reducing toxic concentrations in the gut and ultimately improving health. Metchnikoff's ideas were instrumental in introducing whole new areas of research to the scientific community relative to identifying intestinal microorganisms and their range of health benefits.

Researchers have since found that consuming fermented milks and probiotic bacteria can have the following effects[215]:

Immunologic:

- local macrophages are activated, increasing antigen presentation to B lymphocytes and producing secretory immunoglobulin A (IgA), both locally and systemically
- cytokine (proteins involved in signaling the immune response) characteristics are altered
- sensitivity to food antigens is reduced

Nonimmunologic:

- food is digested and there is competition with pathogens for nutrients
- local pH is altered to create an unfavorable local environment for pathogens
- bacteriocins (toxins produced by bacteria) are produced to inhibit pathogens
- superoxide radicals are scavenged
- epithelial mucin (secretions of mucous membranes) are produced
- intestinal barrier function is enhanced
- competition takes place for adhesion with pathogens
- pathogen-derived toxins are modified

Probiotics can be found in dietary supplements in the form of capsules, tablets, and powders. A few common probiotics, such as *Saccharomyces boulardii*, are yeasts and are different from the typical probiotic bacteria. Examples of foods containing probiotics are yogurt, fermented and unfermented milk, miso, tempeh, some juices, and soy beverages. Most commonly, the bacteria come from two groups, or species: *Lactobacillus* and *Bifidobacterium*. Each species contains subspecies, such as *Lactobacillus acidophilus* and *Bifidobacterium bifidus*, and within these subspecies are further varieties and strains.

Taking precautions

Our environment is chock full of factors which can increase the incidence and production of abnormal cells. Among these many risks is exposure to chemicals of all kinds. Cancer-causing chemicals (carcinogens) can be ingested through the foods we eat or generated by the metabolic activity of microbes that live in the gastrointestinal tract. That is why it is so important to take all the precautions we can to reduce our exposure and, hence, our risk for cancer. It has been suggested that probiotic cultures may decrease the exposure to chemical carcinogens in a number of ways: by detoxifying ingested carcinogens; altering the environment of the intestine; decreasing the metabolic activities of bacteria that may generate carcinogenic compounds; producing metabolic products which improve a cell's ability to undergo apoptosis (to die); manufacturing compounds that inhibit the growth of tumor cells; and by stimulating the immune system to better defend against cancer cell proliferation.

Scientifically speaking...

Studies have shown that lactic acid (milk-based) bacteria has many effects on the body, including the deactivation of carcinogens and the prevention of mutations and DNA damage in colon tissue. Lactic acid bacteria shows potential as a chemoprotective agent and promise in the prevention of human colon cancer.[216] Other studies support both the favorable effects of lactic acid-forming bacteria on intestinal microflora and the immune system, and a statistically reduced risk of breast cancer when combined with a high intake of fermented milk products, including Gouda cheese.[217] In one such study, researchers observed increased immune activity in milk fermented by the culture *L. helveticus* R389 in response to mammary gland tumors. In this case, the milk fermented by *L. helveticus* R389 was able to delay tumor growth and modulate the relationship between the immune and endocrine systems. Researchers found that interleukin-6 (the cytokine involved in estrogen synthesis) and an important component in estrogen-dependent tumors and in the initiation of cellular death, decreased.[218]

In another study it was found that the three-year recurrence-free survival rate for superficial bladder cancer increased significantly in participants who had *lactobacillus casei* bacteria added to their chemotherapy treatments compared to the group of participants who had chemotherapy alone.[219] Researchers have also been studying *Bifidobacterium longum* in relation to cancer treatment. *Bifidobacterium longum* is a harmless, anaerobic bacterium found among normal bacterial flora. In one such study, investigators found that *B. longum* produced an enzyme called cytosine deaminase, which was able to convert 5-fluorocytosine into 5-fluorouracil—a chemotherapeutic agent. Based on this work, researchers suggest that *B. longum* could be useful for enzyme/pro-drug therapy in the treatment of oxygen-deficient, solid tumors.[220] Oxygen-deficient tumors, more commonly known as *hypoxic* tumors, are growths that have been found to be more difficult to treat by external radiation and chemotherapy.

It has also been shown that there is a strain of Bifidobacterium (B. adolescentis) that develops and proliferates in solid tumors. Due to this bacterium's activity, it has been hypothesized that it might be a highly specific and efficient vehicle for transporting anticancer genes into target tumors in cancer gene therapy.[221] Finally, researchers at Harvard Medical School have concluded that probiotics have been shown to have a positive impact in diarrheal diseases, inflammatory bowel diseases, irritable bowel syndrome, helicobacter pylori-induced gastritis, atopic diseases, and in the overall prevention of cancer.[222]

Eating organically

What are organic foods?

Organic foods are agricultural products—foods and fibers—that must comply with certain regulations, as follows:

- Organic foods must be grown and processed without the use of conventional (toxic) pesticides, synthetic ingredients, artificial fertilizers, human waste, or sewage sludge.
- Organic foods must be processed without ionizing radiation or food additives, or through bioengineering techniques.
- Organic meat and poultry is prohibited from the use of antibiotics and synthetic growth hormones.
- Organic foods require 100% organic feed for organic livestock.

Organic food production in this country is legally regulated. Regulations assure consumers that the organic products they purchase are produced, processed, and certified in accordance with the Organic Foods Production Acts standards. Currently, the European Union, the United States, Japan, and many other countries require producers to obtain organic certification in order to market their foods as "organic."

The ability to farm "organically" depends on having healthy, rich soil to produce plants that are resistant to pests and diseases. Organic farmers make use of specific practices and techniques, such as crop rotation (alternately growing different crops to prevent the build-up of pests and pathogens specific to one variety), cover crop planting (to ensure the fertility of the soil and prevent erosion), beneficial insect release, and composting. Farmers who choose to farm organically agree that soil and water conservation are critical for future generations, as conservation works in harmony with nature by providing quality food while preserving and protecting our resources. Organic production also eliminates the use of unnatural, genetically modified organisms and bioengineered products; does not use pesticides or harmful fertilizers that contaminate the soil or seep into water bodies such as rivers, lakes, and oceans; does not pose a health risk to farmers; and ensures a healthier and more sustainable environment.

History

Originally, albeit long ago, all food was organic. Small family farms produced fruits and vegetables (as well as dairy products and meats) for personal consumption. There were no pesticides; there was no irradiation or bioengineered food. Eventually, these small farms began to sell whatever extra produce they had, generally fresh vegetables, to local markets and stores. Over time, with the rise of industrialized farming, corporate entities have decreased the number of small family farms dramatically. This has given rise to the cost-effective mass production of livestock and agriculture, but as a result of this practice, food quality, animal welfare standards, and protection of our environmental resources have been compromised. With the increased demand from consumers for unadulterated whole foods, however, there has been a resurgence of small farms that are returning to the "old ways," and incorporating new business models to stay competitive with corporate farming practices. Since the early 1990s, the demand for organic food has grown at a rate of 20% a year and is expected to keep growing. Supermarkets are jumping on the bandwagon and have become distributors for the organic produce of these farmers.

Regulation

According to the *Nutrition Business Journal*, total organic food sales (anything and everything organic) in the United States reached $24.6 billion in 2008 and are increasing significantly on a yearly basis.[223] Organic food is the largest segment in the organic category, accounting for 93% of all organic sales and totaling $22.9 billion. Fruit and vegetables account for the largest portion of all organic food sales. This one category represents 37% of total organic food sales in 2008. The second largest categories are beverage and dairy, representing just over 14% each.[224] In the United States, the Organic Foods Production Act (OFPA) of 1990 was Title 21 of the 1990 Farm Bill. Its purpose was to establish national standards for the production and handling of foods labeled "organic." OFPA authorized the formation of the National Organic Program (NOP) to establish organic standards and make recommendations to the Secretary of Agriculture for setting these standards.[225] The U.S. Department of Agriculture (USDA) is assisted by the Food Safety and Inspection Service (FSIS)[226] and the Animal and Plant Health Inspection Service (APHIS).[227] Various other organizations and agencies handle other aspects of food regulation in this country. They are the Federal Trade Commission,[228] the Centers for Disease Control and Prevention,[229] the Environmental Protection Agency,[230] the Department of Commerce (controlling weights and measures),[231] and the Bureau of Alcohol, Tobacco and Firearms.[232] These agencies have the responsibility for regulating production and processing conditions, sources, labeling and the claims on labels, distribution conditions, and assignment of liability. To ensure farms meet all the USDA standards required to qualify for the seal of "organic," government-approved certifiers visit each farm and inspect its processes. Companies that handle and process farm produce are also required to obtain organic certification before the produce ever reaches the supermarket. The exception to this rule are farmers whose growth income is less than $5,000 annually. In this case the farmers are permitted to call their products "organic," but are not permitted to utilize the USDA seal (see Figure 4-17 on next page).

The organic seal

Food products are required to accurately indicate their organic content through the use of four different labels, as follows:

1. "100% organic" means that the product contains ONLY organically produced ingredients and processing aids (excluding water and salt). This is generally a single-ingredient food, such as a fruit or vegetable. These products may display the organic seal.

2. "Organic" refers to a product that is made of more than one ingredient and is at least 95% organic. These products may display the organic seal.

3. "Made with organic ingredients" refers to products that contain at least 70% or more organic ingredients. The label may display the list of organic ingredients on the front panel. These products do not display the organic seal.

4. "Contains organic ingredients" refers to products with fewer than 70% organic ingredients. The product's list of ingredients is not allowed to be displayed on the front, but rather must be displayed on the back panel. These products do not display the organic seal.

FIGURE 4-17. USDA Seal of Approval for organic products, 2010.

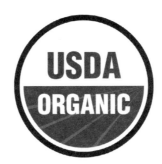

Organic versus conventional farming

When it comes to working the land, there is considerable difference between organic and conventional farming methodologies. They differ in the techniques farmers use to control weeds, feed poultry, and prevent livestock diseases, as well as in the types of fertilizers and irrigation methods they use. In organic farming, farmers use natural fertilizers, such as manure and compost, while conventional farmers use predominantly chemical fertilizers. Organic farmers use birds and insects that naturally feed on pests in order to reduce plant disease and methods, such as mating disruption and/or traps, to catch pests. In conventional farming, farmers directly spray chemical insecticides on plants to kill pests and use chemical herbicides to control weeds. Organic farmers, on the other hand, use methods like crop rotation, tilling, hand-weeding, and mulching to free the soil of its weeds. For livestock growth and maintenance, conventional farmers use growth hormones, antibiotics, and medication; organic farmers feed animals only organic fodder and grains. Methods like rotational grazing provide a balanced diet and keep living areas clean, too, which in turn helps keep animals disease-free.

Organic food statistics

In the United States, research continues to point to the growing appetite for organic foods by consumers. The USDA Economic Research Service (ERS) cites a study by the Hartman Group, the leading expert in organic surveys, where it was found that 19% of consumers bought organic food weekly in 2008, up from just 3% in the late 1990s, and that as of 2008, 69% of adults were buying organic food at least occasionally. In the same ERS report, the Food Marketing Institute stated that organic food was available in 82% of retail food stores as of 2007.[233] In fact, to meet the growing demand for organic products, there has been an increase in both the amount of farmland and the number of farms under organic management in the United States from the late 1990s to the late 2000s. Specifically, U.S. organic farmland increased from 1.3 million acres in 1997 to a little over 4 million acres (or 0.5% of all agricultural lands) in 2005.[233]

Pesticide residue in food

The Pesticide Data Program, or PDP, is a division of the USDA's national pesticide residue database program.[234] This program, along with state agricultural departments, laboratories, and other federal agencies, samples and analyzes the pesticide residue in the food and water supply. During 2008, PDP tested 13,381 fresh and processed fruits and vegetables, almonds, honey, catfish, corn grain, rice, groundwater, and treated and untreated drinking water for various insecticides, herbicides, fungicides, and growth regulators. (For fresh and processed fruit and vegetables, almonds, honey, catfish, and rice, approximately 76.4% of all samples tested were from U.S. sources, 19.8% were imports, 2.7% were of mixed national origin, and 1.1% were of unknown origin. Approximately 20% of the apple juice samples and 29% of the honey samples were of mixed national origin. Corn grain, groundwater, and treated and untreated drinking water were all from U.S. sources.) Excluding catfish, groundwater, and treated and untreated drinking water, 30% of all samples tested contained no detectable pesticides, 24% contained one pesticide, and 46% contained more than one pesticide.[235]

Four different monitoring programs have tested pesticide residue in conventionally farmed foods compared to organically farmed foods. The first monitoring program, the USDA Pesticide Data Program, revealed that pesticide was detected in 73% of conventional produce as compared to 23% of organic produce. The second, the California Department of Pesticide Regulation (CDPR) Marketplace Surveillance Program also detected pesticide residue in 31% of conventional produce as compared to 6.5% of organic, and the third, the Consumers Union Private Residue Testing Program detected pesticide residue in 79% of conventional produce as compared to 27% of organic. Finally, a program in Belgium also detected higher pesticide residue levels (49%) in conventional produce than in organic produce (12%). According to the PDP data, overall pesticide residues are 3.2 times more likely to be found in conventional produce than in organic produce; according to the CDPR data, residues in conventional produce are 4.8 times more prevalent; according to the Consumers Union data, residues are 2.9 times greater; and according to the Belgian data, residues are 4.1 times greater.[236]

Pesticides linked to cancer

Many studies have reported a link between pesticide exposure and serious health problems. These include: childhood cancer,[237] lung cancer,[238] prostate cancer,[239] breast cancer,[240] and neurotoxicity.[241]

Foods with high levels of pesticide residue affect everyone, both adults and children. Children are much less capable than adults of detoxifying most pesticides, however, so the effects can be much more deleterious. Keep in mind that when conventionally farmed produce is tested for residue, it is being tested in the same condition in which it is expected to be eaten when purchased from the grocery shelves. Since testing of this produce consistently shows remaining levels of residue, and since organic foods show much less, if any, residue, we would be best served to consume as much organically grown produce as possible.

You may be surprised to learn that, contrary to popular thought, pesticide residue, in most cases, cannot be eliminated—or even significantly reduced—with prolonged washing or peeling. This is because pesticides have been created to do the precise opposite—to either adhere to the skin of the fruit or vegetable or be absorbed into the edible portion. Knowing that information, and knowing that by avoiding fruits and vegetables with the highest levels of consistent contamination we can reduce our risk of pesticide exposure by 90%, is critical to our ongoing good health.

The following types of produce have been found to have the highest levels of pesticide residue:

- *Fruits:* peaches, apples, strawberries, nectarines, pears, cherries, red raspberries, and imported grapes
- *Vegetables:* spinach, bell peppers, celery, potatoes, and hot peppers

Food items with lower pesticide levels include:

- *Fruits:* pineapples, plantains, mangoes, bananas, watermelon, plums, kiwi, blueberries, papaya, grapefruit, and avocados
- *Vegetables:* cauliflower, Brussels sprouts, asparagus, radishes, broccoli, onions, okra, cabbage, and eggplant

Remember DDT?

In the not-too-distant past in the United States, DDT was the most widely used pesticide on all kinds of plants and produce. In a study published in *Lancet* in 2001, researchers analyzed the concentration of DDE (DDT's "breakdown product") in blood samples from mothers who had delivered babies between the years 1959 and 1966. Results of this study indicated that babies born to these mothers tended to be either premature—a major contributing factor in infant mortality—or of low birth weight.[242] *Silent Spring*, a book by Rachel Carson published in 1962, reports on one of the first major studies that questioned the widespread use of DDT, but it wasn't until 1972 that DDT was finally banned from use in the United States.[243] Furthermore, although the Stockholm Convention banned the use of DDT for agricultural purposes and the United States National Toxicology Program[244] classified DDT as "reasonably anticipated to be a human carcinogen," it is still being used as a pesticide in some countries. The Environmental Protection Agency is responsible for assessing all pesticides and setting what it calls "acceptable risk of exposure."[245] Though the EPA has determined that about 60% of herbicides, 90% of all fungicides, and 30% of all insecticides are "potentially cancer-causing," they are still used in food production and consumed through the foods we eat. Therefore, it is clear that one of the best methods of protection from these carcinogenic chemicals is to eat organic foods.

Is eating organically better for us?

In 2007, researchers at Warsaw Agricultural University found that organic foods contain higher levels of vitamin C, phenolic compounds, essential amino acids, minerals, and total sugars, and have fewer nitrites, nitrates, and pesticide residue when compared to conventional crops.[246] Other research in 2008, involving random samples of commercial late-harvest blueberries in New Jersey, revealed that blueberries grown according to organic standards yield significantly higher levels of sugar (fructose and glucose), malic acid, total phenolics, total anthocyanins, and antioxidant activity (ORAC) than fruit from conventional crops.[247] In still other studies, organic pears and peaches have been shown to have increased polyphenoloxidase activity, and polyphenol, ascorbic, citric acid, and α-tocopherol content, as compared to conventional pears and peaches.[248]

Organic milk also reveals significant differences when compared to conventionally farmed milk. One research study, for example, revealed significantly higher levels of conjugated linoleic acid, linolenic acid, alpha-tochopherol and beta-carotene in organic milk as compared to conventional dairy milk.[249]

In fact, differences have been found in many other areas of research. In one study, researchers compared salicylic acid content in organic vegetable soup to non-organic vegetable soup. Salicylic acid, a chemical compound found in plants, has anti-inflammatory medicinal properties and is commonly found in aspirin. Researchers in this study found that the organic soup had a significantly higher salicylic acid content.[250] In another study, when conventional, certified organic, and omega-3 eggs were examined, it was found that the organic egg yolks contained a higher percentage of palmitic and stearic acids than the conventional yolks and that the omega-3 eggs contained a higher amount of omega 3-fatty acids.[251] "Omega-3 eggs" are produced with the hope of attracting a wider consumer base. To alter the nutrient content of the eggs, the nutrient content fed to the hen also must be changed by adding products high in omega-3 fatty acids such as flaxseed, marine algae, fish, and fish oil.[252]

Eating organic poultry has also been shown to be a healthier way to eat. One reason is because organic chickens are not given antibiotics, vaccines, and growth hormones as conventionally grown chickens are given. Another reason is that in order to prevent disease-producing microbes from growing in conventionally grown chickens, poultry farmers often add Roxarsone, one of many drugs approved by the Food and Drug Administration, to chicken feed. Roxarsone is a chemical compound that contains arsenic and is a known carcinogen. In a study by the Institute for Agriculture and Trade Policy, it was shown that three quarters of the raw chicken breasts, thighs, and livers tested from conventional farmers have detectable levels of arsenic, compared to only one third of certified organic, or other "premium," chicken parts and whole chickens.[253] This is because organic farming requirements do not allow arsenic to be used in organic chicken feed. Instead, organic chickens are fed all-natural grains which are chemical- and pesticide-free.

American Cancer Society guidelines

The American Cancer Society publishes the *Guidelines on Nutrition and Physical Activity for Cancer* to provide recommendations to healthcare professionals and the public regarding dietary and lifestyle practices that help reduce cancer risk.[254] These guidelines are based on scientific evidence relative to the relationship between lifestyle and the risk for cancer. To formulate these guidelines, the ACS acquires results from a combination of clinical trials and observational studies, coupled with a progressive understanding of cancer biology. The ACS guidelines stress the importance of consuming a healthy diet with plenty of food from plant sources and adopting a physically active lifestyle.

Let's take a closer look at "consuming a healthy diet" and what that entails. We know that the best place to start is by consuming food that contributes to maintaining a healthy weight. To accomplish this goal we need to: know and be aware of standard serving sizes, consume smaller portions of high-calorie foods, substitute vegetables and fruits and other low-calorie foods for calorie-dense foods, and choose beverages in the amounts that help maintain a healthy weight. We should also consume five or more servings of vegetables and fruits each day, make vegetables and fruits a part of every meal, and eat different varieties. Our diets should also include whole-grain products such as rice, bread, pasta, and cereals; fish, poultry, and beans; and, on occasion, lean cuts of meat.

The American Cancer Society advises preparing meat by baking, broiling, or poaching, but advises against red meat's excessive consumption, especially in the form of cured and preserved meat. Meat that is preserved has salt added to it in the form of a mixture of sodium nitrite and sodium chloride to prevent the growth of harmful bacteria, called *Clostridium botulinum*. This organism causes botulism, or food poisoning, when we consume the contaminated meat that contains it. When cured or processed, meats are subjected to high temperatures through cooking in the form of frying, grilling, and so on. These cooking processes form certain chemical compounds called *nitrosamines* (such as nitrosopyrrolidine and dimethylnitrosamine): substances which have been found to cause cancer.

The harmful effect of nitrosamines was first discovered by accident in 1956 by two British scientists named Barnes and Magee, while they were screening chemicals for use as solvents in the dry cleaning industry. Their research reported that dimethylnitrosamine produced liver tumors in rats, and their discovery initiated a series of research studies on nitrosamine compounds.[255]

Approximately 300 nitrosamine compounds have been tested and 90% of them have been found to be carcinogenic. N-nitrosodimethylamine has been found to cause liver cancer and tobacco-specific nitrosamines have been found to cause lung cancer.[256] Studies have also linked eating large amounts of red and processed meat to an increased risk for colorectal cancer. In one large case study (a meta-analysis of 13 studies) a daily increase of 100 gm of all red meat was associated with a significant 12 to 17% increased risk of colorectal cancer, and a significant 49% increased risk was found for a daily increase of 25 gm of processed meat.[257] In another study that reviewed published cohort and case-control studies over a 20-year period, an association was also found between nitrite and nitrosamine intake and gastric cancer.[258]

According to researchers of a study conducted by the Department of Biophysics at the University of Toronto and the Ontario Cancer Institute, nitrosamines produced a high incidence of pancreatic ductular tumors in the Syrian golden hamster; the researchers of this study also reported that there appears to be a similarity between these tumors and those found in humans.[259] The risk of ovarian cancer also appears to increase for women who prefer fat, fried, cured, and smoked foods.[260] Diets rich in vegetables and fruits have been found to inhibit the mutagenic effects of such nitrosamines[261] and ascorbic acid has been shown to protect cells from nitrosamines, which damage genetic material.[262]

In terms of alcohol consumption, we are advised to limit alcohol consumption to no more than two drinks (for men) and one drink (for women) per day. One drink of alcohol is equivalent to 12 oz of beer, 5 oz of wine, or 1.5 oz of 80-proof distilled spirits.

For adults, ACS guidelines stress the importance of being physically active as well. First of all, exercise needs to be a part of our daily living. Engaging in at least 30 minutes of moderate to vigorous physical activity on five or more days a week is advised, but 45 to 60 minutes of intense physical activity is preferable. Children and adolescents are encouraged to engage in at least 60 minutes per day of moderate to vigorous physical activity five days or more per week.

Antioxidants

Antioxidants are substances that protect cells from the damage caused by unstable molecules, or free radicals. These are chemicals whose molecular, or ionic, structure includes an unpaired ("free") electron, usually conferring high reactivity in biological systems. Most free radicals contain oxygen.[263] In an effort to gain stability, a free radical looks to "steal" an electron from a nearby molecule. When the invaded molecule gives up its electron, that molecule then becomes a free radical. This causes a chain reaction, which in turn may cause cellular disruption. Types of biologically significant free radicals include hydroxyl, peroxyl, superoxide, nitric oxide, and singlet oxygen radicals.

Free radicals and other reactive oxygen species are derived either from normal essential metabolic processes in the human body or through exposure to the environment. *Oxidation* is also a natural chemical reaction and a necessary component of many processes that take place within the body and in the environment. A car fender that rusts, a copper pipe that turns green, or a banana that turns brown are all examples of the natural oxidation process that occurs in the environment. When the oxidation process occurs in the body, however, even though it may be part of a normal chain of events, it can become harmful when it produces free radicals or reactive oxygen species. This is because in an attempt to gain stability, the free radicals attempt to acquire electrons or donate them to surrounding tissues, and this results in damage to the tissues themselves.

In the body free radicals form in the following ways:

- Free radicals are byproducts of the continuous respiratory and energy-producing processes
- Free radicals are used by the immune system to kill invading organisms
- Free radicals are generated in biological reactions involving trace metals (iron, chromium, cobalt etc.)
- Free radicals increase the generation of other free radicals
- Free radicals develop from cellular injury during the inflammatory process

When free radicals are unchecked, they disrupt and damage proteins, carbohydrates, fats, and DNA. Their destructive effects contribute to many diseases, such as arthritis, cataracts, heart disease, and cancer. If we can render free radicals inactive by supplying our body with antioxidants, we may ultimately live longer and healthier lives.

Certain external sources are also known to give rise to free radicals, including cigarette smoke, radiation, chemicals (drugs, pesticides, and industrial solvents), ultraviolet light, environmental pollutants, and ozone.

A healthy body can handle exposure to free radicals, both on the inside and from the outside. But when too many free radicals are produced and too few antioxidants are available, a condition known as "oxidative stress" develops. This is the way long-term cellular damage occurs. It is therefore worth noting that although free radicals are implicated in a number of health problems, numerous studies have also shown that antioxidants boast protective effects relative to these same health problems. Confirmation of this fact can be found in a report by the Institute of Medicine's Panel on Dietary Antioxidants and Related Compounds, which states, "a dietary antioxidant is a substance in foods that significantly decreases the adverse effects of reactive oxygen species, reactive nitrogen species, or both, on normal physiological function in humans."[264]

More on the antioxidant and free-radical connection

Antioxidant compounds decrease the adverse effects of free radicals in two ways. The first way is through antioxidant molecules that are generally stable enough to donate an electron to an out-of-control free radical. In donating this electron, the antioxidant neutralizes the free radical and prevents any further damage. Simply put, it is the antioxidant's job to scavenge free radicals and convert them into a harmless form which can then be excreted by the body. This process is does not utilize enzymes and is therefore referred to as the non-enzymatic process of inactivating a free radical.

The second way in which antioxidants offset the effects of free radicals is through enzymes, or enzymatic systems, including glutathione peroxidase, superoxide dismutase, and catalase, that decrease the concentrations of destructive oxidants in tissue. Here is the way it works. First, superoxide dismutase converts two superoxides into hydrogen peroxide and oxygen. Then, catalase breaks down the hydrogen peroxide into water and oxygen. Finally, glutathione peroxidase (like catalase) breaks down the hydrogen peroxide and reduces the organic peroxides to alcohols. This provides another route for the elimination of toxic oxidants from the body.[265] The following is a list of some of the plants and other compounds that have antioxidant properties and help counteract free radical damage.

Alpha-lipoic acid is manufactured in the body and is the only antioxidant that is both fat- and water-soluble. This means that it is easily absorbed and transported across cell membranes, providing protection against free-radical damage both inside and outside the cells.

Beta-carotene is a member of a class of substances known as carotenoids. As we know, carotenoids are the chemicals and principal pigments responsible for the red, orange, yellow, and green colors of vegetables and fruits. Similar to the other carotenoids, beta-carotene is a natural fat-soluble pigment found principally in plants. Converted by the body into vitamin A, it acts as a powerful antioxidant and helps support the immune system.

Bilberry. Native to Northern Europe and a cousin to the blueberry, bilberry has been used for centuries, both medicinally and as a food in jams and pies. Bilberry fruit also contains plant pigments, known as anthocyanosides, which have excellent antioxidant properties.

Burdock. Burdock is not only native to Europe and Northern Asia, but is now widespread throughout the United States, where it grows as a weed. In Japan and parts of Europe burdock is cultivated as a vegetable. Burdock consists primarily of carbohydrates, volatile oils, plant sterols, tannins, and fatty oils. Although researchers still aren't sure which of its active ingredients are responsible for its healing properties, this herb is believed to have anti-inflammatory, antioxidant, and antibacterial effects.

Carnosine is another naturally occurring dipeptide with a number of actions. A potent antioxidant, carnosine helps to flush toxins from the body, has immune-boosting properties, and is known to reduce and prevent cell damage caused by beta-amyloid, the peptide found in the brain of Alzheimer's patients. Recent evidence even suggests that carnosine may have an important role in the sense of smell. Carnosine is currently being studied for its part in preventing glycosylation, a long-term complication of diabetes, as well as cataracts, neuropathy, kidney failure, and skin conditions.

Catalase is also produced naturally within the body. Within cells, the major function of catalase is to prevent the accumulation of toxic levels of hydrogen peroxide, formed as a byproduct of metabolic processes, by converting it into water and oxygen. It also helps break down potentially harmful toxins in the body, including alcohol, phenol, and formaldehyde.

Conjugated linoleic acid (CLA) is a natural polyunsaturated fatty acid found in many foods, including milk, cheese, and meats, particularly beef. Once inside the body, CLA is absorbed by phospholipids. These are fats that serve as the principal structural components of cell membranes and act as a strong antioxidant, providing a defense mechanism against free radicals.

Coenzyme Q10 has a structure similar to that of vitamin K and is a fat-soluble quinine. CoQ plays an important role in the production of energy in the mitochondria of the cell. CoQ's reduced form, ubiquinol, also serves as an antioxidant. Ubiquinol inhibits lipid peroxidation in biological membranes and in low-density lipoprotein (LDL), and also protects membrane proteins against oxidative damage.

Cryptoxanthin is a natural caretinoid pigment that is converted to vitamin A (retinol). As with other carotenoids, cryptoxanthin is an antioxidant, which not only helps prevent free-radical damage to cells and DNA, but also stimulates repair of already damaged DNA.

Curcumin is the principal curcuminoid of the Indian curry spice called turmeric and is part of the ginger family. Curcuminoids are polyphenols, and give turmeric its yellow color. The curcumin in turmeric supplies its earthy, bitter, peppery flavor. Curcumin is reported to inhibit fat peroxidation and DNA damage.

Daidzein. Isoflavones have potent antioxidant effects to counteract the damaging effects of free radicals. Besides functioning as antioxidants, many isoflavones can compete with estrogen for the same receptor sites and, as a result, produce nonhormonal effects.

Dehydroepiandrosterone (DHEA) is a steroid produced by our adrenal glands in varying quantities as we age. The adrenal glands convert the DHEA to the major sex hormones, estrogen and testosterone. DHEA is the only hormone to decline with age in both sexes. DHEA has been shown to have an inhibitory effect on free radical generation.

Garlic *(Allium sativum)* is actually a species of the onion family and has been used throughout history for both culinary and medicinal purposes. Garlic contains antioxidant phytochemicals, including unique water-soluble organosulfur compounds, lipid-soluble organosulfur components, flavonoids, and allicin, which prevent oxidative damage.

Ginkgo (ginkgo biloba) Ginkgo is one of the oldest living tree species in the world. Because of its ability to treat a variety of ailments and conditions, its leaves continue to be among the most extensively studied botanicals today. Ginkgo leaves are consumed most often in the form of a concentrated, standardized ginkgo biloba extract (GBE), and in Europe and the United States this condensed version is among one of the best-selling herbal supplements. Ginkgo leaves contain a variety of phytochemicals, including flavonoids and terpenoids, which have potent antioxidant properties.

Grape seed has shown nutritional and medicinal value throughout history from ancient Greece to European folk healers. Polyphenols and resveratrol are some of the powerful antioxidants found in grape seed. Grape seed extract has been shown to treat a wide range of health conditions caused by free radical damage.

Green tea is manufactured from fresh, unfermented tea leaves, thus providing an abundance of polyphenols, notably catechins. Catechins are powerful, water-soluble antioxidants. Recent evidence suggests regular green-tea drinkers may have a lower risk of developing heart disease and certain types of cancer. Green tea is also claimed to be useful for weight loss management.

Genistein is another isoflavone found in plants, specifically soybeans and soybean products. Genistein not only acts as an antioxidant, but also plays a predominant role as a tyrosine kinase inhibitor, the enzyme involved in cell growth and proliferation. Genistein is currently being explored for its potential benefits in chemotherapy treatment.

Germanium. Small amounts of organic germanium are found in some plant-based foods, and inorganic germanium is mined and widely used as a semiconductor in the electronics industry due to its ability to transport electrons. Geranium appears to plays a role as an oxygen catalyst, antioxidant, electro-stimulant, and immune enhancer.

Glutathione. Produced in the human liver, glutathione is a small protein composed of three amino acids, cysteine, glutamic acid, and glycine. Its antioxidant properties are found in the human lungs and many other organ systems and tissues.

Lutein (from the Latin *lutea*, meaning "yellow") is one of over 600 known, naturally occurring carotenoids. It is found in green, leafy vegetables, such as spinach and kale, and is a well-known antioxidant.

Lycopene, another carotenoid supplying the red pigment to fruits and vegetables, is present in human serum, liver, adrenal glands, lungs, prostate, colon, and in the skin in high levels. Lycopene has been shown to possess antioxidant and antiproliferative properties. Fruits and vegetables that are high in lycopene include tomatoes, watermelon, pink grapefruit, and guava.

Manganese acts as a cofactor and catalyst in many enzymatic processes, such as hydrolysis, phosphorylation, and transamination. Manganese is required in several metalo-enzymatic reactions, such as manganese superoxide dismutase (MnSOD), a metalloenzyme used to resolve free radicals by protecting the mitochondria during cellular respiration. Manganese is involved in the health and maintenance of ligaments and tendons and is essential to the synthesis of connective tissue.

Melatonin, a hormone found in all living creatures, plays a role in the regulation of the circadian rhythm of several biological functions, with the particular role of protecting nuclear and mitochondrial DNA. Melatonin is known as a potent scavenger of free radicals.

Methionine is a sulfur-containing essential amino acid. Methionine belongs to a group of compounds called lipotropics, which aid the liver to process fat in the body. Besides fat metabolization, it has been shown that a variety of oxidants react readily with methionine to form methionine sulfoxide, and that methionine residues are efficient reactive oxygen scavengers.

Oligomeric proanthocyanidin (OPC) is a class of flavonoids found in the skin and seeds of grapes and in pine bark. OPCs act as antioxidants in the human body.

Para-aminobenzoic acid (PABA) is considered as part of the B-complex vitamin family. As an antioxidant, PABA provides protection against ozone, smoking, and other air pollutants that can damage other cell structures through oxidative stress. PABA has been utilized extensively as a sunscreen in topical lotions to protect the skin from harmful ultraviolet radiation upon exposure to the sun.

Quercetin is a type of plant-based flavonoid shown to have anti-inflammatory and antioxidant properties. Quercetin has been shown to act as an antihistamine, reducing the inflammatory process. In studies done in cell cultures, quercetin has been found effective against some types of cancer cells.

Selenium is another trace mineral essential to good health, but required in only small amounts. Selenium is incorporated into proteins to make selenoproteins, important antioxidant enzymes.

Superoxide dismutase appears in three forms in humans: SOD1, located in the cytoplasm and in the mitochondrial intermembrane space; SOD2, found in the mitochondrial matrix; and SOD3, which occurs extracellularly. This enzyme metabolizes superoxide radicals to molecular oxygen and hydrogen peroxide, thus providing a defense against oxygen toxicity.[266]

Vitamin C (ascorbic acid) cannot be made by the human body and can only be obtained through the diet or supplementation. It is required for synthesizing collagen, tendons, ligaments, and bone, and plays an important role in synthesizing the neurotransmitter norepinephrine. Vitamin C is a water-soluble antioxidant and protects the proteins, lipids (fats), carbohydrates, and nucleic acids (DNA and RNA) of the body from damage.

Vitamin E is a fat-soluble antioxidant existing in eight chemical forms (alpha-, beta-, gamma-, and delta-tocopherol and alpha-, beta-, gamma-, and delta-tocotrienol). Each form has varying levels of biological activity. Alpha-tocopherol is the form that is most commonly absorbed and found in the largest quantities in the blood and tissue. Vitamin E is uniquely suited to inhibit production of ROS, or reactive oxygen species, formed when fat undergoes oxidation. Alpha-tocopherol is known to inhibit the activity of protein kinase C, an enzyme involved in cell proliferation. Vitamin E is an important cell-signaling molecule involved in the activity of the immune system and modulation of the inflammatory response. Nuts, seeds, vegetable oils, and green, leafy vegetables are among the best sources of vitamin E.

Zeaxanthin also acts as an antioxidant. It belongs to the carotenoid group, of which fruits and vegetables are the most important sources. Carotenoids can be subdivided into carotenes and xanthophylls. Zeaxanthin, a xanthophyll, is the most common carotenoid alcohol found in nature, and it is this compound which gives corn, saffron, paprika, and many other plants their unique color. High concentrations of this compound can be found in the macular portion of the eye's retina; it has been shown to be crucial for good eye health by offering protection against ultraviolet damage, macular degeneration, cataracts, and glaucoma.

Zinc is an essential trace element on which numerous aspects of cellular metabolism depend. Zinc has an important role in the body's growth and development, the immune response, neurological function, and reproduction. On the cellular level, the function of zinc can be divided into three categories: catalytic, structural, and regulatory. In its catalytic role, nearly 100 different enzymes depend on zinc for their ability to catalyze vital chemical reactions, and it has been shown that the activity of antioxidant enzymes is enhanced to counteract oxidative stress in the presence of zinc. In its structural role, zinc is an important component of proteins and cell membranes. In its regulatory role, zinc has been found to bind to DNA and influence the transcription of specific genes, to participate in cell signaling, and to influence hormone release and nerve impulse transmission.

In 2002, researchers analyzed the various antioxidants present in the plants that constitute part of our recommended dietary intake. Their results, published in the Journal of Nutrition, lists the following foods as the best sources of antioxidants:[267]

- *Berries:* dog rose, crowberry, blackberry, black currant, sour cherry, strawberry, blueberry, cranberry, raspberry, cloudberry and rowanberry
- *Fruits:* pomegranate, grape, orange, plum, pineapple, lemon, dates, kiwi, clementine, and grapefruit
- *Legumes:* broad beans, pinto beans, and soybeans
- *Nuts, seeds, and dried fruit:* walnuts, sunflower seeds, apricots, and prunes
- *Vegetables:* kale, chili pepper, red cabbage, peppers, parsley, artichoke, Brussels sprouts, and spinach
- *Cereals:* barley, millet, oats, and corn
- *Roots and tubers:* ginger and red beets

Several studies have revealed the therapeutic value of antioxidants in cancer prevention. For example, dietary intake of beta-carotene and lutein/zeaxanthin has been inversely associated with the risk of renal cell carcinoma,[268] and indole-3-Carbinol (I3C), a specific compound found in cruciferous vegetables (like broccoli, cabbage and cauliflower) has been found to play a role as a chemopreventative agent in breast cancer. In one particular study involving women with an increased risk for breast cancer, it was found that Indole-3-Carbinol expressed itself as a chemopreventive agent through its estrogen-receptor modifying effect.[269]

Other studies have concluded that ornithine decarboxylase, a key regulating enzyme for the synthesis of polyamines, essential for cell proliferation, can be activated by viruses, oncogenes, or carcinogens,[270] and that curcumin, a major active component of the food flavoring turmeric (*curcuma longa*), exhibits anticarcinogenic properties *in vivo*. In this case, research from the University of Texas MD Anderson Cancer Center revealed that the growth inhibitory effect of curcumin against several breast tumor cell lines was correlated with its inhibition of ornithine decarboxylase activity.[271] Quercetin, a flavonoid phytochemical, has also been shown to have anti-cancer properties through its ability to regulate cell cycles, interact with type II estrogen binding sites, and inhibit the action of tyrosine kinase.[272]

Lycopene is yet another phytochemical with anticancer properties. This bright red pigment found in tomatoes and other red fruits has been shown to protect lipoproteins (the "packages" in which cholesterol travels through the blood) and cell walls, the outer portions of the cells, which regulate water, nutrients, and waste products inside and outside the cell. Carotenoids like lycopene are highly lipophilic, which means they have the ability to dissolve in or mix with lipids; carotenoids are commonly found within these lipid components. Researchers contend that the ability of carotenoids to scavenge free radicals may be greatest in a lipophilic environment,[273] and that purified lycopene decreases DNA oxidative damage.[274]

There are increasing numbers of studies that also reveal the beneficial effects of vitamins. Vitamin C, for example, has been documented for its antioxidant properties as well as for its ability to enhance components of the immune system, such as antimicrobial and natural killer cell activities, lymphocyte proliferation, chemotaxis, and delayed-type hypersensitivity.[275] Vitamin E has also been studied for its association to bladder cancer mortality. In one study among 991,552 U.S. adults in the Cancer Prevention Study II, it was found that regular vitamin E supplementation for 10 years or more was in fact a factor in reducing the risk of death from bladder cancer.[276] Vitamin E is also known to block the formation of nitrosamines from nitrites consumed in the diet, and to protect against some cancers due to its ability to enhance immune function.[277] Other less well-known compounds have also been shown to have anticancer effects, such as alphalipoic acid, an antioxidant that protects against oxidative stress and induces apoptosis in hepatoma cells, suggesting that it may prove useful in liver cancer therapy.[278]

The amino acid L-arginine is another compound that has numerous functions in the body and has been found to block the formation and development of colorectal tumors;[279] wheat germ extract (under the brand name Avemar®) has been shown to inhibit growth and induce apoptosis in human lymphoma cells;[280] and ginger, the underground stem, or rhizome, of the plant *Zingiber officinale*, has been used as a medicine in Indian, Asian, and Arabic herbal traditions for hundreds of years. In one study, ginger was found to inhibit growth and modify secretion of angiogenic factors in ovarian cancer cells.[281]

In another study conjugated linoleic acid (CLA), a compound found in meat and dairy products, was shown to induce apoptosis of preneoplastic lesions and inhibit angiogenic factors in mammary cancer. The authors of this study contend that CLA may be an excellent candidate for prevention of breast cancer.[282]

The ORAC method

The different methods that exist to measure the antioxidant capacity of foods and supplements are oxygen radical absorbance capacity (ORAC), ferric ion reducing power (FRAP), and trolox equivalent antioxidant capacity (TEAC).[283] The most popular method is the ORAC determination, developed by the National Institutes of Health, which tests a variety of foods. This method has shown that certain spices, nuts, berries, and legumes rate very highly in antioxidant content. Increased consumption of high-antioxidant fruits and vegetables has been clinically correlated with significantly increased plasma, or "total ORAC" value.[284]

In a report published by The Organic Center for Education and Promotion at Tufts University, scientists have reported that most Americans consume between 1,200 and 1,600 ORAC units per day, less than a third of the preliminary goal for optimal antioxidant activity of 3,000 to 5,000 units.[285] In an effort to assign foods a unit value based on antioxidant capacity, the USDA has established a system using serving size per gram as a baseline. In this system, food groups are rated "very high," "high," "moderate," and "low." The rating of "high" means that foods contain antioxidants in the range of 3,000 to 5,000 units. Using this system, someone who consumes foods in this range—that is, high in antioxidant potential—needs to devote only about 60 calories a day, or just 3% of a typical 2,000-calorie-per-day diet, to their consumption. On the other hand, those who choose only "low-antioxidant" foods require much more, about 312 calories per day, of these foods, again based on a typical 2,000-calorie-per-day diet, and in order to reach the ORAC unit goal of 5,000 units or 15% of daily caloric intake.[285]

Shown in Table 4-23 are the ORAC values for 100 common food items (per 100 gm, or 3.5 oz) consumed by the U.S. population, including fruits, vegetables, nuts, seeds, spices, and grains.

TABLE 4-23. ORAC values of commonly consumed food items (per 100 gm, or 3.5 oz) in U.S. population. (Source: *http://www.ars.usda.gov/sp2userfiles/place/12354500/data/orac/orac07.pdf.*) 2007.

Food	ORAC Value	Food	ORAC Value
Spices, cloves, ground	314446	Spices, paprika	17919
Sumac, bran, raw	312400	Chokeberry, raw	16062
Spices, cinnamon, ground	267536	Tarragon, fresh	15542
Sorghum, bran, high tannin	240000	Ginger root, raw	14840
Spices, oregano, dried	200129	Elderberries, raw	14697
Spices, turmeric, ground	159277	Sorghum, grain, red	14000
Sorghum, bran, black	100800	Peppermint, fresh	13978
Sumac, grain, raw	86800	Oregano, fresh	13970
Cocoa, dry powder, unsweetened	80933	Nuts, walnuts, English	13541
Spices, cumin seed	76800	Nuts, hazelnuts or filberts	9645
Spices, parsley, dried	74349	Cranberries, raw	9584
Sorghum, bran, red	71000	Pears, dried, 40% moisture (Italian)	9496
Spices, basil, dried	67553	Savory, fresh	9465
Baking chocolate, unsweetened, squares	49926	Artichokes, boiled	9416
Spices, curry powder	48504	Artichokes, microwaved	9402
Sorghum, grain, high tannin	45400	Chocolate, Dutch powdered	40200
Apples, Golden Delicious, raw, with skin	2670	Beans, kidney, red, mature seeds, raw	8459
Sage, fresh	32004	Beans, pink, mature seeds, raw	8320
Spices, mustard seed, yellow	29257	Beans, black, mature seeds, raw	8040
Spices, ginger, ground	28811	Nuts, pistachio, raw	7983
Spices, pepper, black	27618	Currants, European black, raw	7960
Thyme, fresh	27426	Beans, pinto, mature seeds, raw	7779
Marjoram, fresh	27297	Plums, black diamond, with peel, raw	7581
Rice bran, crude	24287	Candies, milk chocolate	7528
Spices, chili powder	23636	Lentils, raw	7282
Candies, semisweet chocolate	18053	Apples, Red Delicious, raw, with skin	4275
Nuts, pecans	17940	Agave, dried (Southwest)	7274
Apples, dried, 40% moisture (Italian)	6681	Raisins, white, dried, 40% moisture (Italian)	4188

(continued on next page)

Spices, garlic powder	6665	Baby food, fruit, applesauce, strained	4123
Artichokes, globe or French, raw	6552	Apples, Granny Smith, raw, with skin	3898
Blueberries, raw	6552	Dates, deglet noor	3895
Plums, dried (prunes), uncooked	6552	Strawberries, raw	3577
Beans, black turtle soup; mature seeds, raw	6416	Peanut butter, smooth style, with salt	3432
Sorghum, bran, white	6400	Currants, red, raw	3387
Chocolate syrup	6330	Figs, raw	3383
Plums, raw	6259	Cherries, sweet, raw	3365
Baby food, fruit, peaches	6257	Gooseberries, raw	3277
Lemon balm, leaves, raw	5997	Apricots, dried, 40% moisture (Italy)	3234
Soybeans, mature seeds, raw	5764	Peanuts, all types, raw	3166
Spices, onion powder	5735	Cabbage, red, boiled, drained, without salt	3145
Blackberries, raw	5347	Broccoli raab, raw	3083
Garlic, raw	5346	Apples, raw, with skin	3082
Coriander (cilantro) leaves, raw	5141	Raisins, seedless	3037
Alcoholic beverage, wine, table, red	5034	Pears, raw	2941
Raspberries, raw	4882	Agave, cooked (Southwest)	2938
Baby food; fruit, apple and blueberry	4822	Apples, Red Delicious, raw, without skin	2936
Basil, fresh	4805	Juice, blueberry	2906
Nuts, almonds	4454	Apples, Gala, raw, with skin	2828
Dill weed, fresh	4392	Spices, cardamom	2764
Cowpeas, common (blackeyes, crowder, southern); mature seeds, raw	4343		

Tea

For almost 50 centuries people have been brewing tea. After water, tea is now the second most popular beverage consumed on a global scale. Tea comes from the tea plant *Camellia sinensis*, a plant with dark, glossy green leaves. The finest teas currently come from five countries: India, China, Sri Lanka, Japan, and Taiwan.

Interesting stories abound about how the goodness of this varied beverage was discovered. The first is a Chinese legend crediting the discovery of tea to Shen Nung, or the "Divine Farmer," the legendary Emperor of China, about 5,000 years ago. The Emperor, considered the founder of agriculture and all Chinese medicine, was well known for his love of travel. During Shen Nung's travels he preferred to boil his water before drinking to purify it. Chinese legend has it that Shen Nung first tasted tea when one day a leaf from a wild tea bush landed in his boiled water. Curious about its taste, the Emperor took a sip and immediately appreciated its flavor. The Chinese credit Shen Nung with identifying hundreds of medicinal— and poisonous—herbs by personally testing their properties.

Another tea story tells us about Bodhidharma, the Buddhist monk from southern India and founder of the Chan school of Buddhism, who took a journey to China. Angry with himself for constantly dropping off to sleep while meditating, it is said Bodhidharma decided to inflict self-punishment by cutting off his eyelids. Legend says that tea bushes sprung from the places where his eyelids fell. Yet a third story tells us that Gautama Buddha, or Siddhartha, the spiritual teacher from ancient India and the founder of Buddhism, discovered tea after some leaves fell into a vessel of boiling water and its taste was enjoyed. Wherever the truth lies, the fact remains that China is considered the birthplace of tea drinking, with records of its consumption as far back as 1,000 B.C.

Tea was routinely used as a medicine when the Han Dynasty, which lasted for more than 400 years (206 B.C. through 220 A.D.), ruled China. The Han Dynasty is thought to be one of the greatest periods in Chinese history. Records show that tea became a social drink during the Tang Dynasty (618 to 907 A.D.), but during this time the preparation and processing of tea was quite different from most present methods. Tea leaves in the Tang Dynasty were made into cakes and then dried. Subsequent bricks of tea were ground into a powder in a stone mortar, and then hot water was added. Sometimes powdered tea cakes were boiled in earthenware kettles prior to consumption.

During the Song Dynasty (960 to 1279 A.D.), tea's processing and production underwent a two-fold change, where the Chinese began to pick and steam the tea leaves immediately to retain their color and freshness and tea-drinking became more of a popular ceremonial and social event. Powdered tea and ceramic ware became hallmarks of the Song tea ceremonies, and Japanese monks visiting China during this period returned home with both the tea and the ceremony in hand. Ironically, the ceremonial aspect of drinking tea became nearly extinct in China, but ultimately evolved into the present-day Japanese tea ceremony. The Song tea period also saw the birth of white-tea varieties, such as Palace Jade Sprout and Silver Silk Water Sprout. To produce these types of paper-thin white tea, tea buds are picked from bushes or wild tea trees in early spring and steamed immediately. After steaming, the outer unopened leaf is discarded and the delicate inner part is reserved and then rinsed in spring water and dried.

In the mid-13th century, tea's processing methods evolved where tea leaves were roasted and then crumbled instead of being steamed. During this period extraordinary trade and cultural exchanges between the Chinese and the Japanese Samurai society took place. Tea seeds were imported from China and the Japanese began cultivation. As tea continued to grow in popularity, green tea became a common beverage among people in high society. Soon, in the 16th century, imported tea was introduced into Europe and quickly became popular. Today, automation has taken over, contributing to improved quality control and reduced labor costs. Although tea has undergone many changes throughout history, its pleasures and benefits continue, enough so that many people would agree with the ancient Chinese saying, "Better to be deprived of food for three days than of tea for one."

Tea has a slightly bitter, astringent, but very pleasant taste in most cases. Teas are a rich source of polyphenolic flavonoid compounds, which exhibit strong antioxidant effects both in humans (*in vivo*) and in cell culture studies performed in the lab (*in vitro*). The flavonoid concentration of tea depends on the type of tea—whether it is blended, decaffeinated, or instant, and its preparation—the amount used, time brewed, and temperature. Highest concentrations of flavonoids can be found in brewed hot tea at 541–692 µg/ml. Instant preparations have about 90–100 µg/ml, and iced and ready-to-drink teas have the lowest concentration. Tea is also a natural source of theophylline, a methylxanthine, as is the caffeine in coffee and the theobromine in chocolate. Tea contains the stimulant caffeine as well, which constitutes 3% of the dry weight and up to 40 mg per 8-oz cup of prepared black tea.

Catechins, the antioxidants in teas, constitute about 30% of a tea's dry weight. Catechins are particularly high in white and green teas. This concentration is less in decaffeinated tea due to the decaffeinating process it undergoes. The different catechin compounds include epicatechin (EC), epicatechin-3-gallate (E3G), epigallocatechin (EGC), and epigallocatechin-3-gallate (EGCG). As an antioxidant, EGCG is about 25 to 100 times more potent than vitamin E or vitamin C. Green tea and black tea differ in their chemical content of catechins, where black tea contains a lower concentration due to oxidation during the fermentation process. A cup of green tea prepared at the right temperature contains about 0.5–1.0 gm of catechins per liter (0.5–1.0 gm/33.8 oz), and black tea contains about one third this value.

Catechins have various physiological effects, and there is considerable evidence to support the versatile role they play in protecting against different types of cancer. For example, most tumor promoters inhibit cellular communication and increase cytotoxicity. In one study, for example, researchers showed that catechins may confer their protective effects by antagonizing these qualities.[286] The compounds in tea have been shown to contain a variety of functions, including behaving as antioxidants, antimutagenics,[287] and antihypertensives.[288] Tea has been shown to reduce the risk for many cancers, noticeably colon and rectal cancer,[289] liver cancer,[290] skin cancer,[291] breast cancer,[292] brain tumors,[293] and distal gastric cancer (in women).[294] Tea has also been found to have an antibacterial effect, where frequent consumption of black tea may significantly decrease dental cavity formation even in the presence of sugars in the diet.[295]

Epigallocatechin, the main polyphenol in green tea, has been shown to exhibit anti-angiogenic and anti-metastatic activity, and to inhibit gelatinases, the enzymes involved in breaking down gelatin into subcompounds to be used by the cells.[296] Green tea catechins have also been shown to inhibit the human cytochrome, P450, an endogenous multienzyme complex which is reported to mediate the metabolic activation of procarcinogens into carcinogens.[297] Tea polyphenols have also been found to induce prostate cancer cell death[298] and leukemia cell death.[299]

Tea classifications

Tea is normally classified into different types based on the extent of fermentation (oxidation) to which the leaves have been subjected, and on its quality, preparation methods, and processing. Below are some of the more popular types of teas consumed throughout the world:

White tea. White tea is one of the most expensive varieties of tea. New buds of young leaves are picked and the outer leaf cover is discarded. These buds are protected from sunlight and hence do not have the plant pigment chlorophyll that ordinarily imparts the color. White tea is produced in lesser quantities, but is distributed in many countries, thanks to the advent of tea bags in the early 1900s.

Green tea. Tea leaves undergo minimal oxidation in this variety. Oxidation is arrested by heating the leaves with steam- or dry-cooking in hot pans. The leaves are then left to dry and separate, or are rolled into tiny pellets, called gunpowder tea. The processing of green tea is accomplished within one or two days of harvesting.

Oolong tea. Oolong tea is very popular in China and is processed to result in a tea somewhere between green and black tea. Due to variations in processing, oxidation can range anywhere between 10 and 70%.

Black tea/red tea. In black and red teas, leaves are oxidized completely. This process takes about two weeks to a month. This is the most common form of tea in southern Asia (India, Sri Lanka, Bangladesh, and Pakistan), African countries, Europe, and North America. Black tea may be further classified as orthodox, or CTC—"crush/tear/curl"—based on the method of production.

Pu'erh. Pu'erh tea is also known as *pou lei* (pronounced po-lee) in Cantonese. Pu'erh teas come in two forms: raw/green (*sheng*), or ripened/cooked (*shou*). This "large-leaf" tea is named after the Pu'erh County near Simao, Yunnan, China. Pu'erh may be harvested young, or aged until it is highly mature, and can be drunk immediately or after many years of aging. Today, Pu'erh teas are often classified by year and region of production in the same way that wine is often described. Pu'erh teas are compressed into various shapes, such as bricks, discs, bowls, squares, or mushrooms. Compression of the tea ensures that its quality will remain intact for a long time. People have been known to keep raw Pu'erh up to 30 to 50 years, while ripened Pu'erh can be kept for 10 to 15 years.

Yellow tea. A special kind of tea, yellow tea is processed similarly to green tea. The difference is in a slower drying process, where the damp tea leaves are allowed to sit and yellow. This is a nonfermented, nonoxidized tea. It is also similar in taste to green tea, but the additional step results in the finished tea leaves' natural light-yellow color.

Kukicha. Kukicha, made from the stems, stalks, and twigs of the tea plant during the dormant season, are dry-roasted over a fire. Kukicha is also called "winter tea" and is a popular health beverage in Japan.

Genmaicha. Genmaicha is a green tea blended with dry-roasted brown rice, sometimes called "popcorn tea" because a few grains of rice pop during the roasting process. This tea was originally consumed by the poor in Japan, where the rice served as a filler to reduce the price of tea, but today it is enjoyed by everyone.

Flower tea. Flower tea varieties are processed or brewed with actual flowers. The tea varieties are either green or red, but the flowers for each variety are specific. For example, in jasmine tea, jasmine flowers are brewed with green or oolong tea. Roses, lotuses, lychees, and chrysanthemums are also widely used flowers in this tea's preparation.

Approximately 76 to 78% of the tea produced and consumed throughout the world is black, 20 to 22% is green, and less than 2% is oolong.[300] Almost all the tea bags currently sold are blends of various teas. Tea traders mix the different varieties of tea to maintain the flavor, aroma, and, most importantly, the price of the tea over a period of time.

Tea's therapeutic benefits

Some of the therapeutic effects of tea have been extrapolated from laboratory studies using cell cultures. Tea's principal beneficial effects arise from the antioxidant properties of its polyphenols.[301] Tea polyphenols enhance antioxidant enzyme activity (of glutathione peroxidase, catalase, quinone reductase, phase II glutathione-S-transferase, and others) as well as intercellular communication.[302] Polyphenolic compounds found in tea have also been shown to chelate transition metal ions like iron and copper to prevent their participation in harmful chemical reactions.[303]

Studies confirm that the total antioxidant capacity of green tea is greater than black tea[304] and that green tea is quickly absorbed into the bloodstream, revealing peak increases in plasma at 40 minutes after ingestion.[305] Green tea has been shown to decrease oxidative DNA damage, lipid peroxidation, and free radical generation in both smokers and non-smokers,[306] and green tea catechins have been found to enhance exercise-induced loss of abdominal fat and improve circulating triglyceride levels when 625mg/day is consumed.[307] Consumption of more than three cups per day of both black and green has revealed a 21% lower risk of stroke as compared to results when less than one cup per day is consumed.[308] Furthermore, acute ingestion of green tea extract has been shown not only to increase fat oxidation during moderate-intensity exercise, but to improve insulin sensitivity and glucose tolerance as well.[309]

In addition to all its anticancer effects, tea has also been found to play a potential role in the promotion of oral health, thermogenesis, bone health, and cognitive function. If you add milk to tea you will lower the concentration of flavonoids per serving, but you can always compensate by increasing the size of the serving.

As you can see, a large body of scientific evidence is available to substantiate the fact that tea is very important in our daily lives, most significantly due to its capacity as a potent antioxidant and its ability to maintain cell integrity, prevent DNA damage, and curb the growth of cancer cells.

Tea brewing

The most appropriate way to brew tea is to place the loose tea in a teapot or tea infuser, a device designed to function like a tea bag. The temperature of brewing depends on the type of tea. Green tea, which is barely oxidized, tastes best when brewed in water at temperatures around 80°C or 176°F, while black tea is best brewed at 100°C or 212°F.

Black tea. To brew black tea, warm the pot in which you intend to brew the tea by rinsing it slightly with warm water. The temperature of water best suited to brew black tea is

100°C, or 212°F. Once the water starts boiling, steep the tea in the water. Black tea is best brewed for 30 seconds to five minutes. Brewing the tea for a longer period results in the release of tannins, astringent plant compounds, which contribute to bitter-tasting stewed tea. If you're looking for a "wake-up" tea in the morning, don't let it steep for more than two to three minutes. Brew it, strain it, and serve.

Green tea. Heat the water to around 80°C to 85°C (176°F to 185°F). Temperature in this case is inversely proportional to the quality of the tea leaves; this means that the better the quality of tea, the lower the temperature required. If the heated water is too hot it will produce a bitter taste because the green tea leaves will be overheated.

Oolong tea. Brew oolong tea at a temperature between 90°C to 100°C (194°F to 212°F). Warm your brewing vessel before pouring in the water. Traditionally, brown clay Yixing teapots have been considered the best type of brewing vessels for oolong tea. Due to its pure taste and mineral content, spring water is recommended to generate cups of this flavorful tea.

Tea additives

Some of us like tea straight, with nothing added. Others add flavors like sugar, honey, lemon, milk, or fruit jams. Milk, for example, reduces the tannin content and neutralizes the tea's acidity; white sugar, honey, and fruit jams add sweetener. The correct order to preparing one's tea is to brew the tea, then add sugar, then milk. In cold regions, such as Mongolia and Nepal, the inhabitants add butter to the tea as a means of creating caloric content and resulting in more like a rich broth than a brew. I've heard that you have to acquire a taste for it; admittedly it may not be everyone's "cup of tea"!

Sugar substitutes

Most people I know can't resist the taste of sweets. You know the ones I'm talking about—the piece of cake, the cookies, or the chocolate bar that is so hard to pass up. In fact, I know some people who would prefer to skip meals altogether and go straight for the dessert. But in excess the sugar contained in these foods can take its toll on the body. Eating large amounts of sugar adds extra calories, for example, which can cause blood sugar problems and weight gain over time.

To avoid consuming large amounts of sugar on a daily basis, many people have turned to artificial sweeteners as low-calorie alternatives. Artificial sweeteners are sugar substitutes that provide the sweet taste of sugar, but supply few, if any, calories. Artificial sweeteners are much sweeter than sugar, and generally lesser amounts are needed to provide the equivalent sweetness of sugar. There are two types of sugar substitutes used in the foods we eat: nonalcoholic (artificial sweeteners) and sugar alcohols. Nonalcoholic sweeteners do not add calories to food; sugar alcohols, on the other hand, do contain calories, but fewer than sugar.

Sugar alcohols are found naturally in foods, such as fruits and vegetables. Because they can be found in nature, they are considered natural sugar substitutes; however, they are neither sugar nor alcohols. Sugar alcohols are actually carbohydrates with a chemical structure that partially resembles sugar and partially resembles alcohol, minus the ethanol that alcoholic beverages contain. Sugar alcohols contain from one to three calories per gram and are used to replace the higher calorie corn syrup found in many food products. Sugar alcohols are sometimes combined with artificial sweeteners to enhance a product's sweetness. Examples of sugar alcohols are sorbitol, mannitol, isomalt, and xylitol.

In 2004 alone about 2,000 sugarless and sugar-reduced products were introduced in the United States market by the food industry. These replace the sugar found in food items like gum, candy, cakes, cookies, pudding, salad dressing, jelly, jam, and ice cream, and in beverages like soda and flavored bottled water. Market analysts at Mintel, a market research firm, have estimated that between 2000 and 2005, 3,920 new food products were launched in the United States and that in 2004 alone 1,648 of these products were artificially sweetened.[310] Another market research firm, Freedonia, has revealed that the United States market for artificial sweeteners totaled $189 million in 2008 and that alternative sweeteners will account for 12% of the market by 2013, with sales totaling $1.3 billion.[311]

The two most popular artificial sweeteners are saccharin and aspartame, considered to be 200 times sweeter than sugar. People use sugar substitutes for lots of different reasons. Here are a few:

> **Weight loss.** People who are dieting prefer to use sweeteners with few to no calories in place of high-calorie sugar in order to avoid compromising taste. This allows them to eat the same foods with reduced calories, thus avoiding weight gain.

> **Better dental care.** Ordinarily, sugar undergoes fermentation by the microfloras present on our dental plaque. Sugar substitutes do not ferment and hence are not as detrimental to the teeth.

> **Diabetes mellitus.** People suffering from diabetes mellitus have problems regulating the sugar levels in their blood. Artificial sweeteners help limit their sugar intake, while not depriving them of food choices. Though some sugar substitutes do have some caloric value, they are incompletely absorbed and metabolized by the body and thus do not allow for drastic sugar fluctuations.

Reactive hypoglycemia. Hypoglycemia is a condition that also affects blood-sugar levels, but differently from diabetes. In this condition, the individual produces excess insulin as the system quickly utilizes glucose (sugar) from the bloodstream. As a result, the glucose level in the blood goes below the normal levels, often quickly. People with hypoglycemia use artificial sweeteners to prevent this kind of blood glucose fluctuation.

The following artificial sugar substitutes are compatible to the taste of sugar, but provide very little to no food energy: acesultame potassium, alitame, aspartame, aspartame-acesulfame salt, glucin, neo-hesperidin dihydrochalcone, neotame, saccharin, and sucralose. Because of this energy disparity, the level of sweetness of these substitutes cannot be compared based on energy content.

A sweet history

Saccharin was first discovered in 1879 by Remsen and Fahlberg at Johns Hopkins University.[312] By the 1950s and '60s, saccharin had become a popular calorie reducing alternative to sugar, and is often found in restaurants in pink packets under the popular brand name Sweet N' Low. As time went on, it was no surprise when several competitive FDA-approved alternatives emerged on the market, namely: sucralose, aspartame, acesulfame potassium, and neotame.[313] Controversy first grew around the effects of saccharin when a study by Reuber, et al. showed that saccharin caused bladder cancer in lab rats.[314] Studies like this one did open the door for more animal research to be undertaken on the subject. For example, in 1980, a paper by Taylor, et al. revealed startling results when it demonstrated that first-generation laboratory-bred male rats showed a 30% occurrence of bladder cancer when exposed to a diet comprised of 7.5% saccharin.[315] Furthermore, in the largest study of its kind in 1985, when 2,500 first-generation rats were fed a dietary saccharin concentration of 4%, the results were conclusive that the rats' risk of bladder cancer increased as well.[316]

Based on these results, the sale of saccharin was banned in Canada. In the U.S., however, saccharin stayed on the shelves. In 1981 a law was put into effect that product labels had to include a warning that saccharin can cause cancer in laboratory animals, but this label has since been removed.

NutraSweet® and Equal® are other artificial sugar substitutes that contain the non-saccharide sweetener aspartame. Well-documented studies have shown that aspartame has been associated with increased lymphoma, leukemia, and other cancers. In March 2006, the first article was published that demonstrated a clear link between aspartame and its subsequent carcinogenic effects.[317] "More than twenty years have elapsed since aspartame was approved by regulatory agencies as an artificial sweetener," researcher M. Nathaniel Mead said in a 2006 paper. "But scientists draw conclusions on carcinogenicity based on the evidence available at the time, and new research out of the European Ramazzini Foundation of Oncology and Environmental Sciences bolsters recent calls for reconsideration of regulations governing aspartame's widespread use in order to better protect public health, particularly that of children."[318]

In an interesting twist, a 2008 study has shown that artificial sweeteners actually decrease the ability to perceive caloric intake. In that study, rats given yogurt sweetened with zero-calorie saccharin were found to consume more calories, gain more weight, and add more body fat compared to the group that ate yogurt sweetened with plain sugar.[319]

The Splenda® controversy

Sucralose is another highly popular artificial sweetener, commonly marketed under the brand name Splenda®. Due to Splenda®'s popularity, it can now be found in over 4,000 products in 80 countries.[320] Despite its growth, Splenda® is mired in controversy. According to Dr. Joseph Mercola, osteopathic physician and best-selling author, there have been insufficient human trials conducted with regard to sucralose and its long-term effects. Dr. Mercola states that not only have most of the studies on sucralose been performed on animal subjects, but that the ones with human subjects tend to address only one symptom (such as the study evaluating sucralose in relation to migraine headaches) rather than the overall potential safety concerns related to the compound. In Dr. Mercola's estimation, this means the studies' results are less valid. A case in point, the longest, published sucralose study was only 13 weeks long— meager parameters of examination by experimental standards—and was performed by the manufacturer of sucralose. The manufacturer did submit *unpublished* research to the FDA that studied humans taking sucralose for six months. This study, however, only focused on sucralose in relation to blood sugar in diabetics—again, according to Dr. Mercola, avoiding the subject of overall product safety.[321] McNeil Nutritionals, LLC, the manufacturer of sucralose, or Splenda®, states on its website that "The safety of sucralose is supported by more than 100 scientific studies conducted over a 20-year period." Dr. Mercola vehemently refutes this claim, stating that only 84 scientific research articles have been published; only 15 of those studies were animal trials; only five were human trials; and none focused on the bigger picture of human safety.[321]

The major concern relative to Splenda® is in reference to the nature of sucralose itself.

Sucralose is a substance formed from sucrose and is about 600 times as sweet as sugar. Sucrose is made up of the simple sugars glucose and fructose. However, when Splenda® is manufactured it undergoes a chemical process where three "chlorine" molecules are added. This process converts the sucrose to a class of chemicals called *organochlorines*. Organochlorines are organic compounds containing at least one chlorine atom. Many insecticides, such as DDT and pentachlorophenol, a wood preservative, are organochlorines. The sucralose molecule is almost structurally identical to the sucrose molecule; however, because its glucose rings invert, it becomes a derivative of galacto-sucrose. This new molecule does not occur in nature and our bodies are incapable of metabolizing it.

The makers of Splenda® claim that it provides "zero calories." This is not because the sweetener does not generate calories, however, but because the body cannot identify it as a chemical substance and therefore cannot metabolize it.

The research data from animal studies regarding the metabolization of sucralose reveals that the major portion of sucralose is not absorbed by the body. It is estimated that while 85% of ingested sucralose is excreted in the feces and urine, 15% is absorbed into the upper portion of the gastrointestinal tract.[322] However, given the variability of our digestive capabilities and our ability to absorb nutrients, we can only assume that some of us may actually be absorbing more than the estimated 15%. Furthermore, a variety of consumer complaints about Splenda® include, but are not limited to, gastrointestinal problems, migraines, seizures, dizziness, blurred vision, allergic reactions, blood-sugar spikes and weight gain.

James Turner, attorney and chairman of the national consumer education group Citizens for Health, represents businesses as well as individuals and consumer groups in a wide variety of regulatory matters concerning food, drug, health, environmental, and product-safety matters. Mr. Turner has served as special counsel to the Senate Select Committee on Food, Nutrition, and Health and to the Senate Government Operations Subcommittee on Government Research.[323] Based on his understanding that the use of Splenda® poses a growing health concern, Mr. Turner petitioned the United States Food and Drug Administration to revoke its amendment to be considered a "food additive." In his petition, Mr. Turner stated, "The Agency should ask the Inspector General of the Department of Health and Human Services to investigate consumer health concerns and publicly posted adverse event reports related to the widespread use of sucralose (Splenda) as a result of the Agency's approval of sucralose in 1998 despite serious safety concerns that the Agency originally acknowledged but ultimately set aside." Turner then went on to state, "The Agency should initiate a full-scale public-health investigation (involving U.S. Public Health Service environmental health officers) in and around McIntosh, Alabama, into local residents' reports of environmental exposure effects related to the transport and use of chlorine and the release of cyclohexane, a known toxin, from the Splenda plant in McIntosh, Alabama, looking into health problems than [sic] can be caused by exposure to cyclohexane, including but not limited to: coma; encephalopathy; liver abnormalities; chronic 'painter's syndrome' [sic]; psycho-organic solvent syndrome; organic solvent dementia; difficulty concentrating; dementia; memory loss; mood disturbance;

arrhythmia; confusion; dermatitis; dizziness; fatigue; headache; in-coordination; inebriation; irritability; lethargy; impaired speech; and stupor."[324]

The bottom line here is that there is mounting evidence showing that artificial sweeteners may not be as harmless to the human system as we once thought. Once again, it is always best to consider artificial sweeteners as "food additives;" in other words, not as food substances which enter our body in the form nature intended. As I always recommend, educate yourself as much as possible about your food choices and always try to keep those choices feasible and natural.

Water

Feel thirsty? Never ignore the urge to quench your thirst. How much fluid do we need? Most of us grew up with the adage that drinking eight glasses of water each day was appropriate. However, in 2004 the Institute of Medicine took a closer look at how much fluid the body really needs. Based on the Institute's results and new guidelines, there is no fixed number of glasses of water each of us needs to consume on a daily basis. Instead, the guidelines recommend that a good way to gauge and meet our daily fluid needs is by using our own thirst as guide. While water is the best choice for staying hydrated, other beverage choices such as juice, milk, coffee, and tea can also count toward our daily fluid intake. When the IOM reviewed hundreds of studies from peer-reviewed scientific journals, it concluded that healthy women, ages 19 to 30 (who live in temperate climates), are adequately hydrated when their total water intake is 2.7 l per day. Men, ages 19 to 30, are adequately hydrated when their total water intake is 3.7 l per day. Fluids, in the form of drinking water and other beverages, provide 3.0 l (101 fluid oz, or about 13 cups) for men and 2.2 l (74 fluid oz, or about nine cups) for women and represent approximately 81% of total water intake. The remainder of our water intake, as contained in food substances, provides the rest, or approximately 19%, of our total water intake.[325]

Every day we lose close to 2.1 qts of water through breathing, sweating, urinating, and bowel movements. In extreme conditions, lack of adequate water results in dehydration and organ failure. Typically we require more water when we exercise regularly, during the hot weather months, or when we experience a fever. Generally speaking, our average food intake meets 20% of our water requirements, while the rest of it comes from water and other beverages we drink. Fruits are also a great source of water.

Water is an essential nutrient to all living things. Its chemical formula is H_2O, where one molecule of water consists of a combination of one atom of oxygen and two atoms of hydrogen. Water inside the body is distributed between the water-like fluid inside the cells, called *intracellular* fluid, and outside the cells, the *extracellular* fluid. The body's water content is approximately 60%, of which 40% is intracellular and 20% is extracellular.

In the past, water was pretty much—well, water. But today there are many types on the market. The most common waters are as follows:

Spring water. Spring water is defined as bottled water derived from an underground source from which water flows naturally to the surface of the earth. Commonly found in food stores as bottled water, spring water is regulated by the FDA as a "food." To qualify as spring water, the water must be collected either at the spring itself or by tapping into the underground formation that feeds the spring. Whichever method is used, the water must retain the quality and physical properties of the water that flows naturally from the spring to the surface.

Purified water. Purified water is drinking water that has been treated with processes such as *distillation*, *deionization*, or *reverse osmosis*. These processes remove the bacteria and dissolved solids, making it "purified," and this is the preferred form of water for use in chemical and biological laboratories. This type of bottled water is usually labeled "purified drinking water," but it can also be labeled based on the process it undergoes—hence, "distilled drinking water," "deionized water," and "reverse-osmosis water." Choosing one type of water to drink over another is generally a matter of personal preference. Many brands of bottled water of this type on the market are labeled "Purified drinking water only."

Mineral water. Mineral water contains minerals or other dissolved solids, which can give it a slightly noticeable taste. The FDA classifies mineral water to "contain not less than 250 parts per million total dissolved solids." The levels in the mineral water must be consistent with the levels and relative proportions of the mineral and trace elements from the water's source. No minerals may be added to the water.

Sparkling bottled water. Sparkling bottled water contains the same amount of carbon dioxide it had when it emerged from its source. These waters may be labeled as "sparkling drinking water," "sparkling mineral water," or "sparkling spring water."

Artesian water/artesian well water. Artesian water comes from a well in a confined, or "artesian," aquifer, an underground bed or layer of permeable rock, sediment, or soil that yields water. A confined aquifer is sandwiched between confining layers of impermeable materials, such as clay and sandstone, which impede the movement of water into and out of the aquifer. Because the ground water in these aquifers is under high pressure, the water level rises upward to a level higher than the top of the aquifer without assistance.

Well water. Well water is also accessed from underground aquifers.

Municipal/tap water. Municipal, or tap, water is piped right into our homes. Although tap water is not regulated by the FDA, it is regulated by the Environmental Protection Agency. The EPA's Office of Ground Water and Drinking Water issues extensive regulations on the production and distribution of drinking water, including regulations on source-water protection, the operation of drinking water systems, and the contaminant levels and reporting requirements.[326]

Over the last few years, bottled water—water packaged for retail sales—has become the most popular form of drinking water in the United States. Worldwide sales of bottled water are estimated to be between $50 to $100 billion annually, and retailers are counting on an approximate yearly increase of 7 to 10%.

Water and cancer

Adequate water intake has been linked to the reduced incidence of some cancers. Results of a case-control in-hospital pilot study, for example, have revealed that drinking water has a strong, inverse, protective effect on breast cancer risk.[327] The protective role of water intake has also been found to reduce colorectal cancer risk. For example, in one study researchers found that men who consumed more than four glasses of water per day (in addition to food) compared to men who consumed one or fewer glasses, had a marginally decreased risk for colon cancer. In this same study performed with women, more than five glasses of water per day was associated with decreased colon cancer risk.[328] Although the mechanism for this protective effect is not very clear, it is thought to result from the water and fiber interaction, which dilutes toxic compounds and speeds up the transit time in the bowel, ultimately reducing mucosal contact with carcinogens.

In 1999, Michaud, et al. examined the relationship between total fluid intake and the risk of bladder cancer over a period of 10 years among 47,909 participants. Michaud's study revealed that a high fluid intake was associated with a decreased risk of bladder cancer in men. Researchers in this case demonstrated that concentrated urine or less frequent urination increased the exposure of the cells lining the bladder to carcinogens. Their theory, named the "urogenous-contact hypothesis," is one explanation offered for the inverse association found between the risk of bladder cancer and fluid intake.[329] In 1991, Bitterman, et al. also reported that patients with urinary tract cancer consumed significantly less fluid compared to their healthy study counterparts.[330]

In summary, though research has shown that drinking enough water is important, more than one in three Americans over the age of 60 are not getting enough total water from all sources.[331]

Chlorine and cancer

The relationship between cancer and chlorine, a popular water decontaminant, has been the subject of intense study. When chlorine combines with natural organic matter, it forms trihalomethanes (THMs), or haloforms. THMs are potent carcinogens, such as chloroform, bromoform, bromodichloromethane, dibromochloromethane, and several others. Carcinogens like these have the ability to disrupt cellular metabolic processes and damage cellular DNA. The National Water-Quality Assessment (NAWQA) Program, implemented by the U.S. Geological Survey, has revealed that trihalomethanes and other volatile compounds have been found frequently in test samples of untreated ground water from drinking-water supply wells (1,096 public and 2,400 domestic wells) throughout the country.[332]

In a study reviewed in 1987 it was found that exposure to chlorinated surface tap water for a minimum of 40 years in ten areas sampled utilized in beverages was associated with bladder cancer risk in both sexes. This same risk was not found among long-term users of non-chlorinated ground water.[333]

Harmful water

The Environmental Protection Agency regularly collects data to decide whether regulations for the kinds of substances mentioned above should be required based on their potential to pose a human health risk.[334] The *Drinking Water Contaminant Candidate List* (CCL) is the EPA's principle guideline of contaminants; the contaminants on this list are known or anticipated to occur in public water systems. The Safe Drinking Water Act (SDWA) requires the EPA to publish an updated CCL every five years. The EPA published the first CCL ("CCL 1") of 60 contaminants in March 1998 and the second ("CCL 2") of 51 contaminants in February 2005.

The EPA's latest list ("CCL 3") was published in September 2009 and finalized after evaluating 7,500 unregulated contaminants. This list includes 104 chemicals or groups of chemicals and 12 microbiological contaminants. The list found chemicals used in commerce, pesticides, disinfection byproducts, biological toxins, and waterborne pathogens. Since some of the contaminants on the list are known carcinogens, their levels are closely monitored to ensure that the supply of municipal/tap water is safe for drinking. However, despite the EPA's efforts to monitor the country's water supply, I have always felt that the best method for making sure the water coming into your home from the municipal water supply is safe is to fit water faucets used for drinking with filters which are capable of removing more than 99% of all contaminants. The dichotomy we face, therefore, is obvious, because while we still use chlorine to minimize the risk of illness by water contamination, its use may also increase cancer risk associated with our drinking water.

Our risk of contaminants doesn't stop there. Lead pipes used in water distribution have been around for more than a century based on their longevity (the lifespan of iron pipes tends to be around 16 years versus the lifespan of lead pipes of around 35 years). Lead pipes are also more malleable, allowing for bending around existing structures. Because lead is water-soluble, however, it poses a significant detriment to the health of the public. For example, studies have shown serious health effects in adults at very low blood/lead levels, including cancer, cardiovascular disease, peripheral arterial disease, and death from all causes.[335]

Other compounds used in pipes are not necessarily any better. Polyvinyl chloride (PVC) is a synthetic resin made from polymerization of vinyl chloride. PVC is the largest producer of organochlorines and consumes about 40% of our total chlorine production, or approximately 16 million tons of chlorine per year worldwide.[336] Plastic pipes made from PVC are used for water distribution in and around the home, although it has been shown that during its life cycle PVC causes a wide range of health hazards—in some cases at extremely low doses—including cancer, disruption of the endocrine system, reproductive impairment, impaired child development and birth defects, neurotoxicity (damage to the brain or its function), and immune system suppression.[336]

Water therapy

Water is therapeutic! What do we mean by that? Water has so many benefits it would be hard to state them all. The biggest one, of course, is its life-giving quality: without water we would die. On a subtler level, water is also the primary medium in which all the various chemical reactions in our body take place. It is the solvent in which most molecules are dissolved in the body, and it carries and distributes nutrients, metabolites, hormones, enzymes, and other substances throughout the body. At the same time, water helps in eliminating waste materials from the body through urine and feces, and is an important thermo-regulator, helping to maintain body temperature, keep cells hydrated, and lubricate mucus membranes and joints. The brain and spinal cord also depend on water. Water is the predominant component of the medium that cushions the brain and spinal cord, thus forming a shock-absorber for the body's central nervous system.

While the human body is composed mainly of water, percentages can vary from person to person. This is because different cells in the body contain different amounts of water. For example, because muscle cells are 70 to 75% water and fat cells are only 10 to 15% water, a muscular person will derive a larger percentage of his/her body weight from water.

In his book *Your Body's Many Cries for Water*, Dr. Fereydoon Batmanghelidi explains that lack of water in the body is the cause of many diseases.[337] Dr. Batmanghelidi discusses the role of water in the body and shares his belief that counteracting chronic dehydration can transform the health of society at large. Dr. Batmanghelidi's message is a practical one: "You are not sick, you are thirsty. Don't treat thirst with medication." According to Dr. Batmanghelidi, the relationship between dehydration and DNA damage is easy to understand, as follows: while every cell produces byproducts during chemical reactions, water washes these elements out of the cell and takes them to the liver and kidneys for processing. Lack of enough water to circulate these byproducts out of the cells gradually erodes the transcription patterns in the DNA stored in the cell nucleus. Hence, lack of water can lead to dehydration and drain energy levels, posing health risks for the very young and very old.

Drinking water does all these things:

- improves energy levels
- enhances mental and physical functions
- helps get rid of waste and toxins from the body
- helps maintain healthy skin
- helps in weight loss
- decreases incidences of headaches and dizziness
- aids in all digestive functions
- maintains the body's homeostasis

Drinking enough water is simply one more element proving that our approach to maintaining good health must be multidimensional. In light of the fact that health is not merely the absence of a disease or infirmity, it is necessary to take steps in several directions simultaneously. Adding water to our list of beneficial substances will help us pay attention to an element that plays a significant role in our body's daily chemistry.

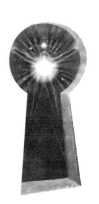

5. Mental Facets of Health

On life and living

I sat on my usual rock on top of the cliffs of the Palisades overlooking the Hudson River in my hometown of Fort Lee, New Jersey. A gentle breeze and sounds of distant traffic on the George Washington Bridge were my only companions.

I was contemplating how thankful I was for the educating experience of having cancer in my youth. Does that sound strange? It would not surprise me if you thought I was crazy, but it's true that I have gained in so many ways from my illness. Cancer created a curiosity in me and guided me in directions I probably would have never pursued under normal circumstances. For example, anyone who has walked the long road of cancer treatment understands how deeply morale is affected during the process of detection, treatment, and recovery—a process that is anything but normal. And at that time, three decades ago, there were no meetings or lectures or support groups to provide help for my ailing confidence. Those of us walking that path had to find our own way to comfort, and it has taken three long decades for support systems for people with cancer to slowly—albeit significantly—improve.

Then, as I continued to sit and think, something dawned on me. Who was in a better position than I to share my experiences and knowledge given my empathy for others, my long-researched understanding of cancer, and the fact that I was someone who had lived with cancer and recovered from it? The fact that I feel so comfortable in this role is evident every time I am given the opportunity to speak at a meeting, at adult education classes, at lectures for the American Cancer Society, or even with patients in my office, and I continue to relate unequivocally to the faces gathered before me. Some of these faces reflect skepticism, some trepidation; some show nonchalance, others show hope; some express interest and others express eagerness and anticipation. I have been there. And I continue to be there every day, and to understand the vast array of emotions you feel.

I know too that it is not easy to deal with grief from a loss, whether that loss is as obvious as the death of a near-and-dear one or is one which comes from severe emotional and physical suffering. Of course grief of any kind is multifaceted in its pain. But the grief from the loss of one's health is no less impactful, no less important, and no less traumatic than the loss of another human being. Ill health, especially ill health related to a life-threatening disease like cancer, similarly causes intense feelings of loss—and the fear of loss. Loss of control...loss of health...the fear of ultimately losing everything we know and love.

This reaction may not always be obvious to those around us, but these emotions are very much a reality for a person experiencing cancer. It is not easy to hear that you have cancer, even if you have tried to mentally prepare yourself for the worst. It is not easy to "accept" a diagnosis of possible death and move on so that you can get through treatment with the ultimate goal of recovery. One thing, however, is clear. Grieving is a natural, ongoing part of the process.

Grief

Grief, or coping with loss, is in fact a completely normal aspect of the process of healing. Grieving is the step that allows us to work toward acceptance and then deal with the problem. Elisabeth Kübler-Ross, a renowned psychiatrist and author of the well-known book *On Death and Dying*, has elucidated the now commonly accepted five stages of grief.[1] I have found that these stages are no different for accepting the loss of health than for accepting the loss of someone you love. The first is a feeling of numbness that sets in as you think, *This can't be true* or *This isn't really happening*. It's a feeling of denial, a natural human reaction that is present even when you are trying to recover from the loss that is simultaneously occurring. This feeling of denial may last for a few moments—or much longer. We may feel paralyzed, distant, or removed from the reality of what is taking place. Some say such numbing is the body's defense mechanism for protecting itself from being overwhelmed by the shock of the loss we are experiencing.

According to Kübler-Ross, this phase is followed by a phase of disorganization when one passes through a range of emotions from anger to bargaining to depression. In the stage of anger we can feel infuriated and frustrated with the situation we face. *Why is this happening to me?* and *What did I do to deserve this*? are natural questions we may ask ourselves during this process. From that stage we naturally transition to a phase in which a desire to bargain takes hold. We want to pull out all the stops, bargain with the universe (perhaps, for some, with God) to get back what we've lost, or to ensure we will never experience such a thing again. For example, *If you take this away, I swear I will do this or that*, or *I promise I'll never...*

Following this stage, depression often takes root, and it is this stage that needs to last as long as it needs to last—basically as long as it takes until feelings of acceptance can ultimately surface. Depression is a strong mood, involving sadness, discouragement, despair, and hopelessness. It affects an individual's thoughts, outlook, and behavior, and can make a person feel tired and irritable and experience appetite changes. During this period, we may experience feelings of sadness and thoughts about those things we may perceive as lost opportunities, and this can easily feed our feelings of depression. Over time, usually in our own time and in our own way, these feelings eventually subside.

Once we move through the phase of depression, we reach a place of reorientation. This is a time when we now accept that we do in fact have cancer. It is when we reach this phase of acceptance, and it is *only* when we reach this phase, that we actually begin to deal with the problem *as it exists*. Thoughts of *I am going to be okay* and *I am going to do what I have to do to get through this* begin to replace the denial, anger, and bargaining that came before, along with the potentially overwhelming depression we once felt.

Each of these phases is natural and the time we spend with each is to a large extent determined by the type of person we are. What is important is that we know that there is no shame in feeling what we feel, or as deeply as we do. On some days it may seem we are stuck in one or another of these phases and will be forever. That is why we need to know that we will not stay trapped in any of these emotions indefinitely and that somewhere in the recesses of our mind we are already aware that these feelings are simply part of the cycle of acceptance. Working to keep them in perspective, trying to understand why we feel the way we do, and feeling free to discuss them with others helps us reach that point of acceptance. We all need to seek the support we require to make this happen, and partly that means feeling free to discuss and work through the stages of our grief in the way that feels the most comfortable. The important thing to recognize is that we are not alone and we do not have to cope with these feelings all by ourselves. Our family and friends can be great supports in dealing with the intensity and gamut of emotions we feel as we work our way through the healing process.

When the unexpected happens

Robert Frost once wrote, "Always fall in love with what you are asked to accept, take what you are given, and make it over your way." My aim in life has always been to hold my own with whatever's going on. Not against: *with*. Many, many years ago, with my newfound acceptance, that is exactly what I set out to do.

My plan to care, cure, and heal my cancer incorporated a pattern of regular visits to the hospital, conversations with my doctors, nurses, and therapists, and regular routines of treatment. This pattern in itself soon became a source of comfort, a source of predictability.

There was always the pattern to rely on, to "look forward to," in a world that had become filled with disillusionment.

Then the unexpected happened. There came a day when I was told that I was "cured" and I was declared "clinically cancer-free." Suddenly I had been given a new lease on life. Of course I experienced the thrill of having survived and the relief of thinking I could now let it all go. But I also experienced a shock when I realized that being cured had created a sudden void in my life. Had I really been freed of nurses, doctors, and hospitals? Had my routine really come to an end? Frankly, I had become so used to this regimen, a routine with which I had identified for so long, that I was unsure what to do next. I floundered for a while, not knowing quite what to do, but I also recognized that this was a good time for some introspection. Ultimately the fact of my new and changed circumstances sunk in. Not only was I now free from medical regimens but I was free to create an entirely new pattern to my life. I could fill my days the way *I* wanted to and do the things *I* wanted to do.

I reflected about my illness and felt thankful that I felt the desire to take the wheel into my own hands. I would be able to move in one direction—or many directions, to do whatever I chose. But as you well can imagine, this sudden renewed freedom brought up all sorts of new feelings, from being excited to being downright scared. My previous routines had been conveniently laid out by others and during my course of treatment I had merely followed the rules. This routine had brought great relief from having to make decisions. Now that I was to be left to my own devices, anxiety and trepidation took hold.

Looking back, I am thankful now for all the signals that were revealed to me after the completion of my treatment. These signs steered a course for a healthier way of living through mental awareness, exercise, diet, and the availability of complementary and alternative health practices. The angst that I felt gradually transformed into the certainty that good would come from all of these experiences. Although I was now officially a "cancer survivor," I did not see myself as someone who wished to merely survive. To me, survival meant, and continues to mean, a kind of limping-along existence, the kind where one barely carries on day to day. To me, survival implies missing something in the pursuit to live. This is why I am not a big fan of labels. If I were to believe that surviving were the most valid truth about my existence, then I would begin to interpret my surroundings through the lens of who I thought I was: "the cancer survivor," simply trying to live day to day. I was definitely not going to allow that to happen. It was when I consciously refused to accept that label that I was able to actively shed the onus of being a "survivor."

It was at that point I found I could use the key I was given, slide it into the keyhole, and open the door to the second chance I had been offered. It was a difficult yet necessary transformation to transcend these limiting beliefs. It meant I had to leave my comfort zone and become less well defined, become label-less—almost rudderless. Soren Kierkegaard, a prolific 19th-century Danish philosopher, once said, "Once you label me, you negate me." In other words, labels serve only to limit us, because we become more focused on the label than on what the experience is trying to teach us.

It goes without saying, at least for me, that it was—and is—nearly impossible to stop wondering if the cancer will come back, if a relapse is just around the corner. As irrational as these feelings may be, I have come to accept that they will always exist to a certain degree. Over thirty years later the feeling has never completely gone away—although the frequency and the intensity of the fear has lessened and the voices of fear have become less audible as time goes on. Now I try to create daily harmony in my life in the things over which I have control and to accept the things over which I do not.

I believe it all begins with our state of mind.

Stevie Wonder is a classic, inspiring example of how it all starts in the mind. Blind from infancy, Stevie Wonder is a brilliant musician with numerous hits to his credit. He has won 25 Grammy Awards, the most ever received by any male artist. He plays a variety of musical instruments: drums, bass guitar, organ, congas, piano, harmonica, and clarinet. Stevie Wonder is the quintessential example of the power of thought, the discipline to implement those thoughts, and the desire to take action to have them become a reality. While he may lack the sense of sight, he certainly has no lack of inner vision, and has used his other senses to compensate and achieve.

Our 16th president, Abraham Lincoln, was born in a one-room log cabin to uneducated farmers, and is another shining example of the power of the mind. Due to economic difficulties in Kentucky, Lincoln's family moved to Indiana, where nine-year-old Abe lost his mother to milk sickness and was then raised by his stepmother. Considered one of the best orators that history has ever produced, Lincoln's formal education was comprised of probably no more than 18 months of schooling from unofficial teachers. Lincoln was predominantly self-educated in his mastering of the Bible, the complete works of William Shakespeare, and English and American history. It was after winning the election to the state legislature that Lincoln came across a copy of *Commentaries on the Laws of England,* which inspired his legal education, and soon he had learned the law well enough to be admitted to the bar. Known to suffer from frequent periods of depression throughout his life, Lincoln continued to guide our country through one of the most distressing experiences in our nation's history, the Civil War. Many historians consider Lincoln the greatest American president ever for both his insight and his single-minded purpose in reaching his goals.

Another inspiring example of an individual whose mind surpassed the obstacles it faced is Helen Keller. Born a normal healthy baby, Helen was left both blind and deaf by an unexplained illness at the age of 19 months. Through her parents she eventually met Anne Sullivan, who played a major role in her life as teacher and friend. Anne Sullivan, who had lost the majority of her eyesight by the age of five, understood what it was like to be a child who had suddenly lost the gift of vision; she understood the need for hope. With patience and time a miracle took place, where Helen not only showed an advanced ability to learn, but was soon reading with raised letters and later with Braille. Helen, through sheer perseverance, willpower, and hard work, became the first deaf-blind person to enroll in Radcliffe College and the first deaf-blind person to earn a Bachelor of Arts degree in 1904. Helen Keller toured the world raising funds for the blind and was eventually awarded the Presidential Medal of Freedom, the nation's highest civilian award, by President Lyndon Johnson.

After hearing about these highly accomplished people, you begin to realize that anything is possible. The mind has an unlimited supply of potential, including the potential the ability to generate thought, and from those thoughts, behaviors…and from those behaviors the action of accomplishment. Having the right frame of mind is a by-product of having the right thoughts, and the right frame of mind allows us to cope with the problems of everyday living. Good emotional health, therefore, has a direct impact on our physical health and wellbeing. This is why I felt the need to learn more about the implications and importance of the mind as it relates to health.

Emotional and mental health

Dr. Martin Seligman is the director of the University of Pennsylvania's Positive Psychology Center and founder of Positive Psychology, a new branch of psychology which focuses on the study of such things as positive emotions, strength-based character, and healthy institutions.[2] Seligman's definition of "being happy" revolves around three components which he believes provide a strong foundation to sound emotional and mental health. The first component is pleasure, or the "feel good" part of happiness. Things like casual conversation fit into this category because conversation invites individuals to talk about the past, present, and future, something that stimulates short-term positive emotions. Seligman refers to the second component as engagement, which refers to being involved with activities we find gratifying, particularly because they absorb us fully. Seligman states that for something to absorb us fully it requires us to draw on our character strengths, such as creativity, social intelligence, sense of humor, perseverance, and an appreciation for beauty and excellence. The third component of Seligman's triad of happiness is the involvement with something larger than ourselves. This includes the interest in or the pursuit of knowledge, goodness, family, community, politics, justice, and/or a higher spiritual power. Whatever it is that captures our involvement, it is that thing which has meaning and satisfies our longing for purpose in life.[3]

A study published in the *Journal of Personality and Social Psychology* also suggests that happiness is important, where the researchers state, "A pattern of emotional expression that accentuates a positive affect undoubtedly has behavioral correlates that could enhance or disrupt the positive effects on physiology and health."[4] Furthermore, where researchers at UCLA have found that optimism is related to strong immune cell function,[5] the reverse has also been found to be true—that psychological depression may be associated with impairment of mechanisms that prevent the establishment and spread of malignant cells.[6] Among persons with a cancer diagnosis, it has been found that depression occurs at a significantly higher rate, a rate approximately three to five times greater than in the general population, and the severity of psychological stress has been associated with lower NK cell activity in ovarian cancer patients, a decline found in peripheral blood as well as in tumor-infiltrating lymphocytes.[7]

The medical cost involved in investigation and diagnosis of illness is overwhelming. In 2002, for example, Abbass, et al. documented that there would be a huge cost savings to the general healthcare system if patients were referred for even short courses of emotionally focused psychotherapy.[8] A number of small-scale trials have supported this work in revealing that psychotherapeutic interventions (especially cognitive behavioral therapy) have been shown to alleviate depressive symptoms in cancer patients,[9] supporting the relationship between emotional and physical health—in other words, the relationship between mind and body.

The World Health Organization defines *mental health* as "a state of wellbeing in which the individual realizes his or her own capabilities, can cope with normal stresses of life, can work productively and fruitfully, and is able to make a contribution to his or her community."[10] Another definition as described in the U.S. Surgeon General's Mental Health Report is "the successful performance of mental function, resulting in productive activities, fulfilling relationships with other people, and the ability to adapt to change and cope with adversity."[11]

Mental health has been analyzed by many experts with varied opinions, but the one thing on which we can all agree is that no matter the individual's race, gender, country of origin, or political party, certain common characteristics signify the presence of good mental health.

Of course, it is evident that assessing mental health is a lot more complicated than measuring physical health. There are no scales and no endurance or "happiness" tests capable of rating mental fitness with any kind of precision. There are, however, many tools that focus on identifying and qualifying an individual's state of mind relative to his overall mental health. These tools can help us reflect on our own unique strengths and identify areas where we can improve our level of "mental fitness." These are tools that help cultivate our strategies for living. As I see it, the end goal is to help us cope with life's ups and downs so we feel better about the way we live our lives every single day.

There are a few ways we can assess our mental outlook. The first way is to gauge our "ability to enjoy life." Do we celebrate the good things, including our future's potential? Enjoying life means knowing that although there will be challenges, we will not let them overshadow the pleasure and satisfaction we feel.

The second is to gauge our "resilience." This means that in times of frustration or anger we are able to put the situation in perspective so that emotions do not overtake us and make us do things we may later regret. Resilience gives us the power to recover so that we do not remain in a reactive state.

Do we feel our life has balance? Have we designated the right proportion of time for work and family? If we spend our time making excuses for not spending enough time with family and friends, it may be time to look at restoring the balance in our life. A "sense of balance" is also a good sign of mental health.

Next, we can look at how "flexible" we are, whether we can "roll with the punches" when things get tough. For example, if a romantic relationship ends, do we assume that we will never be able to trust anyone ever again or, instead, spend time considering what we really want in a relationship and what we may want to change in ourselves to make that happen?

When we look at our overall mental health meter, yet another valid way to test the waters is to ask, *Am I "fulfilled"?* Being fulfilled means doing the things that have meaning to us—whether in the form of acting, writing poetry, volunteering, or exercising. It means doing things that make us feel good about life and about ourselves.

Neuro-Linguistic Programming (NLP) and good mental health

One of the ways for an individual to make the changes he or she wants is by acquiring the mental skills to facilitate those changes. One of those approaches is through Neuro-Linguistic Programming, or NLP. NLP is a field of study that uses a set of guiding principles, attitudes, and techniques to affect the subconscious mind, thus eliciting positive patterns of behavior and psychological experience. NLP modeling attempts to change the patterns of our behavior in order to "model" the more successful parts of our self. The Empowerment Partnership, founded in 1982, is a recognized authority of NLP. This organization's members are highly skilled facilitators who operate under the direction of Matthew B. James, M.A., Ph.D. Their mission is to "empower students to transform their lives and to encourage transformation in others using holistic, complementary, alternative, and integrative approaches to psychology and human understanding."[12]

The premise of NLP, according to The Empowerment Partnership, is that it "allows you to change, adopt, or eliminate behaviors as you desire, and gives you the ability to choose your mental, emotional, and physical states of well-being." NLP is described as a "pragmatic technology based on an ability to produce your desired results, thus allowing you to become proficient at creating your future."[12]

One NLP model, called the Meta Model, has been developed to help individuals uncover unspoken information in order to challenge their generalizations and other potentially distorted messages that involve restrictive thinking and beliefs. Language serves as a representation of our experiences, explaining our reality with words. Because it is common to delete, generalize, or distort information from its deeper meaning, the intent of this approach is to reconnect a person's language to the experience and, as a result, develop new choices in thinking and behavior. By listening to and carefully responding to these types of distortions, deletions, and generalizations in the individual's sentences, practitioners seek to respond to the *form* of the sentence rather than the content itself.

In contrast to the Meta Model, the Milton Model has been described as "a way of using language to induce and maintain [a] trance [state] in order to contact the hidden resources of our personality."[10] This model's three primary goals are: to assist in building and maintaining rapport with the client; to overload and distract the conscious mind so that unconscious communication can be cultivated; and to allow for interpretation in the words offered to the client.

NLP practitioners believe that internal mental processes, such as problem-solving, memory, and language, consist of visual, auditory, and kinesthetic factors that become engaged when we think about or participate in problems, tasks, or activities of any kind. These internal sensory responses are constantly being formed and activated. NLP techniques generally aim to change behavior through the modification of such internal responses. This is accomplished by noticing the way we represent a problem and then by establishing new, more desirable responses to achieve alternative outcomes or goals. In this way, the patterns of behavior we attempt to change form a basis for learning. In understanding our responses we can begin to understand what kinds of results we want and this enhanced understanding can teach us to develop the flexibility we need to achieve those results.

Because NLP helps us learn to handle our responses to our situations differently, it can easily be applied to help us influence the way we react to disease and illness. In this regard, NLP reconditions both our self-image and our attitude toward our illness so that we can begin the process of healing.

Two good examples of utilizing NLP are to "establish rapport" and to "anchor" an emotional state.

Rapport. NLP uses a number of simple techniques to help establish rapport between individuals. Building rapport is an approach founded on the concept of creating a sense of similarity; it is this similarity that reduces differences, and hence, builds empathy.

Often, when the behaviors of one individual are matched and mirrored by another, an unconscious bond is initiated which can lead to feelings of familiarity and responsiveness. Acquiring this ability includes *matching* and *pacing* non-verbal behavior, such as body posture, head position, gestures, and voice tone, and matching the speech and body rhythms of others, such as breathing and pulse. *One of the most critical elements in circumstances of illness and disease is to be able to establish rapport with others. This contributes to more successful treatment through our relationships with caregivers, family, and friends.*

Anchoring. An *anchor* is a stimulus that influences an individual's state of mind and locks that response in place, much like a ship's anchor prevents it from shifting its position. The skill of anchoring, therefore, incorporates the idea behind Pavlovian stimulus-response conditioning, where one observes how a particular stimulus will influence one's state of mind. This response may be associated with unique gestures, voice tone, or touch.

Our minds are continually processing thoughts, and thoughts are responses caused by other thoughts and experiences that have occurred in our past. In essence, these thoughts and experiences serve as "anchors" because they are "anchored" in our psyche. The NLP method of anchoring helps us create new responses to stimuli or elicit old unwanted states in order to create a new, desired state. Subsequently, these new and different responses can motivate us to manifest change and move in healthier directions. *Anchoring positive states, such as calmness and relaxation or confidence in the treatment of a disease or illness, is considered helpful in reconditioning responses and better preparing us to cope with the situations we face.*

The mind can be a powerful tool not only when it comes to general health, but in surgical outcomes as well. In one study at Mount Sinai Medical Center in New York City, for example, 200 women scheduled to undergo either surgical breast biopsy for diagnosis or lumpectomy for treatment of breast cancer were recruited for participation. When researchers randomly assigned participants to either the hypnosis group or a control group, it was found women undergoing surgery for breast cancer who received a brief hypnosis session before entering the operating room required less anesthesia and pain medication during surgery and reported less pain, nausea, fatigue, and discomfort after surgery than those women who did not receive hypnosis. The overall cost of surgery was also less for those women who underwent hypnosis.[13]

A study by Dr. Cynthia McRae at the University of Denver's College of Education also provides clear evidence of the mind-body connection in patients participating in a Parkinson's surgical trial.[14] Thirty patients from across the United States and Canada volunteered to participate in this quality-of-life surgical transplant study, where 12 patients received an actual transplant and 18 were randomly assigned to either undergo a "simulated surgery" or take a placebo. *Placebo*, Latin for "I shall please," can take the form of anything from a sugar or starch pill to, in this case, a surgery that does not really occur. In this study, researchers found that even patients who had received the non-surgical, or "placebo," treatment reported an improvement in their quality of life (although the improvement was not as much as the group that actually received the transplant). In other words, because the patients believed that a procedure to improve their condition had been undertaken, their bodies responded in kind—with a documented improvement in their symptoms.

We cannot separate our minds from our bodies, just as we cannot overestimate the mind's influence on the body. Our minute-by-minute reactions to life's never-ending stimuli have an immense impact on our overall physical health. Whether we recognize it or not, we are constantly reacting to the circumstances around us, consciously and unconsciously, and in ways that affect the ability of our bodies to function. It is also true that with better insight we can become less *re*active and more *pro*active in how we live our daily lives. Life has its inherent hills, bumps, and detours; we all have memorable moments that bring happiness and joy, as well as those that cause unhappiness and which we'd rather forget. Learning to embrace the moments of laughter, delight, and contentment, while learning to tolerate the moments of grief, loss, and sadness with grace, is a goal well worth pursuing.

One of the significant keys to "being happy" is achieving balance; this balance arrives through the understanding and awareness that such a dichotomy exists in all of us. The art of handling life is an ongoing learning process, one that involves constant monitoring in the attempt to stay balanced in mind, body, and spirit. Sigmund Freud said, "Thought is action in rehearsal." With this in mind, and with my *conscious ability*, I much prefer to choose handling life rather than life handling me, much as I would rather be the pinball player than the pinball itself.

As Freud implied, our actions are based on thoughts generated by our mind. Our mind provides direction based on our current thoughts and our subconscious thoughts, both past and present. In a sense, our mind has also been trained by past experiences and perceptions to react in certain ways. Wanting to change is the first step toward healthy mental evolution. I think most of us desire to make changes in ourselves for the better. Understanding *what* to change, *where*, and *how* become the bigger considerations.

The psychology of winning

Winning and defeating cancer starts with an attitude and needs to be a way of life. Most importantly, defeating cancer starts with the concept of believing in yourself. One acknowledged authority on self-development is Denis Waitley. Waitley's book, *The Psychology of Winning*, discusses how optimism and a positive attitude are the two major components on the path to success.[15] Waitley puts forth a relatively simple approach that may be as helpful to you as it has to me. Waitley speaks of ten simple aspects for winning in life. He calls these facets the "secrets of success," and they have been successfully utilized by leaders, athletes, students, doctors, educators, managers—people just like you and me. Waitley's secrets to success are:

- positive self-expectancy
- positive self-motivation
- positive self-image
- positive self-direction
- positive self-control
- positive self-discipline
- positive self-esteem
- positive self-dimension
- positive self-awareness
- positive self-projection

The key word here is POSITIVE. When something is "positive" we are to infer that it will automatically have some kind of constructive effect.

Positive self-expectancy. Before we can understand the quality of positive self-expectancy we need to understand the nature of expectation. *Expectation* is anticipation, a mental picture or a belief one has of the future. *Self-expectation* is what we expect ourselves to achieve. Before, during, and after our diagnosis and treatment of cancer, for example, we can expect that we will continue to be healthy. Waitley says, "Belief is the ignition switch that gets you off the launching pad." Armed with an attitude of optimism and enthusiasm to accomplish a task makes it far more likely that one will find the task simpler, or less daunting, and feel more confident. Because the mind works according to our expectations and human beings have an innate ability to rise to meet their expectations, we can conclude that positive expectations will indeed have positive outcomes. The aim of doing something should not be simply to complete it, but to derive joy from it, so that the result of our actions, the outcome, is directly proportional to the joy and enthusiasm of our input and expectations.

Positive self-motivation. The world around us continues to undergo rapid change with each passing year. With unavoidable change it becomes more and more important to plan and strategize our lives and schedules, something that takes motivation and direction. *Motivation* has been defined as the drive or desire to achieve something. It can be compared to the inner energy that drives our work and life. Motivation is converting the *knowing* into *doing*, which serves to create intention and transform that intention into goal-seeking acts. To become effective, successful, and happy we not only have to be able to motivate those around us, but more importantly, we have to be able to motivate ourselves. We need to set goals and aspirations and to want to work hard to achieve them. We need to convince ourselves that we can be leaders and trendsetters, because at that point more than half the battle will be won. When we motivate ourselves positively we affect those with whom we interact as well.

In terms of health, when there is a disease in the family, feeling motivated to make changes makes a tremendous difference in finding solutions for all involved. Positively motivated individuals act in ways that reduce the upheaval naturally associated with the advent of ill health, thereby aiding the healing process. In a working environment, motivated individuals inspire others around them; they get more work done more efficiently. Simply put, motivation motivates.

Positive self-image. Brian Tracy, the well-known self-help author, has said, "The person that we believe ourselves to be will always act in a manner consistent with our self-image."[16] Sit alone with yourself, check in, and ask yourself what you see. Do you feel good? Or do you feel there's room for some positive changes? *Self-image* is the mental image that we have of ourselves. That perception, however, can be very different from the perception others have about us. Regardless of what other people think, a positive self-image helps us develop qualities so that the world ultimately reflects those impressions back onto us. It's like standing in front of a mirror, smiling, and having the reflection smile back at you. Having a positive self-image is reflected in and by our outlook toward life, our performance, competence, attitude, popularity, and our way of living. Denis Waitley put it very aptly when he said, "First we make our habits and then our habits make us." With a positive self-image we first change the aspects that need changing; as a result life begins to reflect our changes in a more positive light. It may sound basic, but the truth is when we think well about ourselves, the world begins to align with our values.

Self-image is an ever-evolving process of learning that is dynamic in its effects. As we learn to develop a healthier view of ourselves and the world around us, an increasingly positive self-image can affect the quality of our relationships and reinforce what we think and feel about ourselves on all levels: physical, mental, social, emotional, and spiritual. "Accept your body for what it is and love it," states Waitley. "When you love yourself, you are better placed to give and receive love!" Once you accept your body the way it is, the process of healing unfolds naturally.

Positive self-direction. I've heard it said that "no wind blows in favor of a ship without a destination." Certainly direction determines destination, and without a bearing it is impossible to end up where you want to be. Therefore, focusing on the direction you want to go so you can achieve the goals and objectives you have set for yourself is the first order of business. It is all about knowing *who you are, where you are,* and *where you need to go.* Bear in mind, however, that simply taking a direct effort and then using more effort does not necessarily constitute a "positive" approach. It is the enjoyment factor that counts. Going about doing what you do with a *joie de vivre*, or love for life, will be reflected in your ultimate success and pleasure at achieving that success. Dr. Waitley takes this concept to the next level by postulating that not only is self-knowledge the key to achieving our goals, but that failing to plan is synonymous with planning to fail. So, let the power of your self-directed ambitions take you where you need to go.

Positive self-control. Self-control refers to the ability to control impulsivity. It is knowing that we have the ability to exert our will to bring about the specific behavioral change we want. If we believe that on some level we can depend only on ourselves for our happiness, fulfillment, and growth, then it makes sense that we need to exercise the power of self-control to change our own lives. In the 1960s, Walter Mischel, a personality psychologist from Austria and a professor at Stanford University, implemented what he called a Marshmallow Test to study the responses of four-year-olds when being tempted to eat a marshmallow. The children were given a single marshmallow and promised another one only if they waited 15 minutes before eating the first one.[17] Needless to say, some children were able to reign in their desire, while others could not. Interestingly enough, when follow-up studies were done years later on the same children, the tendencies that surfaced during the Marshmallow Test were the same tendencies that were revealed to exist in their lives years later. For example, the children who originally waited more patiently in the test appeared to be better at coping as they aged, were found to get higher S.A.T. scores, to be socially more competent, self-assertive, and dependable, and to be more successful overall. In contrast, the children who had failed to show restraint at age four continued to be viewed as "stubborn" and "easily frustrated" as adults. It seems the very act of self-restraint can help us learn to develop in a more positive manner and grow in non-impulsive ways.

By inculcating self-control, we can train our mind to radiate strength, know peace, and commit to health. Recognizing our true nature gives birth to our highest potential in terms of personality traits or qualities. Developing mental calmness, controlling impulses, exerting patience with forbearance, having faith with devotion, experimenting with creativity, and enjoying fearlessness are just some of the basic qualities of a pure, developed mind. Importantly, self-control contributes to our ability to control a situation, rather than allowing the situation to control us. *This means that when we are dealing with an illness like cancer, rather than allow cancer to control our life, we can put our efforts into controlling the cancer.* There are many who believe that positive self-control can win the battle over the cancer or any other life-threatening disease.

Positive self-discipline. To be disciplined is to follow a certain order of conduct to aid in modeling behavior. The health and welfare of the body has rules, and having positive self-discipline enforces those rules. This means where there is no discipline there is no health. Without the one, the other is not possible. Nothing materializes and no one succeeds without proper planning infused with discipline. Imposing self-discipline brings about positive changes in all aspects of life—our personality, work, relationships, and activities. We must be able to sacrifice spontaneity to some extent so we can effectively follow self-imposed guidelines in our daily lives. How we go about our day and how we strategize our goals is naturally not without personal challenges, because to follow a code of self-management asks that we try to further our understanding of self, of our capabilities, and of our unfolding emotions.

According to psychologists Hom and Murphy in 1985, "When students work on goals they themselves have set, they are more motivated and efficient, and they achieve more than they do when working on goals that have been set by the teacher."[18] I feel this theory applies to all of us, not just to students. Realizing what values we hold and growing in awareness helps us set goals and achieve those goals through a plan brought about by self-discipline.

For example, the idea for writing this book had been with me for many years. When I finally undertook its writing, I committed to giving it my best. No one told me to write down my experiences. I was inspired to do it, and hence have felt good working on it and feel good about the result. You can decide to give your all in any situation, whether dealing with a disease, starting afresh after a broken relationship, or excelling at work. The test of true self-discipline is knowing that the most important time to practice winning is when you aren't winning—yet.

Positive self-esteem. Self-esteem describes the esteem in which we hold ourselves and how we feel about ourselves; it is our reflection of ourselves back to ourselves. The level of this esteem is born of self-appraisal, an examination of our emotions, beliefs, and behaviors, and it is a basic human need. A positive self-esteem bolsters self-confidence and contributes to our overall happiness, and being happy stimulates more positive actions and behaviors that affect not only us, but everyone around us. Highs and lows are a part of everyone's life; the difference is that those of us with positive self-esteem are able to treat them as temporary phases, whereas those of us with lower self-esteem can find ourselves caught up in the emotional drama, feeling we are unable to affect our situations in the way we want. This attitude can easily adversely affect us as well as the lives of the people with whom we interact.

The inner voice that lives within each of us can be heard to speak either positively or negatively during the course of any given day. Those with positive self-esteem hear more positive messages on a more regular basis, so no situation seems too unmanageable. It is that inner voice that guides us to the decisions and judgments we make throughout our lives. If, however, the voice is overly critical or negative, we may find ourselves making decisions that aren't necessarily the best for us, and that can bring up less than constructive feelings about ourselves. The most important judgment we can make is the one we make about ourselves, so we must always honor and respect ourselves first.

There are a number of ways our self-esteem can get a boost. Changing the way you perceive yourself and your life is a good first step to increasing self-confidence. The best place to start is to recognize what needs to change. Implementing these changes can be done on a personal basis or with the help of a professional.

The Mayo Clinic has outlined five steps to move toward a healthy self-esteem.[19] The first of these five steps is to identify troubling conditions or circumstances that may contribute to depressing your self-esteem. Poor relationships, unsatisfying employment, death of a loved one, and illness are some examples of situations that can weigh heavily on the psyche. The second step is to become aware of your beliefs and thoughts. Your thoughts may be positive, indifferent, or negative; however, knowing that they are *your* thoughts—and that they can diminish your self-esteem based on what types of thoughts they are—is what matters. The third step is to pinpoint negative or inaccurate thinking. Notice thoughts about which you feel negative and situations about which you have definite opinions. These negative thoughts and beliefs about something or someone can have physical, emotional, and behavioral ramifications. Physical responses to such negative thoughts and beliefs can cause symptoms such as musculoskeletal pain, sweating, and stomach problems; emotional responses can create anxiety, worry, and depression; and behavioral responses can surface as under-eating, over-eating, spending more time alone, and blaming others for your problems.

The fourth step in gaining a healthy self-esteem is to systematically challenge any negative or inaccurate thinking. Many habitual thoughts and beliefs may feel totally legitimate to you, but are actually distorted perceptions. Inner thoughts, such as all-or-nothing thinking, mental filtering (focusing on the negative), converting positives into negatives, jumping to negative conclusions, mistaking feelings for facts, and constantly putting yourself down, are likely to wear down self-esteem. The fifth and final step to increase self-esteem is to change your thoughts and beliefs to the degree where a higher self-esteem can once again reemerge. Constructive thoughts mend and replace habitual, distressing, and irrational thinking with ones that align us with the truth. Intuitive thought patterns, such as being hopeful, forgiving yourself, avoiding "shoulding," focusing on the positive, redefining upsetting thoughts, and always encouraging yourself help heal a battered self-esteem. Remember, there is nothing wrong with giving yourself a nice pat on the back, even if it's with your own hand! Enjoy the reward; you deserve it.

Positive self-dimension. When we speak of the *dimension* of something, we're talking about its characteristics and facets. When we talk about *self–dimension*, we are looking at the way in which we define ourselves, our knowledge, and our capabilities. The better we know ourselves, the more confidently we feel about implementing our thoughts to produce the best results. When we incorporate various modalities to get to know ourselves better, we enhance our ability to understand our own body, mind, and spirit. Modalities can include anything from yoga and meditation to learning more about our physical bodies through research. Wherever learning is involved, it allows us to expand our awareness of ourselves and the world around us. Expanding our awareness provides many opportunities for growth, and hence leads to the option of saying "no, thank you" to certain options and "yes, please" to others. In some ways we might feel we actually increase our own "dimensionality" or become "bigger" as we expand. As Dr. Waitley says, "There are two primary choices in life, to accept conditions as they exist, or accept the responsibility for changing them."

Positive self-awareness. *Self-awareness* in its truest sense is having an honest opinion of self. If we are able to reach the point where we have an unconditional belief in our capabilities, we will be thinking optimistically, and as a result, continue to move in a positive direction. In order to do this, we need to have ongoing conversations with ourselves, building awareness one moment at a time. Talking to oneself is not an act of madness either. "Self-talk" increases awareness of our thoughts, patterns of behavior, and beliefs, which might otherwise remain forever suppressed. Once we start to really listen to our own inner voice and address it with conscious "talk," we may actually surprise ourselves with capabilities and aspirations that have previously gone untapped. Self-awareness allows us to better understand why we feel what we feel and why we do the things we do. That understanding then gives us the opportunity and freedom to change those things we would like to change about ourselves and create the life we want. As Tao Tzu once said, "Knowing others is wisdom; knowing yourself is enlightenment."

Positive self-projection. *Self-projection* is that ability to project our best selves every day in the way we look, walk, talk, listen, and react. It is having the capacity to care about how and what we communicate to others, as well as to have an internal space that welcomes the process of listening to others. It is knowing the value of the impression we make on others and repaying value to others. The fact is that words actually make up only a small percentage of the total communication we have with other people. The majority of our communication is non-verbal, expressed by posture, body movement, gestures, and voice tone. Through these elements of body language we "project" a true reflection of what we are really offering from inside. Feeling comfortable to express what we are feeling in the form of a warm smile, through eye contact, or by extending a hand allows us to be at ease with ourselves and those around us, and to put our best foot forward every day in every way.

During an illness like cancer, this kind of self-projection can help us manage treatment procedures more proactively, allow us to focus on understanding the procedures with more attention, and communicate with healthcare providers more successfully. I remember during my own cancer treatment seeing a man wait for his chemotherapy treatment armed with an arsenal of jokes to share. He told one joke after another. You could say that he was "projecting" pure joy in that he had the joke gene, or that his self-projection was one of laughter. All the nurses and doctors looked forward to seeing this man because his self-projectional humor filled the halls with laughter. He was a self-generating inspiration who helped the rest of us face our treatments with a smile.

Not having the right means to deal with mental distress can have a negative effect on health outcomes. For example, in a study involving 302 healthy male Japanese workers, a correlation was found between "unstable introverts" and "stable extrovert" personality types and cancer, where emotionally unstable introverts had decreased NK activity along with higher plasma levels of noradrenaline. The researchers of this study state that the emotionally unstable introverted men had a decreased capacity for the host's immune system to defend against cancer, possibly based on two factors: an unhealthy lifestyle and a high sensitivity to mental stress.[20]

Relative to breast cancer outcomes, a number of studies have reported that various psychological factors and other influences, such as having a fighting spirit, having a social support network, and feeling emotions such as anger, joy, guilt, depression, fatalism, and stress, have both positive and negative impacts on both survival and recurrence rates.[21] In one study, for example, Eysenck et al. found that personality types can be predictors of death from cancer and heart disease. In this case, where the individual's personality type was defined in terms of coping with interpersonal stress, it was found that stress was a significant factor in his or her cause of death, where stressed individuals had a 40% higher death rate compared to those that were non-stressed.[22]

As John Steinbeck once said, "A sad soul can kill quicker than a germ." Becoming aware of our thoughts and feelings helps us change the things we want to change and begin to create the healthy life we deserve. The clearer we become about our ever-expanding multidimensional self, the more certain the path to health becomes, and a positive personal image invariably lays the path to self-growth and success.

The mind

The mind is one of the greatest creations gifted by God to humanity. It creates and generates thoughts, actions, and reactions. To understand the mind, we need to look to both our conscious and unconscious minds. The conscious mind has been described as the state of being aware and responsive to our surroundings; in essence, it is the part of us that is constantly processing an ongoing accumulation of mental events. This awareness may involve moods, emotions, thoughts, sensations, and perceptions. The unconscious mind, on the other hand, is the part of the mind that processes *without* our awareness. This portion of the mind holds a collection of repressed memories, emotions, and urges. Both the conscious and the unconscious together form a basis for who we have become—who we are in the now. Exploring both our conscious and unconscious thoughts helps us take steps to better understand ourselves.

I call exploration of this nature performing a "personal evaluation." During different periods in my life, I have taken the opportunity to sit down and write out a list of my values, beliefs, and goals. I ask myself: *Am I living up to the standards I believe I hold in my mind?* And then I listen for the answers that come. Questioning who we are, how we live our lives, and what we believe helps develop our sense of who we are as individuals, something that can be invaluable when dealing with cancer and its aftermath. As I said at the beginning of this chapter, I felt more than a little lost after the verdict that I was "cured" of my cancer and I had many unanswered questions, such as, *What would the future hold?* and *How could I plan and anticipate when the future held so many unknowns?* Questions like these began to appear in my thoughts on a regular basis. It was only when I began to concentrate on the present and to live moment to moment, with all my attention concentrated on that moment, that I realized my future—my tomorrow—was in fact taking shape, and that the shape it was taking was growing more and more concrete everyday. Using my imagination creatively, deepening my faith, and looking at the bright side helped me persevere against the obstacles I knew still lay ahead.

How do we set about accomplishing so much in seemingly so little time precisely when we may be going through one of the most difficult periods of our lives? There are many ways to proceed. In fact, the options are endless. That's why I want to take the time here to go through some of the tools that helped me and that may also help you in experiencing a better today and a brighter tomorrow.

Affirmations

I call it "healthy-speak": the conscious declaration of the truth as you know it in order to support and empower; the recitation of words and statements that provide sustenance for the mind just as food provides sustenance for the body. When we are supportive of ourselves and our abilities, we allow positive energy to flow through our physical being. I think of this energy as mental goose bumps that bathe each and every cell with a constructive force. Saying—as well as repeating and affirming—positive statements to ourselves everyday reinforces and reaffirms our self-worth, makes us feel strong and revitalized. I personally derive strength from their repetition because of my belief in their meaning.

An affirmation can be comparable to an oath or a grave declaration with a specific purpose in mind. As human beings, we understand on some level that everything contains both the positive and negative, good and bad, beautiful and ugly, the yin and the yang, and so on. In this knowing we are also able to call forth the ability to see more of the positive than the negative, more of the beauty than the ugliness, and more of the good than the bad—should we so desire. This ability can be brought about by affirmation simply because if we tell ourselves something over and over again, it can be made possible by sheer conscious willpower and the seeding of the unconscious. If I feel good about myself, surely there will be many more able to see the good in me. If I am worthwhile and lovable in my own mind, surely I am much more likely to be seen in the same light by those around me.

Inspirational words for us are like water to a plant, going deep into our roots to help us grow and flourish. Inspiring words arouse our spirits. They stimulate us in positive ways, mentally, physically, and spiritually. They fortify and awaken the nurturing self within us, giving us hope, confidence, and the strength we need to persevere. If there is no one around to encourage you in this way, do it for yourself with "healthy speak." This is how the daily practice of "affirming" begins.

We all have choices and we all make choices. There is a lot to be said for choosing a healthy outlook. Healthy words build resistance and strength by creating in us a constructive belief system. Since our mind directs and dictates our beliefs, it follows that if we believe on some level that we do not deserve to be healthy, or cannot be healthy, we will continue to act in self-fulfilling ways that validate those feelings about ourselves. Conversely, if we can develop a daily ritual of reciting positive dialogue, then a positive outcome will prevail. How we talk to ourselves is just as important as how we treat ourselves. We can either build ourselves up or tear ourselves down. I don't particularly like to admit that I have days when I have less-than-encouraging thoughts and feelings. But when I allow them to fester by playing them over and over in my mind, it only makes things worse. In no time I find I am dwelling on the negative, and soon depression can overcome me. When I reach that point I can be lulled into a state of apathy, where eventually I feel forlorn and lonely to the degree where I end up muddling through my day, not actively living it. I try to remind myself that if I stop for a moment and make a conscious decision to *think* differently, I may end up *feeling* differently, and that one decision could turn my day around. It's the old adage: Do I see my glass as half empty or half full? In other words, *Will I be prey or predator to my feelings?* and *Do I realize that I have a choice?*

Fearing the worst

Once you have had an illness, experienced a recurrence, or been in remission, it's common to feel that those negative doom-and-gloom feelings will never quite go away. So, let me again share what we talked about earlier: this is NORMAL. It is normal to have feelings of despair and impending catastrophe after a major illness. I would be concerned if you didn't; it just wouldn't be human. It is the nature of human beings to fear and expect the worst; it is how our brains are wired. I will give you an example. Let's just say you and two friends have a dinner date at 7:00 PM. You are done with work early, and decide to go to the restaurant and wait there. You know based on past outings that your friends are always on time. While waiting for your friends, you glance down to look at your watch and notice that it is now 7:05. You begin to look around, wondering if perhaps you are standing where you can't see each other. You start to wander away from where you were standing to look around. At 7:15 you start to worry. Your mind begins to play games. The dialogue within you begins. *We said 7:00—didn't we? Maybe I misunderstood. We did say this restaurant—didn't we? Gee, I hope everything's okay.... What if something happened? I hope they weren't in an accident. They're never this late; something bad must have happened!* At that moment your friends walk in. You instantly feel relieved. You tell yourself how silly you were to worry. They apologize for being late. They'd stopped because they had seen a beautiful candle in the window of a store on the way to the restaurant. They thought you'd really like it and wanted you to have it, so they went in and bought it for you. In the meantime, you had created a whole scenario based in worry and fear—totally baseless in reality. Your mind distorted reality in a negative, counterproductive way.

Why do we seem to lean toward fearing the worst about things? I think that fear comes up the most when we feel unable to manage things over which we have little or no control. We all experience these kinds of thoughts sometimes. They can creep up on us or grab us unexpectedly from behind, but it's all a part of being human. It's when we take a moment to recognize them for what they are that we begin to be able to reassess our thinking and cope with the fatalistic thoughts in a new way. It helps to understand that being pessimistic or anxious is for many the first line of defense. But however natural it may feel to think these thoughts, they are not necessarily based in truth. In fact, often it's just the opposite; we have created an alternate reality that has caused us further distress, or fear, or unhappiness.

It takes a certain level of awareness to decipher what is truth and what is trickery; what is real and what is not; what our version of reality is compared to the reality of others. Our reality is nothing more than how we choose to view the outside world and ourselves. It is our interpretation of everything we are, do, see, learn, and believe. Naturally, because our perceptions come from our unique personal point of view, we imagine what we don't know—or choose not to see that there is more of the story than we can access at any given time. We can never know what other people are thinking and feeling unless they tell us or we ask. Even then, we can never know all the facts about every situation, even if we were to try. Bear in mind that at times our perceptions may be skewed and create confusion, and that the illusions which we accept as reality without further inspection can cause self-inflicted discomfort without any real basis. When we allow these illusions to take over, we often start accepting the first convenient reasoning that comes to mind.

Affirmations, on the other hand, can help us build positive images and strengthen our sense of self. They give us fortitude and a sense of renewal in the process of healing. We must remind ourselves that we are on a journey, one where healing is a marathon, not a sprint. Healthy dialogue (and self-talk) works best when it is practiced every day just the way a marathon is best run after lots of practice to establish strength and persistence. Affirmations are a way of conditioning the mind, just as exercise conditions the body. When we practice affirmations day after day, week after week, month after month, year after year, it doesn't take long before the practice becomes as much of a habit as breathing. Our words naturally become a part of us. Just as we pick up skin moisturizer to tone up our skin or a barbell to tighten our muscles, affirmations influence the mind in ways that keep us healthy.

There is absolutely no doubt in my mind that a healthy state of mind is instrumental in the ongoing journey to maintaining good health and preventing disease.

How to affirm

Affirmations show gratitude for what *is*, and for what can be, and help to remind us of the things for which we are thankful. A time-honored approach to creating your own affirmations is to listen to what others have already created. There are many people from all walks of life who have spoken words of wisdom. You don't have to make up your own right away, and this can ease the way to learning. Listen to a CD you like. Repeat the affirmations aloud. Say them quietly in your mind as you're driving, riding a bus, on a break from work, awakening from sleep, or before you settle in at night. You can read them or write them down. With a keyboard or paper and pen in hand, write what you would like to affirm each day.

Here are some helpful hints when practicing affirmations:

Stay in the present. I find that affirmations work much better when I stay in the present about things. Here is an example. Recite, "I am healthy and happy," with belief and conviction. Speak, write, recite, and listen to it as if you own it in your mind and heart. Avoid saying the following: "Someday I will be healthy and happy," because using the future tense only sets us further apart from what we believe we want. Another good example is, "I am and will continue to be disease-free. Avoid saying, "Eventually I will be disease-free," or "I want to be disease-free." Referring to the future implies that you are not already healthy and happy and disease-free. This can be construed by the mind as being a negative affirmation—an affirmation that we expect only the "bad stuff" to happen. It is therefore imperative that when we do our affirmations we stay in the moment.

Be specific. To condition the mind you must be specific in your intent. You want to accurately relay your thoughts and feelings so you move in the right or most positive direction. Here is an example to which I think we can all relate. Just look at how efficient most of us become when the holiday season arrives and we want to exchange gifts with friends, coworkers, and loved ones. What's the first thing we do when there are a number of people for whom we want to buy gifts? We make a list. We write down all the specific things we want to buy for each person and where to go to purchase those gifts. From that list, we become an automatic guidance system. Our brain now has specific goals and like a homing device we make the necessary adjustments in our daily lives to accomplish what's on the list. If one of the gifts on your list is a ball for your son or daughter, that is not a precise enough piece of information to move you in the correct direction. Your brain must know the specifics to search out and bring home the right thing. Do you want a football, or maybe a baseball, or a volleyball? Your mind needs to know exactly what to look for to send you in the right direction and achieve your objective. To be healthy a mind needs direction. Without a map, we float aimlessly out to sea. Reciting, "A simple arm stretch revitalizes me," rather than "Moving around makes me feel okay," will condition you to move in the exact way that will make you feel better.

Use repetition. Someone once said that repetition is the mother of learning. Repetition conditions the mind, building strong anchors that unconsciously remind us of all the good that is within. As any athlete will tell you, daily practice is equally as important as the game itself. Affirmations work best if you can schedule them into your day, for example in the morning, middle of the day, and then again in the evening. But you can't overdo them. As many times as you like, for as many days as you want, continue them until you feel a change is in order. Then write and say new ones. There's no such thing as being "too positive," after all. The only side effect from the continued reciting of affirmations is good health, so it helps to be disciplined and repetitive in your recitations.

Be personal. When doing affirmations use "I" or your name (or both) in the reciting of your proclamations. For example, "I am strong and healthy," "Douglas Levine is strong and healthy," or, my own favorite, "I, Douglas Levine, am strong and healthy." Remember these words are *your* words, for you and about you and *only* you. They are meant to be personal and intimate. If you stop for a minute to think about the word *intimate*, it usually means something that is essential and private. When I am saying words that are intimate, they are words exclusively for me, "into me," for only me. This is because my illness, and now my health, is about me and nobody else. No one can help me with this mental restoration except me. It's entirely personal.

Keep it simple. If you're new to affirmations, it can help to start with one or two. Write down, read, or listen to these one or two affirmations every day, easing the ability of the mind to absorb them better. I'd like to share an incident relative to this concept that happened when I used to play baseball. I love the game, although when this incident happened, it was the first time I had put on my baseball mitt in about 10 years. Despite my apprehension and awkwardness, I decided to play anyway. When I got to the field, I greeted many of my soon-to-be teammates who were tossing the ball to one another. Realizing I was a newcomer, several of them decided to greet me by throwing the ball to me. Suddenly, unintentionally, they all threw balls in my direction at the same time. The next thing I knew, four balls were being hurled at me at once. At that moment, without thinking, I just stuck my glove straight in the air, hoping that random act would catch one of the balls. Well, it didn't work. I got so confused and was so panic-stricken that I didn't end up catching a single ball, and all four soon littered the grass around me. But as I looked down at the balls at my feet, I did learn a valuable lesson. I had had several balls to choose from. Had I focused on catching just one I would certainly have had the opportunity to catch the one of my choice. The mind is the same way: it can generally only handle one thing at a time. If you overwhelm it by too many affirmations at once, you won't catch the ball. Simplicity in mastering a singular phrase or phrases in the beginning is key to allowing the mind to use these declarations effectively.

Be realistic. When you do your affirmations, make sure what you are reciting is genuine. Be down to earth when sharing these sentences or thoughts with yourself. A major component of affirming is continuing to state the truth about things. Nothing grates on the soul more than when what is being said does not have an ounce of truth to it. Inflated or exaggerated remarks will hinder you, not help you. One of the goals of affirmation is to remove the grandiose beliefs some of us may have and simplify our belief systems about ourselves. Here is a good example. This statement can be defined as a truth: "I deserve to be happy and fulfilled." It is straightforward, positive, and encouraging. This next statement is pompous and egotistical: "I deserve to be happy, have all the riches in the world, and be fulfilled at any expense or the expense of others." While exaggerated, this may be a statement based on some unconscious grandiose wish, and it lacks the support and self-love that make simpler affirmations more understandable and nurturing. So keep it honest and keep it simple.

Be positive. A healthy, winning outlook is the first step toward achieving any goal. Let your words be decisive, upbeat, and encouraging. Allow them to be expressions of faith, not fear. Speak as if you are certain of the outcome. Tell your mind in a definite way how you are. Positive feelings will then continue to reinforce and reconfigure your attitudes and beliefs about yourself. It's similar to cleaning out your closet. The other day I was getting dressed for work. I was looking for a particular shirt that I knew went just right with the pants I had chosen. I opened my closet and pushed shirts to one side and then back to the other side, feverishly looking for that blue shirt, the one I knew was in there. During my search, I pulled out other shirts and extended them toward the light to see if they would work. I even tried on one or two. The first shirt I tried was stained, discolored, and the cuffs were frayed. I immediately unbuttoned it and took it off, hurling it at the end of the bed. I then took the second shirt off the hanger, which also looked as if it had been in my closet for some time. I stood in front of the mirror and began buttoning the shirt. Staring into the mirror, I noticed that my fingers were continuing to fumble in the same area. I looked down and noticed that two buttons were missing from the shirt. When I dropped my arms down, I realized that the sleeves were way too short. Feeling thoroughly annoyed, I took off the shirt and threw it next to the other one to be bagged and given to Good Will. This then inspired me to go through my entire closet and discard clothes that were old, worn, or just weren't "me" anymore. This newfound space afforded me the opportunity to change and replace the clothes I would be giving away with new ones.

This is precisely what affirmations do on a mental level. They purge out the old worn space occupying negative feelings and bring in the new, encouraging, empowering, and constructive forces. This is not to say that we do not already have some positive beliefs about ourselves in our mental closets. I believe we all have them, but we also have old belief systems that have been in place—potentially for a long time. Over the years, due to our experiences, our upbringings, and other forces, some of these negative beliefs continue to haunt us, and some of our more positive dogmas become tarnished. When any of these ways of thinking no longer serve our highest good, they are best let go, or revised to suit our current lives. This may also be regarded as an opportunity to reconsider some of the ideas we rejected in the past, to look at them in a new light. It is possible that these "transformed" ideals can be positively incorporated into our lives. Once that happens, new thoughts and beliefs naturally begin to energize.

Be patient. The expression "Rome wasn't built in a day" has just as much validity as it ever did. Healing is a process that takes time. A friend once told me, "It ain't the getting, it's the going that's good!" So concentrate on the process, not the goal. While goals are important, and planning (as we've discussed) is certainly important, practice is what allows these subtle changes to take place. We can reach our goals by permitting them to naturally unfold simply by undertaking the process of affirmations on a daily basis.

Unfortunately, we have become brainwashed into thinking that most everything can be resolved or achieved instantaneously. From instant cash to pills for pain relief, we expect results to be easy and quick. Turning on the television or reading the newspaper reveals an endless barrage of advertisements for "fast" food, how to be an "instant" millionaire, or how to get "immediate" relief from a cold, pain, or depression. These ads would have us believe that all our problems can be resolved in a matter of minutes. But while these claims may be true occasionally—yes, we can eat more quickly if we are willing to trade good health for fast-food products, and yes, sometimes a pill can alleviate headache pain—the only sure road to mental and spiritual clarity is the one that requires more patience. This is not necessarily a "bad" thing either. When we enjoy the journey, appreciate our daily lives, the process simply becomes part of the enjoyment, and we forget that we were aiming for a quick fix in the first place.

Try to be patient doing your affirmations. Some days you will remember to do them, some days you might forget. Other days you may not think you are doing them "correctly." There may be times when you say or read a statement that triggers negative feelings. I'm not sure anyone really knows why, but in this case it could be that emphasizing the positive reminds us of how far we have to go, or how we've mishandled things in the past. But it doesn't really matter *why*. What matters is that if you find yourself saying, "This is nonsense, it will never work, I feel ridiculous doing these. Why am I wasting my time?" that you just keep plugging along, recognizing that having these thoughts *and overriding them* is the key to progress. So, be forewarned: when you are cleaning the closet, you may get scratched by hangers, get dust in your eyes, or be just plain frustrated that you have to spend time getting things in order. In the end, though, I can say unequivocally that the outcome will give you a sense of accomplishment and a potentially greater sense of peace than you've ever experienced before.

Getting started

Enough theory. Let's look at the many different ways we can do affirmations. After we look at some of the step-by-step methods for performing them, you will be able to do them however you want, whenever you want, and wherever you want. Remember, doing affirmations is about *you* and only you. It's about your relationship with yourself and with your higher consciousness. Finding your path may take some practice, but whichever way you feel comfortable doing them will be the way for you. There is no better way! Are you ready to get started? Great, then let's get to it.

Read your affirmations. I find one of the simplest and easy ways to do affirmations is to read them. They can be read aloud or quietly to yourself. They can be your own words of understanding or someone else's. If the affirmations you wish to recite are your own words, I find writing them and keeping them in one place such as a journal is helpful. Some people choose to jot down one or two sayings on a small piece of paper that they can keep with them. The bottom line is to do whatever makes you comfortable and fits in with your daily life. There are scores of books available on this subject, both at local bookstores and libraries, for those who wish to be inspired by writings or teachings of others. There are individuals from all walks of life who have written and been quoted throughout the centuries. You may be surprised to find that some of their words coincide with your own feelings, so feel free to share their contributions. If you find a book that really speaks to you, carry it around with you, leave it on your night stand, or bring it to work to keep it easily accessible.

Listen to affirmations. Hearing affirmations on CD or MP3 is also an excellent way of getting into the habit. For example, carrying an MP3 or a disc of affirmations with you will turn your commute time into productive time. The streets of New York are filled with people with headphones in their ears. They remove themselves from the hustle and bustle by concentrating on what they want to hear. Instead of listening to music or the news of the day, try listening to a recording of either your own voiced affirmations or someone else's. If you drive to and from work, the privacy in your car gives you the opportunity to listen and recite affirmations without distraction.

On the subject of distraction, it needs to be said that there is no question that we all need some distraction in our lives. Distraction serves as an important component to our sanity; sometimes we need to shift our focus outside ourselves, away from our own thoughts and concerns. But society has produced so many ways we can distract ourselves that we can easily manage to avoid ourselves altogether. And the ways in which we can be distracted are so inviting—the news, television, Internet, music, movies, games: these are just some of the ways we are constantly bombarded with external information.

Of course, there is always plenty of high drama available to us if we choose to stay distracted, on the periphery of consciousness. Again, this is where balance is so important. Being entertained, for example, being able to relax by reading, watching TV, or playing a game, is just that—entertaining and relaxing. But having one foot engaged in the outside world of information, news, sports, gossip, and play, while the other foot is firmly planted in a world of self-development, is really the only healthy and balanced way to go, and it is the place where true healing begins.

Finding that happy medium may take some effort and seem like sacrifice. By that I mean you may feel you have to give up something to get something else. You may have to listen to 10 fewer minutes of radio to complete 10 more minutes of affirmations. You will have those days when the pull to stay outside yourself—in other words, engage in distraction—is very strong and prevents you from engaging in other more thoughtful pursuits. These are days where the latest tragedy, love affair, or weather report competes for your time and energy and convinces you to avoid looking within. The truth is, though, that we can only run away for so long, because sooner or later we all need to "go home." And since home is where the heart is, we need to make time to listen.

Post your affirmations. Placing sayings in and around your home or office is also a helpful way of continuing to reaffirm your beliefs. Attaching notes on the refrigerator, inserting them into pop-up screens on your computer, or pinning them to the corkboard at work can serve as quick jolts of inspiration through the day. Between work and home, most of us feel the pinch of time constraints that prevent us from always affirming in the manner we might prefer. That's why using "shortcuts" that we place in front of us can be small yet effective references to encourage a change in direction when we may need it the most. I think this is one of the reasons I like desktop calendars so much. Besides taking up very little space and giving you the date and day, many have insightful sayings on each day of the year. At a glance, you can take a minute to reflect. Even such a little thing can be an oasis in the desert of daily living when things are tough, a cool drink of water when you're feeling emotionally thirsty. Pausing for a bit of introspection can be very rewarding—an additional tool on your continued quest for a healthy life.

Imagine affirmations. Imagination, someone once said, is the birth of all invention. Everything that surrounds us at one time began in someone's imagination, and represents someone's fantasy that reached fulfillment. The car we drive, the building we inhabit, or the book we are reading was at one time just an idea; that idea became an image and, eventually, reality. Vividly imagining what you would like to see affirmed in your life is your mind's practical way of restating your beliefs. In this case, you may be someone who prefers to create and listen to your own mentally generated affirmations, a process which can be just as helpful as reading or listening to the CDs of others.

Let me give you an example. The other night I woke up from a dream and rolled over. With one eye open, I glanced at my alarm clock and noticed that it was only 5 AM. Being half asleep and half awake, I rolled onto my back and put my hands firmly under my head. I aimlessly stared into space, trying to decide what to do. I then quietly asked myself, "Should I get up or should I go back to sleep?" It was useless to pretend that I was seriously entertaining the possibility of getting up, so I decided to turn over and go back to sleep. I didn't have to wake up until 6:30 and within minutes I had drifted back to sleep, knowing that I would have another hour and a half of rest. As the morning changed the darkness into light in the bedroom, I woke up. Looking over at the alarm clock, I saw that it was much later than it should have been. I wondered why I hadn't heard the clock radio go on. I peered through one eye at the clock, and saw that the alarm *had* gone off, but I had slept right through it! Realizing that I had overslept for almost an hour, I frantically ripped the covers off my body and raced bleary-eyed into the bathroom and jumped in the shower. Feeling discombobulated, I quickly dressed and ran out the door to go to work. It felt like the quintessential morning from hell.

As you might imagine, this was a morning that I didn't have the mental space or time to read or listen to my affirmations for the day. Knowing I was agitated and feeling restless, I decided the best thing to do was to put my imagination to work while I drove. I turned off the radio, went into the recesses of my mind, and asked myself the following question: What could I say to make this day a better one, since the morning hadn't started out so well? I began searching for the right words as images passed through my mind. At that moment, my focus changed from feeling restless to concentrating on finding the words that would help put me in a better place. After a few moments I settled down and began silently reciting over and over to myself, "Slow, deep breathing relaxes me." As I continued to repeat these five words, I began to feel my respiration deepen and slow. My neck muscles began to relax and my abdomen began to feel less rigid. As the minutes passed, I began to feel easier and a calmness gradually replaced my self-inflicted high anxiety. My thoughts continued to assist me in letting go. I began to feel much less harried and I felt better with every breath I took. In the absence of a typical start with a book, CD, or journal, I went within and used my innate gift of imagination to redirect me to a more peaceful place. Soon I arrived at work, a bit late, but none the worse for wear.

Equally important as how and what to do is *when* to do your affirmations. Since affirmations are such a personal conveyance, it is difficult to give you a definitive answer on when to do them. It's up to you, really, and when you feel most comfortable to "receive." I do have some suggestions that may be helpful.

Be alone. A quiet room, a car, or a park are all good places where you can take the time to say what you want to say. I always feel that time alone is time well spent. This may sound selfish, but time you spend in developing your inner consciousness can be just as important as making time for others. I know many people who effortlessly and willingly find time to share and, in fact, will generously do anything for other people. But when it comes to themselves they seem to have great resistance. For many of us, the habit of doing something for ourselves has become less important than doing something for someone else. *The truth is that you are no less important and deserve the same kind of care and consideration that you give to or have for anyone else.*

To some, the idea of being *alone* may have a negative connotation attached to it. The very word may conjure up feelings of loneliness and abandonment or may bring up feelings of isolation and alienation. I can tell you from personal experience that this phenomenon is particularly common among cancer survivors. The last thing I want to identify with is feeling isolated and disconnected. For me, the idea of "being alone" tends to bring up all sorts of heightened irrational emotions, like feeling forsaken and in despair. It's odd, then, that what I've learned is that the more I am alone doing affirmations, the more I know that I am *not* alone. "Alone time" has become "oneness time." It is the time I have given myself a moment to connect with my inner self in order to connect with something greater than myself. So, if you find being alone feels awkward, I invite you to stay with it, do your best to believe there is something more, and have faith that a great relationship (with yourself and with the universe) will come of it.

Be prepared. I find a certain amount of mental readiness is required to do affirmations on a daily basis. By "readiness" I mean deciding for yourself when you feel at your best to receive "the good." In general, I have come across two types of people: morning people and night people. We all know them—people who don't seem to really wake up until the day is half over and people who wake up raring to go first thing in the morning. I have a friend who comes to life after 10 PM. He says he does all his best reading and writing late in the wee hours of the night. I have another friend who feels she is most productive in the early morning hours when she first wakes up and is the most energetic and clear-minded. So a good question to ask yourself might be, *When do I think I would receive the maximum benefit from my affirmations?* And then go with your innate biological flow to let that perfect harmony unfold.

I would also like to take a moment to address those individuals who might not have the luxury of choosing a "right" time of day due to personal or professional constraints.

Some days it's just impossible to find the time to listen while you're driving, to glance at posted quotes, or to read at lunch. As in other areas, in this one too I am a firm believer that doing something is better than doing nothing. Even a phrase repeated once or twice helps. Over time, your body will take the total sum of your self-instruction and put it to good use.

Affirmations and your state of mind

Besides evaluating our best time of day to do affirmations, what about taking into account our state of mind? Doesn't it make a difference how we feel about doing our affirmations at any given point in time? Of course it does. But remember, the process of affirming can have a profound effect on our state of being.

The two most common feelings we experience are on opposite ends of the same spectrum: calmness and distress. And though these two words may contain some of the same letters and the same number of letters, that's about all they have in common. When we are feeling calm, we invite fertile ground for cultivating our belief systems. This is an excellent time to listen, write, recite, and imagine. Doing affirmations when we are calm is naturally conducive to experiencing further feelings of wellbeing, a state which then helps us feel more accomplished. This effect further contributes to an ongoing commitment to continuing with our affirmations.

Then there is calm's evil twin, as I like to put it: distress. When the feeling of distress comes barging in, calmness can go right out the door as if it were never there at all. Sometimes when the emotion of distress takes over, it can make you feel totally out of control. I've been known to feel anxious, irritable, and overwhelmed, robbed of the day's strength. When it has a real grip on me, I can be consumed to the point where I cannot focus on anything except my distress. I crave sugary snacks, but then after eating them feel guilty about gorging myself. I over-stimulate myself by watching too much mindless television, even knowing that I'm being self-destructive. Believe it or not, affirmations in times like these can be a life preserver to get you back to the shores of calmness—an energy saver allowing you to temporarily catch your breath and regain your footing. Remember my earlier story of sleeping through the alarm and starting the day off frazzled? I used an affirmation to assist me in calming down so I could gain my composure and get back in control of the things I *could* control. This is a prime example of how to use affirmations when you are feeling distressed to help you stop feeling that way. There is no shame in seeking help *from* yourself, *for* yourself. Pause, talk to yourself, and trust that your higher power will give you the answer you seek.

Types of affirmations

Affirmations come in all different sizes and shapes. Which kind of affirmation you choose will depend on which part of your self you are addressing. The "self" is who we think we are and what we have come to know about ourselves. It is normal to develop perceptions about ourselves as we grow and develop, but it is also important to be aware that while some of these perceptions may be true, others may not be as true. Somehow we come to believe both the truths and the untruths. We have all had the experience where someone (it could be a friend, a family member, or even a stranger) says something about us that makes us question our own beliefs. Before we know it, without blinking an eye, we automatically process it as something that must be true. It could be about our looks, our intellect, or our personality, but for some reason, without really thinking it through, we believe it. If we accept such statements as truth, it may well be only a short step to incorporating them into our consciousness, into our perception of ourselves. Ultimately, if we accept them fully, we will soon believe them to be more real than what we originally knew to be the reality. If this happens, it won't take long before we have believed them for so long that we no longer question their validity at all. In essence, they become who we are, who we believe ourselves to be. We soon forget how they have gotten there because over time they have become "our own" strong beliefs.

Strong beliefs of this nature naturally spawn self-fulfilling prophecies, loosely based on nothing more than what we think we believe. I can give you a personal example, one which has had a profound effect on me for as long as I can remember. When I was growing up my parents told me that I was not as smart as my sister. This general observation was based on the scholastic outcome of a *single* test. Through elementary school and high school my sister was the model student. She got As, all the teachers loved her, and she made the National Honor Society. I, on the other hand, had come home with a low grade on a math test in the fourth grade. "You're lazy! You will never be as smart as your sister!" my father declared as he looked at me with my test paper firmly grasped in his fist. Being young, impressionable, and already fairly insecure, it never occurred to me not to believe what my father said to me on that winter day. With my head down to hide my tears, I turned and retreated to my room quietly, saying to myself, "He's right." And from that day onward, I subconsciously set out to prove my father had indeed made the correct assessment of my abilities.

As the years progressed, I continued to do poorly in school. I never even tried to study and continued to barely pass test after test. I was placed in remedial reading classes during the summer, and my cousin Jamie was lassoed into tutoring me in math on Saturday mornings. I was unwittingly becoming the version of myself I had taken on. It was my own self-fulfilling prophecy: What you believe, so shall you be. And all it took was one cold winter day in the fourth grade, when vulnerability led to self-sabotage. When I was out of the house and began college my self-perpetuating failures only continued to reinforce what I now believed unquestioningly. Over and over again, my dismal grades reminded me on some unconscious level that my father was right. For many, many years I did not doubt for one second that what my father had said to me was true.

It wasn't until my second semester of college life that I began to question my beliefs about things. Sometimes you need to distance yourself from the old to start anew. It was here that I decided to re-evaluate my situation, perhaps create some new beliefs about myself. Feeling totally inadequate and never quite as smart as everyone else, I would simply change some things about myself that I felt needed changing. I took a break from studying in the library one day and started jotting down the things I believed about myself. I wanted to see how the "good" things about myself would measure up against the "not so good" things. It wasn't one of my happiest moments, I assure you, but I knew it was something that needed to be done. I needed a clearer understanding of who and where I was. It was then, in a moment of absolute clarity, that I realized the only thing holding me back was the opinions I had formed about myself. As soon as I started writing my list, it was clear that I had plenty of beliefs about myself, but I wasn't sure exactly where I had gotten them. They were thoughts and feelings that dealt with everything from my appearance to my motivation. They were thoughts of poor self-esteem and misguided self-direction. I continued to write down the ideas that came to me, regardless of what they were or if they made sense. My task at that moment was to get all my impressions out on the table. Once I knew what I was dealing with, maybe then I could introduce new ideas. Once I identified my real beliefs, maybe I could challenge those that didn't feel right, and then find ones that would be more consistent with who I really was and, more importantly, who I wanted to be.

I was not fully aware at that time that I was beginning my own personal revolution—and evolution. From that time on, I began to unlearn those beliefs that were self-limiting and replace them with a whole basketful of new core beliefs. It turns out that using affirmations was a method that helped me become the person I am today.

If you think this kind of exercise would be helpful for you to identify what types of affirmations you might like to introduce to yourself, jot down on a piece of paper all the things that you believe about yourself. They can be things about health, relationships, appearance, intellect, or personality—basically anything at all that starts with "I think I am…" or "I believe that…." Whatever comes to mind is important enough to write down. There is no "right" way or "wrong" way. The exercise is just a way to get these thoughts out in the open. If you experience some emotional pain, shame, or embarrassment associated with what you are writing down, simply acknowledge it and write it anyway. Pay special attention to any particularly self-limiting beliefs. These are the negative notions with which you have lived your life in the past, but are now ready to be discarded once and for all.

Below are some of the many affirmations I have used from time to time; you may find them helpful too.

- *The water I drink nourishes and cleanses my body.*
- *The fruits and vegetables I eat are health-giving.*
- *I am breathing healthy, fresh air that delivers life-giving oxygen to my cells.*
- *I am strong and healthy.*
- *I love to exercise; it makes my body strong and my mind alert.*
- *I continue to find time for myself everyday.*
- *I am healthy and happy.*
- *Sleep revitalizes me.*
- *Laughter lifts my spirits.*
- *I respect my body and accept who I am.*
- *I have a healthy self-expectancy.*
- *I am my best friend.*
- *Good will always come out of my actions.*
- *Fear of recurring illness is just that: FEAR.*
- *I am loved and I enjoy making time for family and friends.*
- *I enjoy peace of mind.*
- *Faith brings me closer to hope.*

I am not implying that your affirmations should look like or be limited to these statements—in fact, quite the opposite. The only limit to what you come up with is the limitation of your imagination; in other words, the scope is limitless. Set your mind free, make your decision, and begin without constraints or limits of any kind.

Assertiveness

Medical Dictionary Online (www.online-medical-dictionary.org) defines assertiveness as a "strongly insistent, self-assured, and demanding behavior."[23] This includes the ability to protect one's rights and to have one's own ideas, while respecting the rights and thoughts of others. When diagnosed with a serious disease it is only natural to feel confused, not to mention devastated, depressed, and, quite possibly, angry. Loving family, well-meaning friends, and healthcare professionals can provide meaningful assistance in lifting our emotions to make the road to recovery as easy as possible. However, at the end of the day, after all the advice and well-meaning gestures, *you* are the only one who can make the decisions about how to live your life, how to think about yourself, and how to look at the world. In the words of Canadian personal-growth trainer Leland Val Van de Wall, "Thinking creates an image. Images control feelings. Feelings cause actions, and actions create results."

Assertiveness has become an important added dimension in personality development. Because assertiveness is directly related to self-esteem and is helpful in boosting self-confidence, experts say that developing our assertiveness quota can reap great results. The ability to be assertive is considered an important communication skill, one that should not be confused with aggression, as is often the case. The ability to assert one's self is not at all synonymous to dominating; on the contrary, it is a way to express your views while at the same time respecting the personal opinions of others by choosing to exchange ideas in a cooperative manner. It is the art of presenting thoughts and ideas without imposing them. Practicing the capacity to exert assertive behavior during illness and treatment not only helps the recovery process, but also helps us to be stronger people.

I could write pages on the subject of how assertiveness helps and hardly get started, but, in a nutshell, I'll just say that assertiveness increases our coping abilities and gives us some semblance of control over a situation. It can help us be more open to new and positive thoughts and ideas, boost feelings of self-confidence and internal security, and bolster our sense of involvement in the decision-making process at hand. The Mayo Clinic states assertiveness has many benefits which can help us:

- understand and recognize our feelings
- earn respect from others
- improve communication
- create win-win situations
- improve decision-making skills
- create honest relationships
- gain more job satisfaction[24]

Asserting our rights with others

Asserting our rights with others might imply forcing our point of view on other people or constantly feeling the need to be right. But asserting our rights appropriately simply means having a say about what's happening so that we get the right thing done for our own greater good with the help of others. It signifies guiding people to understand our questions, thoughts, and feelings about a situation en route to the achievement of disease-free living. To assert means to insist on personal recognition, knowing that whatever you have to say should be acknowledged, respected, and valued. This means that what I say and how I feel matters—during all the stages of the process, including diagnosis, treatment, and recovery from cancer. Never forget that you, the person, and you, the patient, always have rights about your care and treatment. Never be afraid to exercise those rights.

Here are a few of the ways to exercise your right to assert:

Educate yourself. The more you know about your disease, the better off you'll be. Doctors deal with many types and sub-types of the same disease everyday. In doing so, they are experts in this field. Read, browse, talk, and listen all that you can, to *become as knowledgeable as possible.*

Enquire and ask questions. Do not hesitate to ask questions. Asking questions does not imply that you are ignorant; it is evidence only that you are interested and intelligent enough to come up with the queries. If you can't understand all the nuances of the information you receive in one shot, do not think twice about asking a second or a third time. Trying to gain an understanding will add some semblance of control by providing you with a more thorough knowledge of the process.

Feel free to change your mind. Exercise your freedom to change your mind and move to another health professional if you are not getting the care you need. Communication is an important and integral part of your recovery process; if you feel communication is lacking, you should feel free to move on to a relationship that meets your needs. It is your life, and the choices are yours.

Identify your goals and objectives. Now that you have educated yourself and found a practitioner with whom you are comfortable, go on to identify an overall goal for your treatment. While some may choose a potentially longer life, others may choose a higher quality of life...although let's face it, both would be nice. Some go for short-term goals, while others take the approach of a longer-term perspective. I remember someone who chose to make multiple short-term goals for herself. She needed to take one step at a time before she was ready to take on things for the long term. She was an inspiration to many who watched as her insight and ongoing attempts to know herself better not only saw her through her treatment, but also made the process more manageable and less daunting.

Be unswerving and consistent. Prolonged treatment is never easy to endure, especially with cancer, which weakens us physically and emotionally. Choose your goal and work on achieving it. The road might be rocky and you may feel shaky, but when you keep an eye on the summit the path doesn't appear as difficult as it might otherwise.

Put yourself first. You need to come before anyone else. Knowing that and carrying it out is an essential requirement during the course of your treatment. Don't think of what others are doing or thinking. Go on with a focused approach that has one aim: to improve your health and the quality of your life. Don't waste time and energy on the opinions of others. You are responsible for yourself and have a responsibility to yourself—so go ahead and help yourself achieve your goals.

Care for yourself to assure your cure. You need proper care to get strong and stay strong. In essence, taking care of yourself makes it possible for the cure to occur. Work on replenishing your lost nutrients by way of consuming a healthy diet, work on exercising your body to gain strength and endurance, socialize to lead a happy life, and always keep your target in sight. Work on achieving your goal with a combination of any measures that you think will make you feel good about you.

Continue your education and find new ways to help yourself. The world is evolving, and we are evolving along with the world with advancement in all facets of health. New discoveries in treatment and medications are changing people's lives and improving their quality of life. A cure should not be the end of your education; it should be the beginning. As you continue learning about what both conventional and alternative medicine have to offer, you will continue to benefit from new ideas, discoveries, and breakthroughs.

Visual imagery: The imaginative force

"There is a law in psychology that if you form a picture in your mind of what you would like to be, if you keep and hold that picture there for long enough, you will soon become exactly as you have been thinking."
- William James (1842–1910)

Visual imagery can be defined as a flow of thoughts that includes sensory qualities like smell, touch, hearing, taste, and motion. Visual imagery is the ability to create a realistic mental scene by using the imagination in the absence of physical stimuli. Aristotle called the imagination "a window to the soul"—to our inner thoughts, ideas, and feelings. Imagination has created art, literature, science, and mathematics, and has led us to cultivating crops, harnessing electricity, and flying to the moon. In summary, as mentioned previously, imagination makes the impossible possible.

Visualization is synonymous to creation. It is the creation of thoughts in the mind to accomplish something, where hidden capabilities are suddenly brought forth by the mind's applied influence. Visualization helps create, build, simplify, and lay down a defined path toward attainment of an objective. These objectives can vary from person to person. For some it might be the attainment of peace of mind, while for others it might be success at work or good health and happiness. Visualization has been defined and explained by great minds throughout history in different ways, but its essence remains the same.

For example, artist Paul Gauguin said, "I shut my eyes to see"; for Albert Einstein, imagination was "more important than knowledge." Author Ingrid Bengis once said, "Imagination has always had powers of resurrection that no science can match." Imagination is a tool that permits us to appraise the past, envisage the future, and perform certain actions that might not have been thought possible. Visual imagery as a methodology has been growing in popularity, recognized for its effects on psychology and, thereby, physiology. Through the process of imagery, it has been proven that we can enhance the mind-body relationship to improve both our physical and mental health.

Improving visual imagery's inner representation means creating realistic images that the body can perceive and to which the body can respond. The flow of thoughts can be so vivid that it is almost as if we are actually seeing, hearing, feeling, smelling, and tasting the images we imagine. Nikola Tesla is a great example of imagery in action. When he first arrived in America as a young man, Tesla dug ditches to survive, but his mind never stopped fomenting his future inventions. It has been said that his immense contributions to the fields of electromagnetism, nuclear physics, and theoretical physics are significantly due to his powerful visual abilities, abilities he used to problem-solve his theories before he ever committed his ideas to paper or conducted the experiments to prove them. Tesla is known for vividly conceptualizing the workings of his inventions to the minutest detail prior to implementation. In his autobiography, he describes that he often experienced moments of inspiration, sometimes accompanied by illusion or visions which manifested first into concepts, then into step-by-step procedures, and then, finally, into real form. In fact, more often than not, Tesla credits his successes to the precision of his imagination.

Albert Einstein said that when he was 16 he used to imagine the feeling of riding alongside a light beam. His conclusions, based on these images of light, later became one of the two principles of the theory of relativity. Einstein also is known to have said that he seldom thought in words, that instead he generally "thought" in images and pictures that guided his innovations and discoveries. Musician Wolfgang Mozart is reported to have composed music through visualization as well. Mozart said that when he was alone, his musical notes revealed themselves with clear definition in his mind, allowing him to hear the resultant work of art, complete and beautiful. For Mozart, the spontaneous link between his senses manifested itself in the form of music, written down only after he had visualized an entire composition in his mind.

Imagery and complementary medicine

Visual imagery is one component of the array of complementary medical approaches we have today. In complementary medicine, visual imagery is best known for its direct effects on the body's physiology because it stimulates change on different levels. Through imagery we can elicit changes in the body in ways that are usually considered inaccessible by conscious direction. Even the ancient Greeks, including Aristotle and Hippocrates, had their patients use forms of imagery to encourage the healing process. These great physicians not only believed that images release forces in the mind that stimulate the heart and other parts of the body, but that a strong image of a disease is sufficient to cause its actual symptoms. Western medicine began to notice the advantages of visual imagery in the late 1960s when biofeedback research incorporated imagery in its studies. In the early 1970s, for example, Drs. O. Carl and Stephanie Matthews-Simonton started experimenting with imagery for cancer patients at a time when people undergoing treatment were beginning to express an interest in complementary therapies to ease pain and nausea and to reduce depression and anxiety.

Dr. O. Carl Simonton was a radiation oncologist, originator of the Simonton Method, co-author of the book *Getting Well Again*, and founder of the Simonton Cancer Center in Calfornia.[25] As far back as 1969, the Simontons' research isolated certain techniques that enabled individuals to influence their own internal body processes, such as heart rate and blood pressure. The Simontons' programs focused on ways to promote balanced health and enriched lives through influencing beliefs and belief systems. According to Carl Simonton, "Essentially, the visual imagery process involved a period of relaxation, during which the patient would mentally picture a desired goal or result. With the cancer patient, this would mean his attempting to visualize the cancer, the treatment destroying it and, most importantly, his body's natural defenses helping him recover." Although there are many who have attempted to discredit the Simontons' research and methodologies, stating that they provide no evidence that guided imagery helps reduce disease or even influences the conventional treatment of serious disease, the Simontons maintained that "understanding how much you can participate in your health or illness is a significant first step in getting well."

In his book *Guided Imagery for Self-Healing*, Martin Rossman, M.D. explains that when illness occurs it means that something is out of balance and needs adjustment, needs to be adapted, or needs to be changed.[26] Dr. Rossman states, "Using imagery in this way allows illness to become a teacher of wellness. Imagery can allow you to understand more about your illness and to respond to its message in the healthiest imaginable way."

In my mind, those of us who undergo painful experiences of fear and physical discomfort owe it to ourselves to explore every way we can to feel better. One way is to use autosuggestion, where the subconscious mind can be trained to believe something with the purpose of bringing about positive results. For example, a cancer patient can use this tool to reinforce the belief that he is getting better and is fully capable of dealing with the lows commonly associated with disease and treatment.

Let's take a look at some examples from studies conducted through the years.

In the first, 80 women undergoing multimodality treatment (surgery, radiotherapy, chemotherapy, and hormone therapy) for large or locally advanced breast cancers participated in a randomized controlled study to evaluate the immuno-modulatory effects of relaxation training and guided imagery. Results showed that those patients who participated in relaxation and guided-imagery sessions had a significantly higher number of mature T-cells following their chemotherapy and radiotherapy than those patients who underwent medical treatment alone. Furthermore, those women who rated their imagery practices highly showed elevated levels of NK-cell activity at the end of chemotherapy and at follow-up.[27]

In another study, psychological distress and coping methods were examined in postsurgical patients with malignant melanoma over a six-week period. This study consisted of providing health education and psychological support to participants, which included enhancing problem-solving skills and teaching relaxation techniques. Researchers in this case found that the group of patients receiving intervention showed significantly lower depression, fatigue, confusion, and total mood disturbance, as well as a higher level of vigor than the participants who did not receive this support methodology. Specifically, the patients who received educational techniques and support tools were shown to utilize significantly more active-behavioral and active-cognitive coping than the study's control group.[28]

In other research in the same field undertaken at St. Mary's Hospital in London, 139 women with stage I and stage II breast cancer were instructed to practice relaxation and guided imagery along with their outpatient radiation therapy. In this case, researchers found that moods were better in the patients who practiced a combination of relaxation and imagery compared to those who practiced relaxation alone, and that the women who benefited the most from this approach were 55 years of age and older.[29]

Furthermore, according to researchers at the Guided Imagery Program at the Miller Family Heart and Vascular Institute at Cleveland Clinic, the positive role of guided imagery in medicine has been determined significant in its ability to help patients cope during medical and surgical procedures, chemotherapy, dialysis, *in vitro* fertilization, and other treatment procedures.[30] As the Cleveland Clinic's website states, "Over 200 research studies in the past 30 years have explored the role of mind-body techniques in helping prepare people for surgical and medical procedures and helping them recover more rapidly." These studies have shown that guided imagery may significantly reduce stress and anxiety before and after surgical and medical procedures. In addition guided imagery has proven to help people:

- dramatically decrease pain and the need for pain medication
- decrease side effects and complications of medical procedures
- reduce recovery time and shorten hospital stays
- enhance sleep
- strengthen the immune system and enhance the ability to heal
- increase self-confidence and self-control

There are endless ways to use imagery to relax, ease pain, and alleviate virtually any kind of suffering. Studies have shown that suggestion techniques can actually increase the period of survival for people with disease. In one study published in *Lancet* in 1989, for example, Stanford University psychiatrist David Spiegel reported that women with breast cancer who participated in weekly support groups along with self-hypnosis for pain at the time of their regular treatment lived twice as long as women who received only conventional treatment.[31] Spiegel's findings rocked the medical community because although doctors had begun accepting the notion that psychological intervention could reduce anxiety and fatigue, many were skeptical that it could actually help people live longer. Since Spiegel's study, numerous similar findings relative to the usefulness of visualization techniques have been reported. In one, when investigators at Cincinnati Children's Hospital Medical Center conducted a randomized, controlled clinical trial investigating the effectiveness of imagery on patients undergoing tonsillectomy and/or adenoidectomy, research showed that when visual imagery was added to routine analgesics the participants' pain and anxiety, both after surgery and at home, was significantly diminished.[32]

Guided imagery has also been shown to be a useful tool in combating depression. In one study that examined 60 short-term hospitalized depressive patients, intervention via guided imagery was shown to effectively enhance patients' comfort and decrease their symptoms of depression.[33] Clearly, there is no longer any doubt that imagery can create a bridge between mind and body by linking internal perceptions and emotions to psychological, physiological, and behavioral responses.

In individuals with illness, it has also been found that the "grief that is not spoken" can commonly contribute to a downward spiral in both mental and physical health. For example, according to the National Cancer Institute, "Depression is a disabling illness that affects about 15 to 25% of cancer patients. It affects men and women with cancer equally. People who face a diagnosis of cancer will experience different levels of stress and emotional upset."[34] Often, specific issues facing a person with cancer naturally include the fear of death, an interruption of life plans, changes in body image and self-esteem, changes in social role and lifestyle, as well as monetary and legal concerns. This represents an indication not that depressed patients get cancer, but that cancer patients get depressed, and that depression increases the likelihood of hardship.

Visualization and color

Whether in nature when the leaves change or in the paintings of great masters, colors literally color our world by having an impact on our minds and emotions. So, it makes sense that color is also instrumental in aiding positive visualization techniques. We already know that our minds, thoughts, and beliefs affect the state of our mental health. Given the fact that imagery is so important in this mind-body equation, it's not surprising that different colors have been shown to have different effects on our mental wellbeing. Our moods and actions have always been affected by colors in the environment, and research has shown that this is partially due to the fact that color triggers the endocrine system, a response which has a beneficial impact on both the immune and nervous systems as well.

For example, it's no wonder that the color blue is a favorite for many because blue has an overall calming effect, and feeling calm assists in easing physical and emotional tension. Staring up at a big blue sky on a beautiful day, for instance, is as calming as you can get. The color red, on the other hand, affects the endocrine, pituitary, and adrenal glands and can act as a stimulator. Because red is associated with high energy, visualizing red can give us a charge of energy when we need a boost. These are just two examples of how adding the element of color to your visualization or guided imagery techniques can positively affect your health and wellbeing.

How to use visualization techniques

We all visualize all the time, so there is really nothing new to learn on that score. When we speak of "techniques" in visualization, then, we are simply drawing attention to something we already do in order to create awareness and conscious realization around it.

To visualize, therefore, simply begin. Focus on the goal you want to achieve or the feeling you want to have. If looking at a picture helps you get an image in your mind, choose one to contemplate and immerse yourself in it. Then close your eyes and imagine it. You not only want to *see* the image in your mind, but *feel* the feelings you are choosing to generate, such as healing, happiness, and strength. The more you repeat this exercise, the easier it will be to conjure up the associated images and feelings quickly and effectively.

Visualize in the first person. It's always more powerful and effective to feel yourself in your imaging; in other words, to *feel* yourself going through each motion as you imagine yourself doing it, as opposed to seeing yourself from a third-person perspective—as if you're watching a movie of yourself. Being in the first person means that when you go through the actions of your imagination, it will feel more like a personal experience.

Look forward to the process of visualization. Setting aside a bit of time, no matter how short, when you know you can visualize provides you with something to look forward to. It's a time to spend living joyful moments you expect to achieve and a time when you know you can create anything you want to create. Moments like these can help bring feelings of hope and expectation back into your life. Since you are completely in charge of what you create, there are no boundaries. There is no such thing as a monotonous routine when it comes to imagining.

Use physical participation in your visualization. If you have difficulty walking, picture and *feel yourself* getting up out of that chair and moving, taking steps across the room. Next time you might picture and feel yourself walking right out the door. Perhaps you could see and feel yourself being with loving friends and family who support your endeavors. Actually *feel the energy* involved in visualizing the process and know that on some level you are actually experiencing the images you are creating in your mind.

You can visualize yourself at home alone, or with a family member or friend. It always helps to "set the scene" to be the most conducive environment for you. Take the time everyday to visualize your goals—whatever they may be. Goals vary from person to person and from moment to moment. Some goals last years or even a lifetime. Remember, your goals are *yours*, and that's what makes them so important to pursue. They can be anything from wishing to change a lifestyle to healing a disease. Athletes train themselves to visualize their winning ways, whether sinking a winning free throw in basketball or making a 20-foot putt in golf. Visualization allows for inward action in rehearsal so that the outward world becomes a reality of our thoughts. So, as they say, be careful what you wish for!

"Formal" visualization

Although visualization is something you undertake of your own free will and can do totally on your own, in your own time, and at your own convenience, you can also choose to undertake a more formal approach. As more and more people have become aware of this school of alternative thought, certified instructors have become available to guide individuals in the techniques of visual imagery to achieve the best possible results.

Instructors teach visual imagery techniques in which participants use various positions: either sitting, standing, or lying down. Instructors use calm, low, well-modulated voices that allow time between each suggestion as they guide the class through various steps of visualization. Many instructors encourage participants to take the time after class to jot down their experiences in writing to discuss in subsequent classes. The focus of these classes is to direct the mind by way of suggestions so that one's physiology responds to those suggestions.

Remember, we cannot separate the mind from the body, so whatever our thoughts and beliefs, the body naturally follows. With clear, specific purpose, visualization gradually takes shape to the point where we begin to "own" the messages we have created. Experts advise that the process does take time and that very often it can take about six weeks before "visible" or "concrete" results can be appreciated. However, many people have reported they feel improvement relatively quickly as they continue their attempts. This feeling is again a prime example of the process being as important as the goal itself.

Prepare your surroundings and "be one" with them. It's pretty obvious that it's a lot tougher to relax and concentrate on goals if you are surrounded by chaos. Most of us need quiet. While there are people who are lucky enough to be able to close out the outside world to the degree where they can visualize easily on a crowded bus or during their commute on the train, I can tell you from personal experience I am not one of them. For me, it's necessary to find a time and space that is relatively calm and peaceful. If I am visualizing on my own, I then picture a calm, serene environment, one not necessarily indoors...perhaps a place by the ocean or a running stream with the wind rustling in the trees. I usually begin with a prayer that I hold close to my heart or by stating a belief or faith. Having faith in our beliefs generates the trust and optimism we need for visualization to make things happen.

Think of a clearly defined purpose. The only way I find I can focus on a specific purpose is when I am confident about my wants and goals. Confusion or lack of clarity clouds intention. Visualize about your specific need. If you are sick, visualize being healthy. If you have family problems, visualize the problems are solved, and all concerned are relaxed, together, and having a good time. If you have problems at work, visualize a functional, healthy, competitive working environment.

Relax and focus. Close your eyes to clear your mind and relax your body, and then begin to focus on your purpose. Concentrate on the thought. Know you will have other thoughts passing through your mind. Try to ignore those intruding external thoughts and just focus on *your* thought and feel the energy behind your picture. During a relaxation session at a yoga class I once took, we were told to imagine our aches and pains leaving our bodies through our limbs. Following along with the voice of the teacher, I began to imagine the pain in my aching body leaving me, flowing outwards through my arms and legs. Soon a soothing calm had infused me, both my mind *and* my body, totally renewing me. Because it was such an enriching experience, I continued when I got home. I lay on my bed in solitude with soft soothing music playing in the background and made a conscious effort to relax my body with comforting visual imagery. Soon my body relaxed, any pain I had subsided, and the tension in my body dissipated. Once my body had totally relaxed, my mind was calm and my thoughts were focused. In a moment my breathing had become even and peace was my only companion.

Imagine and feel your body healing. First comes imagination and then comes reality. After a while you won't have to *imagine* your body healing because you will *feel* it healing; intuitively and instinctively you will just know. The clearer the imagined picture, the better the technique of visualization will work. Picture a healthy self. Picture yourself having a healthy vitality, optimally utilizing the hours of the day and your energy. I know you will discover as I did that when you feel better about yourself, you automatically begin to feel better in the presence of others. As a result your life will continue to improve.

Make autosuggestions. Self-suggestion can absolutely induce changes in both the mind and body, and it has been proven that the powers of the subconscious mind influence our actions as well as our "non-actions." The subconscious mind can be a compelling tool, one unparalleled in strength for achieving our goals. Simply repeating suggestions or affirmations to ourselves day after day can begin the cycle of change. Over time the subconscious mind gets the message and will automatically support these thoughts through actions.

We can relate this verbal message to anything at all. A common goal might be losing weight. By repeating, "I will have lost 10 pounds by the end of this year," we have begun the focus on our ability for weight loss. You may find that the resistance that has kept you away from exercise and submitting to negative eating patterns finally disappears and that you can finally go from inaction to action. Slowly but surely autosuggestions compel us to take measures toward the achievement of our goal.

Don't judge your autosuggestions. Acknowledge, welcome, and accept the suggestions you make to yourself without criticism. Let the process unfold in its own way. As I said before, there is no right or wrong way; there is only *your way*. Give yourself the freedom to allow yourself to be you and experience the process and approach that feels comfortable.

Keep up your momentum and do not expect instant results. As discussed earlier, many of the best things in our lives take time to come to fruition. In this case, the process is just as important as the end results because you will find tremendous satisfaction in the moments themselves. Patience improves with time, maturity, and understanding. The ability to endure delay, and to wait without frustration, will take continued self-discipline. Knowing that you are building success and contentment with every step will be incentive enough for your willingness to continue on this path.

Be enthusiastic. Enthusiasm for what we do can be introduced into every single facet of our lives. Enthusiasm motivates us to feel enjoyment, passion, and excitement. When we are passionate about something we have the motivation to achieve it.

Enjoy your accomplishments with humility. Accomplishment of even the smallest feat can bring unprecedented exultation. Savor that success the way a baby who takes his first steps does—with pure joy, abandonment, and an appreciation for all that has taken place. In short, acknowledge what you are attempting to do, recognize none of us are perfect, and don't compare yourself to anyone else. Don't be afraid to make mistakes or be afraid to ask for help, and always retain your sense of wonderment. Keeping these suggestions in mind, the feeling of being humble will intuitively appear.

Meditation

Meditation refers to a state of mind in which the body is consciously relaxed and the mind is calm and focused. It involves a suspension of the usual stream of thoughts in order to calm the mind and generate relaxation on physical, mental, and spiritual levels. It is often one or more levels deeper than the one we access for visual imagery. Meditation is about getting back to the quiet that already exists in the center of each of us. Originating in the East and practiced for over 5,000 years, the concepts and techniques of meditation exist in various forms among most peoples, including Jews, Christians, Muslims, Buddhists, and Native Americans. Different meditative disciplines encompass a wide range of spiritual practices that emphasize different objectives—from achieving a higher state of consciousness or creating greater focus, creativity, or self-awareness to simply trying to acquire a more relaxed and peaceful frame of mind.

The word *meditation* originally comes from the Indo-European root *med-*, meaning "to measure," and entered English through the Latin word *meditatio*, which indicated physical and intellectual exercises of all kinds. Eventually meditation came to mean "contemplation," as we continue to interpret it today.

Meditating supports the coexistence of thought without judgment or distraction of any kind, allowing us to connect with the ever-expanding universe in all of us. Although many assume that meditating is born of a spiritual or religious conviction or belief system, in reality meditation practices can arise simply from an interest in learning how to quiet one's mind and concentrate more fully. I agree with Sogyal Rinpoche's book, *The Tibetan Book of Living and Dying*, which states, "Devote the mind to confusion and we know only too well, if we're honest, that it will become a dark master of confusion, adept in its addictions, subtle and perversely supple in its slaveries. Devote it in meditation to the task of freeing itself from illusion, and we will find that, with time, patience, discipline, and the right training, our mind will begin to unknot itself and know its essential bliss and clarity."[35] Also in the *Book of Living and Dying*, it is said that learning to meditate is the greatest gift you can give yourself in this life, because it is only through meditation that you can undertake the journey to discover your true nature, to find the stability and confidence you will need to live—and die—well. Rinpoche goes on to explain why here in the West our culture has not embraced meditation as a way of life. In his words:

> *"We are so addicted to looking outside ourselves that we have lost access to our inner being almost completely. We are terrified to look inward, because our culture has given us no idea of what we will find. We may even think that if we do, we will be in danger of madness. This is one of the last and most resourceful ploys of ego to prevent us from discovering our real nature.*
>
> *So we make our lives so hectic that we eliminate the slightest risk of looking into ourselves. Even the idea of meditation can scare people. When they hear the words egoless or emptiness, they think that experiencing those states will be like being thrown out the door of a spaceship to float forever in a dark, chilling void. Nothing could be further from the truth. But in a world dedicated to distraction, silence and stillness terrify us; we protect ourselves from them with noise and frantic busyness. Looking into the nature of our mind is the last thing we would dare to do."*

Meditation is said to be the road to enlightenment. Buddhism centers around the practice of meditation, and Buddha himself is known to have achieved enlightenment through meditation under a Bodhi tree. Hindus have multiple forms of meditation, some practiced widely, others relatively unknown. The Baha'i faith also believes in spiritual growth through meditation. Their prophets say, "Meditation is the key for opening the doors of mysteries to your mind. In that state man abstracts himself; in that state man withdraws himself from all outside objects; in that subjective mood he is immersed in the ocean of spiritual life and can unfold the secrets of things in themselves." Whereas Christians follow meditation through prayer and contemplation, as do the Catholics with use of the rosary and the practice of adoration, Native Americans use flute-playing as a common form of meditation and spiritual ritual. Believers in Islam, whose prophet Muhammad spent many hours in contemplation to gain the insight and revelation for their holy book, the *Qur'an*, attribute powers of healing to the practice of meditation. History shows that Judaism also incorporates meditative practices throughout the *Tenach* (the Hebrew Bible) and the Kabbalah in various forms of deep thinking and contemplation.

Dr. Ainslie Dixon Meares (1910–1986) was an Australian psychiatrist, an authority on stress, and a prolific author who lived and practiced in Melbourne, Australia. Dr. Meares' work reveals an interesting relationship between meditation and cancer. In one study, for example, his research showed that with meditation advanced cancer patients exhibited a 50% chance of having a greatly improved quality of life, a 10% chance of slowing the rate of tumor growth, and a 10% chance of a less marked, but still significant, slowing.[36] Dr. Meares' research also suggested that regressing normal human function to a more archaic level of mental function ("atavistic regression") during intensive meditation caused a similar physiological regression. Based on this work, Dr. Meares believed that the relationship between mental and physiological function likely involved the immune system. Involvement of the immune system would suggest a further influence on an individual's natural defenses against cancer. In the doctor's own words, "There is no suggestion that all cancer patients, or even a majority of cancer patients, who practice intensive meditation will achieve some kind of miraculous cure. The purpose is to suggest to colleagues the possibility of an effective alternative treatment of cancer, either as an adjunct to orthodox treatment or as a form of treatment in its own right."[37]

Dr. Meares also wrote a number of books on this subject, including his best-seller *Relief without Drugs: How You Can Overcome Tension, Anxiety, and Pain*.[38] *Relief without Drugs* emphasizes an approach encouraging mental relaxation and mental stillness that "restores harmony and function," rather than an approach of physical relaxation, as is so common in many other types of meditation techniques.

In other work focusing on meditative approaches, Dr. James Austin, a neurophysiologist at the University of Colorado, reported in his 1999 landmark book, *Zen and the Brain*, that Zen meditation has a decided effect on the brain, one which has been confirmed through EEG studies which examine brain activity.[39] Slow, meditative breathing is one technique that changes brain activity due to its ability to reduce the volume of air flow. This reduction in air flow results in quiet, prolonged expiration, muting the firing activity of nerve cells in the brain and aiding in the production of a more relaxed state.

According to Dr. Austin, Zen emphasizes meditation as a way to enlightenment, a spiritual awakening to the knowledge that we and the universe coexist. Using the phenomena of meditation, Dr. Austin ties the latest insights of neurology to the most important technical and psychological notions of Japanese Zen, and his work is considered the most thorough attempt to date to confirm Buddhist theories of knowledge and self-consciousness through the lens of Western neurophysiology.

Meditation in daily life

How does meditation help us in our daily lives? Since meditation is looking within, it gives us a chance to further understand ourselves, our thoughts, our dreams, and our goals. When we meditate we drive all conscious thought from the mind, and in this "resting state" we can gain in outlook and dimension by becoming a part of the infinite space that exists in that vast realm. Meditation brings stability where there is fear and rockiness and induces a calmness and clarity, to result in an increased overall sense of wellbeing. Worldwide, doctors are recommending meditation as a means of improving health by lowering blood pressure, easing breathing problems, reducing anxiety, and lessening stress. Numerous articles and books have been written expounding the incredible benefits of meditation. Increased productivity, delaying of the aging process, a reduced need for medical care, an increased strength in self, improved memory function, a greater sense of peace, and increased creativity are all positive manifestations of the meditative process.

For meditative success, the most important thing is that it be practiced regularly and adopted as a lifestyle. There is no instant coffee of meditation; this brew must be steeped slowly and enjoyed daily. Dr. Joan Borysenko, leading expert on stress, spirituality, and the mind/body connection and author of *Minding the Body, Mending the Mind*, defines meditation as any activity which keeps the mind pleasantly focused on the present.[40] Dr. Borysenko states that retraining the mind through mediation teaches us to surrender and allow ourselves to embody the meditation experience. She states, "These two paths—taking action where required and surrendering where no further action is possible—are the paths to stress hardiness." To this point, it can be helpful to encourage cancer patients to make the effort to let go and take one day at a time. Attempting to focus on the present—without contemplating prognosis, the process of treatment, or potential survival rates—can help improve the outcome relative to any type of treatment undertaken.

Meditation classified

There are basically three classifications of meditation: *concentrative, mindful,* and *analytical.*

- As the name implies, concentrative meditation means focusing on one particular thing, be it your own breathing or a sound, chant, or image. The simplest way to perform concentrative meditation is to sit quietly and focus your attention on the natural rhythm of your breath.
- Mindful meditation involves an awareness of sensations, images, thoughts, sounds, and smells without being actively involved in them. Here the field is broader as the mind does not concentrate on one thing but on an array of things in the immediate environment. The meditator is focused *on*, but is not involved *in*, the sensations he experiences; needless to say, it takes practice to induce calm and peace in the midst of stimulus. The Buddhists call this kind of meditation *vipassana.*
- Analytical meditation is quite different from mindful meditation and concentrative meditation in the sense that it involves analytical skills. Here, the individual engages in rational thinking, investigates an emotion or thought, and analyzes it from different viewpoints.

The point of this kind of meditation is to understand a particular thought or emotion so it can be resolved, thus reducing its impact on the mind. In doing so, transformation can occur, and feelings of love, affection, kindness, and compassion can begin to surface.

It's helpful to set the stage for your meditation with: a clean and quiet place to meditate, a comfortable posture, an object on which to concentrate, and a relaxed attitude. For beginners it is especially ideal to have a secluded place with good ambience to encourage concentration. After perfecting the art and science of meditation, theoretically one could perform it anywhere.

It also helps to adopt a comfortable physical posture. The classic postures in Hatha yoga, for example, create balance conducive for meditative practice. The Hindus and Buddhists believe in keeping the spine straight, while the Christians prefer the posture of kneeling. Most people find sitting is the best posture because lying down may induce unintentional sleep. Eastern thought encourages sitting in lotus posture, where the legs are crossed; though difficult initially, this posture is perfected with practice. Focusing on an object or a chant or a mantra can help us avoid distraction; to that end, a *mantra*, a religious or mystical syllable, poem, or phrase, can be repeated over and over during meditation. For this purpose, instructors will sometimes offer various mantras to individuals to suit their temperaments and preferences. Finally, having a relaxed attitude means just letting go, recognizing that nothing can be gained by force or compulsion to do it a certain way. By definition meditation requires one to relax in order to do it!

Meditation can be further delineated into subtypes:

- meditation by way of breath-watching
- meditation in a vacant mind
- meditation in motion
- mindfulness meditation
- mantra or concentration meditation
- contemplative meditation

Breath-watching meditation. This is a simple procedure of concentrating on one's breath, both inhalations and exhalations, to oxygenate the lungs and exhale the carbon dioxide in order to focus the mind. Get in a comfortable position and focus on your breathing with your eyes closed. Feel the breath being taken in and flowing out of the body to achieve a complete state of relaxation.

Vacant-mind meditation means making all conscious thought absent by choosing to empty the mind of all thoughts, feelings, and objects. This practice takes persistence and patience because it can be challenging for most of us to "turn off" all the chatter that tends to fill our minds every minute of every day.

Meditation in motion. This type of meditation involves movement, such as walking in a room or outside in a natural setting, such as a garden. Motion meditation involves timing your breath with the movement of your legs and arms. It also involves being mindful and focused on sensations, such as the pressure being exerted on your knees as you walk or the feeling of your foot touching the ground. Concentrating on the finer aspects of walking helps us gain control of the wanderings of our mind.

Mindfulness meditation. As discussed before, meditating with mindfulness means focusing on the many variables in the environment to heighten awareness. Try to be aware without feeling, analyzing, or judging.

Mantra or concentrative meditation. Concentrating on a specific object or feeling and staying focused on it is one of the best ways to try to meditate. If you like the idea of adding sound to your experience, many people chant, or listen to chanting, as a way to help them focus further. The vocalization and vibration can also help make it easier to connect with one's inner self.

Contemplation meditation. Meditating on a visualized landscape, scenario, or a thought is considered contemplative. A lush forest, blue sky, or vast ocean are examples of contemplative landscapes that can be vividly pictured.

Meditative processes are differentiated through origin, technique, benefits, and feasibility, and there are too many to discuss here, so we'll look at just a few of the more common variations whose benefits have been proven through research.

Transcendental Meditation (TM™) was introduced by guru Maharishi Yogi and has become so popular that it gave birth to the Maharishi University of Management in Iowa. Maharishi has said, "Through Transcendental Meditation™ the human brain can experience that level of intelligence which is an ocean of all knowledge, energy, intelligence, and bliss."

Guided meditation. As the name suggests, meditation is guided toward achieving a specific goal. This can be done with an instructor or alone using your imagination, or by listening to a prerecorded CD or MP3.

Zen meditation. Through Zen meditation, one's body and mind achieve a calmness where the heart rate slows down, breathing becomes regulated and rhythmic, and the body is attuned to the surroundings, all without being affected by outside elements. The classic posture for Zen meditation is called the lotus position. This involves sitting cross-legged with the left foot on top of the right thigh and the right foot on top of the left thigh.

Chakra meditation. This form of meditation focuses on cleansing the body and soul by opening the focal points of energy, called *chakras*, and then channeling the positive energy into the body to build and maintain a healthy balance of energy.

Why meditation is so helpful

It would be easy to dedicate a whole book to the vast benefits of meditation, and many have indeed been written, but for our purposes we'll be listing the three most generally significant: physical, psychological, and rehabilitative.

Numerous physical benefits of meditation on the body include:

- decreased metabolic rate, lowered heart rate
- lowered levels of stress-related chemicals, such as cortisol
- reduced numbers of free radicals that can cause tissue damage and are associated with aging and diseases
- stabilized blood pressure
- higher resistance to diseases
- reduced cholesterol levels
- improved flow of air to the lungs

Psychological benefits of meditation include:

- increased brain wave coherence, leading to greater creativity and improved moral reasoning
- decreased anxiety, depression, irritability and moodiness
- improved learning ability and memory
- increased feelings of vitality
- increased happiness and emotional stability

Meditation has also been found to help with rehabilitation of all kinds, with:

- changes in attitude toward life
- insight into inner self and the ability to establish connections
- creation of a foundation of self-awareness
- better understanding and comprehension of all situations

Medical meditation research

Dr. Herbert Benson of the Mind-Body Medical Institute has been working in the field of meditation and studying meditation's effect on the body for over 30 years. Dr. Benson's many research studies have reported that meditation induces a host of biochemical and physical changes, collectively referred to as the body's "Relaxation Response," or RR.[41] This Relaxation Response includes changes in metabolism, heart rate, respiration, blood pressure, and brain chemistry. Dr. Benson states, "My goal has always been to promote a healthy balance between self-care approaches and more traditional approaches—medical and surgical interventions that can be magnificent and lifesaving, when appropriate. However, self-care is immensely powerful in its own right. The elicitation of the Relaxation Response, stress management, regular exercise, good nutrition, and the power of belief all have a tremendous role to play in our healing."[42]

Dr. Benson's work has proved that not only does the RR affect physiology, but also produces changes in gene expression, as in one study where the whole-blood transcriptional profiles of 19 practitioners of long-term daily relaxation response techniques were compared to practitioners who practiced no techniques and those who practiced short-term RR techniques. "This study provides the first compelling evidence that the RR elicits specific gene expression changes in short-term and long-term practitioners," said Dr. Benson about the findings. "Our results suggest consistent and constitutive changes in gene expression resulting from RR may relate to long-term physiological effects. Our study may stimulate new investigations into applying transcriptional profiling for accurately measuring RR and stress related responses in multiple disease settings."[43]

In another study by Sharma, et al., biochemical activity was measured in 42 practitioners who performed Sudarshan Kriya, or SK, a type of breathing method that elicits a relaxation response. When these practitioners were compared to 42 individuals who did not practice the technique, it was found that the SK practitioners showed better antioxidant status at enzymatic and RNA levels and better immune status due to the prolonged life span of lymphocytes.[44]

Mediation has also been shown to slow the aging process. The cerebral cortex is that part of the brain known as the "gray matter," which is responsible for sensing and interpreting information from various parts of the body as well as maintaining cognitive function. As we age, the cerebral cortex undergoes a thinning out. In a study by Lazar, et al., magnetic resonance imaging showed that when participants undertook the regular practice of meditation, an increased cortical thickness of the brain was observed.[45]

In yet further research published in the American Journal of Cardiology, vital statistics obtained from the National Death Index revealed that participants who practiced Transcendental Meditation™ showed a 23% reduction in the rate of death from all causes, a

30% reduction in the rate of death from cardiovascular disease, and a 49% reduction in the rate of death from cancer, compared to participants of the study's control group.[46]

Spirituality

The process of meditation, like visual imagery, forges a natural ongoing communication between the mind and the body. In working with the mind, the spiritual self automatically begins to reveal itself...because it is always there and ready. Joel S. Goldsmith (1892–1964), teacher and author of *The Art of Spiritual Healing*, once said, "The world is not in need of a new religion or a new philosophy. What the world needs is healing, and regeneration. The world needs people who, through devotion to God, are so filled with the Spirit that they can be the instruments through which healings take place, because healing is important to everybody."[47] After his father's recovery from sickness, Goldsmith began studying Christian Science, but it was when he fell ill with tuberculosis and was given three months to live that his belief in spiritualism and God strengthened. With no hope of a medical cure, Goldsmith sought help from a Christian Science practitioner, and at the end of three months had made a complete recovery. People were skeptical when Goldsmith spoke about this experience, but his x-ray convinced even the most doubtful when it revealed that although he had only one lung, and only a wall of muscle remained where the other lung should have been, he had experienced a complete recovery.

Goldsmith's writings focus on prayer and meditation. His belief was that wellbeing is the result of awareness of God and he felt strongly that aligning oneself with spirit improves all circumstances. According to Goldsmith,

> *"To receive the word of God or spiritual sense, we need to feel rather than reason. This is referred to biblically as receiving the word "in the heart." Note here that the development of spiritual consciousness results in a greater gift of feeling the harmony of being. We understand that neither seeing, hearing, tasting, touching, nor smelling will reveal spiritual truth or its harmonies to us; therefore, it must come through a different faculty, the intuitive faculty which acts through feeling. Heretofore, we have sat down to pray or to meditate and immediately a stream of words and thoughts start to flow. Perhaps we began to affirm truth and deny error. You can see this is wholly in the realm of the human mind. In cultivating our spiritual sense we become receptive to thoughts which come to us from within. We become hearers of the Word rather than speakers. We become so attuned to the Spirit that we feel the divine harmony of being; we feel the actual presence of God. Having transcended the five physical senses, our intuitive faculty is alert, receptive and responsive to*

things of the Spirit, and we begin our new existence as a result of the spiritual rebirth."[48]

The pursuit of spirituality is indeed gaining recognition in the medical field, albeit only recently, in light of its potential effects on both emotional states and disease. According to authors Margaret Burkhardt and Mary Gail Nagai-Jacobsen in their book *Spirituality: Living Our Connectedness*, spirituality is an inherent part of our being, one that requires a place of importance in health practices. The authors' intent is to bring awareness to nurses and students that, "The spiritual core is the place that is closer than our own breath, yet unlimited in its expansiveness. Spirituality impels us to seek and to discover the more of who we are and calls us to enter the depths of our own being, where we discover our intrinsic connectedness with all of life and with the eternal Oneness and Sacred Source of our being."[49]

We don't really know why, but it appears to be true that people who go through periods of suffering—whether mental, emotional, or physical—often experience growth on a spiritual level. It is no wonder Kahlil Gibran wrote, "Out of suffering have emerged the strongest souls; the most massive characters are seared with scars." After experiences of extreme suffering, it is not unusual to find people getting involved with things bigger than themselves, as if their hardship has inspired them to become more compassionate and understanding toward others. I have been fortunate to know many individuals who, after dealing with their own illness and recovery in hospital settings, return to do many types of volunteer work, perhaps in the form of counseling or simply to spend some time with those who need support.

Laughter

"A cheerful heart is a good medicine; but a broken spirit drieth up the bones."
- Proverbs 17:22

Laughter: *The best medicine.* I support this message wholeheartedly, appreciating personally how good it feels to let loose with a belly laugh when the mood strikes. I wasn't surprised in the least to read definitions of the word "laughter" and see it commonly associated with a sense of wellbeing. Laughter: "To express certain emotions, especially mirth, or delight, by a series of spontaneous, usually unarticulated sounds, often accompanied by corresponding facial and body movements," and "to feel a triumphant or exultant sense of wellbeing" (*www.dictionary.com*). Clearly, the effect of laughter, cheer, mirth, and general happiness on health and wellbeing is a welcome inclusion in the process of recovering from an illness or disease.

The word "humor" is derived from the Latin word *umor*, meaning "fluid." One of the earliest mentions of the health benefits of humor is in the book of Proverbs in the Bible. As early as the 13th century, some surgeons used humor to distract patients from the pain of surgery.

Laughter has lasting effects, too. For example, the other day I got together with a group of friends. One of them is a real character, full of jokes, who kept us in stitches the whole time. The buzz from all that laughter lingered on much after we had parted for the evening. I kept on chuckling to myself, thinking about the jokes and the conversation. I then thought about how I often remember the small secrets I shared with my sister during our childhood, and how I always chuckle inwardly at those pleasant memories and am invariably left with a pleasant afterglow.

Why does laughter make us feel so good? The benefits of laughter have been well researched, and laughter has achieved a standard of recognition as a therapy in and of itself. Studies conducted by Drs. Lee Berk and Stanley Tan of Loma Linda University in California, for example, have shown that laughter causes biochemical changes, such as reversing neuroendocrine and stress response hormones.[50] Berk's and Tan's research found that laughter induced an increase in the levels of natural killer cell activity, B-cells, and T-cells, and several immunoglobulin effects (in the form of cytokine interferon and several leukocyte subsets) lasting 12 hours after the initiation of humor intervention.[51] Research has also cited that laughter releases endorphins, the body's own "natural painkillers."[52] Furthermore, laughter, especially belly laughter, has an aerobic function because it provides a complete workout for the diaphragm. The more air moves through the lungs, the more the body's ability to use oxygen is enhanced.

Studies have led to the differentiation of laughter into several categories based on the types of events that cause the laughter. They are:

- *Nervous laughter,* in response to an impending threat
- *Slapstick laughter,* in response to an awkward situation
- *Sadistic laughter,* in response to the misfortunes of competitors or enemies
- *Mocking laughter,* directed at competitors to show a sense of superiority
- *Surprise laughter,* in response to an unexpected turn of events
- *Social laughter,* used to become a part of a social gathering or group
- *Humor laughter,* in response to pure happiness, many times based on jokes or funny anecdotes[53]

A most amazing story is that of Norman Cousins, a prominent political journalist, author, professor, and world-peace advocate, who was diagnosed with the crippling, degenerative disease of incurable ankylosing spondylitis, also known as Bechterew's disease. Informed that he had little chance of surviving, Cousins developed his own recovery program, which included large doses of vitamin C, an emphasis on the need for a positive attitude, love, faith, and hope, and lots of laughter, often induced by the famous Marx Brothers films. He said, "It worked. I made the joyous discovery that ten minutes of genuine belly laughter had an anesthetic effect and would give me at least two hours of pain-free sleep." Cousins then reported that, "When the pain-killing effect of the laughter wore off, we would switch on the motion picture projector again and, not infrequently, it would lead to another pain-free sleep interval."[54]

William James, psychologist and philosopher, once said, "We don't laugh because we are happy but we are happy because we laugh." This statement reminds me of Patch Adams, a medical doctor who became famous for his unconventional approach to introducing humanitarian clowning to medicine and who founded the Gesundheit! Institute in West Virginia, a community hospital aimed at changing society by injecting generosity and compassion into the doctor-patient relationship. When Dr. Adams realized that he could forget his own problems by helping others and that laughter, joy, and creativity formed an integral aspect of the healing process, he began his work toward a model healthcare system that would adopt all these expressions as part of its program. It is Dr. Adams' belief that the health of an individual is closely linked to that of his family, his community, and the world. I support Patch Adams' philosophy that the most revolutionary act we can commit is to be happy—and to strive to make others happy as well.

There is also a branch of yoga—yes, yoga—which focuses on laughter alone. This type of yoga is called Hasya yoga. Practicing Hasya yoga involves breathing exercises, stretches, and laughing games, where laughter is broken down into syllables in a chant form. William Fry, a psychiatrist at Stanford University, is known for his breakthrough work in the growth and development of the field called therapeutic humor. In his book, *Life Studies of Comedy Writers: Creating Humor*, Fry shares the importance of humor in our daily social interactions and individual life experiences.[55] Dr. Fry states that the impact of humor is powerful and that "students of humor have given, and still are giving, serious thought to the many variables and issues related to humor. These scholars have gone beyond the veil that I have called the 'invisibility' of humor. There is this expeditionary force of scholars who no longer take humor for granted, but are recognizing its importance." In his book, Fry establishes that humor assists health by affecting the physiological systems of the body, as it involves "the entire physical being" of the person engaged in levity. As psychologist Ellie Katz once said, "Warning: Humor may be hazardous to your illness."

Learning to laugh

How do you start to laugh if you haven't been feeling much like laughing lately? It appears that the more we laugh the more likely we are to laugh and the less we laugh, the less often we find things that tickle our funny bone or inspire us to laugh. Are you a serious person by nature? Are you going through a difficult time that has taken your sense of humor with it?

Sometimes we need to activate our own funny bones. If we've been doing more crying than laughing, it certainly doesn't help to play tragic tear-jerking movies over and over again. Watching a comedy instead can make us laugh despite ourselves. And "tricking" ourselves into laughter may be the best thing we could ever do to reverse that cycle of feeling lousy. Do you like to make faces in front of the mirror? Do you crack yourself up? Go for it! Will spending time with your best buddies do the trick? Give them a call. Read a funny book, go to a stand-up comedy show—whatever it is you like to do, there are plenty of outlets for your own brand of humor and your own laughter. In fact, there is laughter in the air, so reach out and find it. Let's laugh those blues away!

Whether it's giggling, guffawing, or chortling, laughter has many therapeutic benefits, such as:

- boosting the immune system
- generating a sense of wellbeing
- providing a workout for the diaphragm and increasing our ability to use oxygen
- reducing stress hormones
- reducing and distracting from pain
- providing an internal workout
- improving respiration
- reducing high blood pressure

One of the best things about laughter is that it is infectious. We've all gotten the bug at one time or another when we end up laughing so long and so hard that our sides hurt. Doesn't it feel fantastic? The bond created through laughter makes it one of the best ways to connect with other people, especially since it elevates moods, reduces stress, and improves just about everyone's overall quality of life.

Laughter and illness

During a time of illness or when undergoing painful therapy for diseases like cancer, laughter can help us look at the brighter side of things. An oncologist once said that an important characteristic of those cancer patients who do better than others is their ability to "put cancer in the background" for periods of time. With this in mind, the Mind-Body Medicine Department of the Cancer Treatment Centers of America (CTCA) uses laughter therapy along with conventional cancer care for all their patients.[56]

Art

The conceptualization of art is the result of many things, including love, creation, and living life. In essence, it is a sum total of all the human activities in which we engage, and is not restricted by age, religion, ethnicity, or country. Crayons, pencils, paints, clay, plaster of Paris, collage, songs, musical instruments, cameras, and vocal cords are just some of the instruments used in the creation of music, painting, sculpture, and literature, but all art is born of our desire to uninhibitedly express our inner thoughts, attitudes, emotions, and desires.

Art therapy is a branch of art that encourages creativity to help in the management of physical and emotional symptoms. Recognized worldwide as a viable treatment initiative, art is often used as a diagnostic tool, particularly with children who have undergone trauma, where drawing becomes an expression of their emotional state. In these situations, drawing often becomes a child's preferred method of communication. Creativity can be therapeutic, replacing fear with hope and helping to rebuild confidence. For those suffering with serious illness, art can also serve as a way to express conflict, fear, dissatisfaction, and depression, and can also help reconnect patients with feelings they may have put aside, such as joy, faith, anticipation, and hope.

The capacity of art to heal is recognized by the medical community at large and is increasingly being used to supplement conventional medicine. In one study conducted at Northwestern Memorial Hospital in Chicago, for example, when an art therapist and interdisciplinary team investigated the impact of art therapy on cancer symptoms of an inpatient cancer population, they found that the use of art therapy showed statistically significant reductions in most of the participants' cancer symptoms, along with significant decreases in fatigue and anxiety.[57]

Paoli Hospital's Cancer Center in Paoli, Pennsylvania has also introduced an outstanding practice for patients undergoing chemotherapy and radiation, where they are offered "no talent required" art therapy. It is not a rare sight at Paoli to see patients going for treatment armed with paints, pastels, puzzles, and paper. Time spent in the hospital can now become quality time as well, nurturing a hobby and discovering hidden talents. This particular hospital employs its own art therapist who is often seen spending time with patients, encouraging them to focus on creativity rather than cancer.

Most art therapists work either independently or as a member of a team of caregivers in hospitals like Paoli, and in clinics and outpatient facilities. In these circumstances, cancer patients can be found making collages, painting, and sculpting—activities that contribute to helping them feel more like creators and less like victims. As Mary Donald, resident art therapist at Paoli Cancer Center says, "No one in the art therapy program asked for illness. Art therapy opens the door to creative flow. You're able to be free of the past and the future—to live only in the present." Art has become accepted as a viable addition to regular treatment protocol, as evidenced by the Arts and Humanities Medical Scholars Program at Stanford University, where students are encouraged to explore the strong relationship between art and science, and the Narrative Medicine Program at Columbia University Medical School in New York, where doctors are supported in the practice of writing "parallel charts," where they can present their own interpretations outside the realm of strict medical assessment to their patients.

Art as a healing tool

Other artistic forms, such as the Buddhist mandala and Native American sand painting, are also now recognized as effective healing tools. In Tibetan tradition, the *mandala*, or religious work of art, is considered support for the three bodies of enlightenment: body, speech, and mind. The word "mandala" originates from the Sanskrit for "circle," but the concept behind the mandala is much deeper than its shape. The mandala represents wholeness, a relationship between the infinite and all of us. Embraced by the Eastern religions many centuries ago, the mandala is now recognized as a form of art in Western and secular cultures as well. Buddhist scripture says that sand mandalas emit positive energy into the surroundings and to the people who view them. A good example of this belief in action is when His Holiness the Dalai Lama called on Tibetan monks to construct a sand mandala equivalent to a sacred painting at the Sackler Gallery in Washington, D.C. after the September 11th tragedies. The resultant seven-foot-square mandala, presented for the healing and protection of America, is one of the largest ever created in the West. Work in this field is slowly gaining popularity as a spiritual art of healing in the United States, as drawing mandalas and witnessing their creation is known to be an exercise in healing, creativity, and prayer. Many individuals report that they find creating mandalas, in whatever form, to be inspirational in that it encourages relaxation and calmness of mind and aids the body to heal on all levels—physical, mental, and spiritual.

In her book, *Mandala: Luminous Symbols for Healing*, award-winning author Judith Cornell talks about the healing power of her personal discovery of mandalas. Cornell states, "I created mandalas when I had cancer and experienced a spiritual awakening. This creative process helped me to integrate the reductionism of the scientific world view with my intuitive experiences of wholeness and luminous states of consciousness. The sacred symbol of the mandala not only helped me find the healing power within myself, but also to recover from a sense of psychological fragmentation."[58] From her experience Cornell created the *Mandala Healing Kit*, a learn-at-home program that covers every aspect of mandala practice so that others may benefit from the process.[59]

For cancer patients, working with mandalas is a process that helps them focus less on diagnosis and treatment and more on developing consciousness and inner awareness. For many who have never explored this facet of human growth, this is a step toward the profound understanding that we are all much larger than our physical bodies; in other words, that we constitute a divine soul—a life force—that goes far beyond our healing on a physical plane.

I will share a personal experience to demonstrate how healing can indeed be expressed through art. One day I found myself in some serious need of soothing. I remembered what I had read about how writing was considered cathartic and figured, *What the heck, I'll give it a try.* I got a piece of paper and a pen and sat down. I was sure the thoughts would come pouring out. But nothing happened. I proceeded to wait for the magic I thought was on its way. I waited and waited...but still nothing happened! What was wrong? Wasn't something brilliant supposed to take place?

I took a minute to think about everything I'd read about the process. An important component was supposed to be to "relax," to let your thoughts and creativity flow. So this time I took a deep breath, closed my eyes, and let myself unwind. Eventually, I opened my eyes and found my pen making its way to the paper. It was a while later when I looked at my watch. To my amazement, I found that it had been close to an hour since I'd started. I kept going until the time felt right to stop, and when I was finished I read what I had written about my feelings regarding my bout with cancer. I was surprised at how much lighter I felt after that. I had put my innermost feelings on that paper and I actually felt better. Had I "created art"? Some might say no, but I would have to disagree, for I had indulged in an art form as a type of therapy through writing, and the act of creating something from my thoughts had brought me relief, solace, and even feelings of contentment. This relatively short exercise had provided me with a way to feel differently about the past, so much so that I was now feeling more at peace with all that had occurred. I found no residual hidden bitterness, no feelings of self-pity, remorse, or unhappiness. I was stunned by my reaction. I actually felt a healing had taken place, just the way others had suggested it might. I share this relatively small but significant incident with you to help you realize that whatever you create matters. Keep the creative juices flowing, open your mind, and throw away your inhibitions...because emotions often go unidentified until they find expression.

Art therapy may be safely undertaken without side effects along with conventional treatment. Although it does not provide a cure, art therapy can significantly augment the quality of one's life. To sum up the benefits of all forms of art as therapy, it has been found to help in:

- treatment of anxiety and depression
- treatment of substance abuse and addiction
- treatment of family problems and relationship issues

- treatment for stress reduction and enhanced relaxation
- treating for development of a positive attitude

Music

The use of music as a healing medium dates back to ancient times. Historical writings of ancient Egypt, China, India, Greece, and Rome reveal its use for centuries. The profession of music therapy in the United States began to develop during World War I and World War II when music was used in hospitals as an intervention to address traumatic war injuries and doctors, nurses, and therapists witnessed the beneficial effect it had on the veterans' psychological, physiological, and emotional states. Since then, colleges and universities have developed programs to train musicians how to use music for therapeutic purposes. The first music therapy degree program in the world was initiated at Michigan State University in 1944. Since then the profession has grown considerably. The American Music Therapy Association was founded in 1998, as a union of the National Association for Music Therapy and the American Association for Music Therapy, to train therapists to assess emotional wellbeing, physical health, social functioning, communication skills, and cognitive skills through musical interaction. Therapists are also trained to design music sessions for individuals and groups based on patient needs, using listening, song-writing, lyric discussion, musical imagery, musical performance, and learning through musical interaction.

The therapeutic effects of music can be heard around the world. The Bristol Cancer Help Centre in the United Kingdom, for example, offers a fully integrated range of complementary therapies, psychological support, spiritual healing, and nutritional and self-help techniques to address the physical, mental, emotional, and spiritual needs of cancer patients and their supporters. In 2001, researchers at Bristol performed a pilot study to evaluate the influence of music therapy on positive emotions and the immune system in cancer patients. In this study, 29 cancer patients, age 21 to 68 years, were asked to relax while listening to music and to play musical instruments while at the facility. Results of this study showed that the participants not only felt an increased sense of wellbeing and relaxation, but higher energy levels as well. Physiological data also revealed benefits in terms of increased salivary immunoglobulin A in the listening group and a decrease in cortisol levels (the "stress hormone") in the bloodstream of both groups.[60]

In another study conducted at Memorial Sloan-Kettering Cancer Center, 62 cancer patients undergoing the psychologically stressful procedure of autologous stem cell transplantation were randomly assigned to receive either music therapy or standard care. In this case, anxiety, depression, and "total mood disturbance" scores were found to be significantly reduced in patients who received the music-therapy approach compared to those patients who received only standard care.[61] The use of music has also been shown to help reduce anxiety in women with breast cancer undergoing chemotherapy treatment[62] and to reduce anxiety and increase comfort levels in pediatric cancer patients.[63] As author Hans Christen Andersen once said, "Where words fail, music speaks."

Faith

For many, faith is an act of trust and reliance in God. It can also be a conviction and a knowing of truth. The Bible says of faith that it is the "substance of things hoped for, the evidence of things not seen." The faithful believe we must act on what we believe and that no proof is required, and operate from a secure belief in God and that all things happen through God. Faith is often credited for providing humans with the strength and inclination to take risks, to change, to discover, and to innovate. Faith may be the underlying impetus that spawns emotions, such as love and trust, and is often considered the basis of the very foundation of the world and the existence of the universe.

Why, then, does it appear an inherent part of human nature that we struggle to maintain our faith in difficult times? Why does it seem that when anger or unhappiness rides in the front seat, God is relegated to the back? And why is there such a tendency to fall back on the "Why me" syndrome when things get tough? *Why me? Why did I lose all that money in the stock market? Why do I have to suffer? Why am I having such pain in my relationships? Why am I the one who got cancer?* Difficult situations often have many questions and few answers, but I suspect life has a way of teaching us the lessons we need the most. For me, my own experiences have made me appreciate life all the more through the undeniable, ever-present, environment of faith.

Examples of faith are everywhere, in life and in the Bible, as per a few Christian orientations:

"The kingdom of God is within you."
(Luke 17:21)

"Blessed is the man that trusteth in the Lord and whose hope the Lord is."
(Jeremiah 17:7)

"In the Lord, put your trust."
(Psalms 11:1)

It is my sense that faith means believing that God has a great plan for us, no matter what happens. We all know of Isaac Newton, genius and innovator. But did you know that Newton studied biblical numerology, among many other subjects, and felt that God was vital to the nature and entirety of space in the great system of physics? In *Principia*, Newton said, "The most beautiful system of the sun, planets, and comets could only proceed from the counsel and dominion of an intelligent and powerful Being."[64] This is but one of many quotes that support the idea that faith is of God, not of man. So, every day be sure to keep your faith, in whatever form it manifests, as it is a gift from God.

Prayer

Prayer has been said to be an act of communion with God, or toward any object of worship with faith and devotion, for the purposes of guidance, praise, gratitude, or confession. Many find prayer fosters comfort and peace due to this sacred covenant. Examples are seen in the Bible, as follows:

> *"And whatever you ask for in prayer, having faith and believing, you will receive."*
> (Matthew 21:22)

> *"But certainly God has heard me; he has given heed to the voice of my prayer."*
> (Psalms 66:19)

> *"Be unceasing in prayer."*
> (Thessalonians 5:17)

Some believe in praying first thing in the morning, while others believe in having their own divine conversations with God before going to bed at night. Just as we can practice affirmations and relaxation exercises anywhere and anytime, so too can we pray whenever the urge strikes. We can pray while we drive, cook, walk, or take a short break at work. Since many of us find solace and renewed confidence during and after praying, it is an important moment for which to make time. I personally feel a sense of oneness when I converse with God. I often feel a weight has been lifted off my shoulders, and I am told many others feel the same way.

Sometimes circumstances are such that another human cannot empathize with our situation. As a result, we turn to God to seek blessings. At such times, the act of prayer and God can help lift our spirits. In *The Infinite Way* Joel Goldsmith said, "Prayer is an awareness of that which is by 'seeing' it—not making it so." In other words, allow it to happen, but do not force it to happen. The Dalai Lama once said that prayer was his "simple religion; [that] there was no need for temples, no need for complicated philosophy, [and that] our own brain, our own heart is our temple, the philosophy is kindness." Many wise men and women have stated that the human spirit grows stronger with prayer, and I believe that statement is as true as it gets.

I read somewhere once that prayer is when you talk to God and meditation is when you listen to God. In this regard, Joel Goldsmith said, "To pray is to become aware of the harmony without the mental effort." Many agree that "true prayer" is addressed to the inner self without any expectation from the outside world, and is based on the belief that since God is within us, there is no separation between us and God. In this way of thinking, God is the life, mind, and body in each of us. Prayer leads to a conscious awareness that God is forever manifested and has already bestowed on us everything that we require before we even ask for it. I will cite the simplest of examples. When I return from a long day at work and my daughter welcomes me, jumping up to receive me with a squeal of delight, the combined feelings of love, affection, security, and tenderness that overwhelm me are too deep and profound to put into words. My connection with God feels exactly the same way. I simply thank God for all that He has given me. I thank Him for answering my prayers for love, for my family, and for my health.

The impact of faith on health continues to be an interesting topic to researchers, scientists, and doctors. For example, the Alameda County Health and Ways of Living Study is a program designed to study the influence of health practices and social relationships on physical and mental health. In 1997, when researchers on the panel analyzed the long-term association between religious service attendance and mortality over 28 years for 5,286 respondents, it was found that participants who attended frequent religious events of one kind or another had lower mortality rates than infrequent attendees. These respondents were also found to be more likely to stop smoking, increase exercising, increase social contacts, and stay married. The investigators of this study concluded that the lower mortality rates could be partly explained by improved health practices, increased social contacts, and more stable marriages occurring in conjunction with attendance.[65]

Other studies have also revealed the significant mark that spirituality and religious services can make on our health and wellbeing. In an exploratory study of 112 women with metastatic breast cancer, for example, the relationship between spirituality and immune function was examined. Researchers in this case found that those women who rated "spiritual expression," that is, a greater link with spirituality as an important part of their lives, had greater numbers of circulating white blood cells and total lymphocyte counts, as well as both helper and cytotoxic T-cell counts, all important elements of immune system functioning.[66]

Seeking a "higher" purpose

Without purpose we would drift like a boat without a competent navigator, subject to the winds of change. Finding our life's purpose provides focus, direction, and clarity, so we can reach our objectives. As Helen Keller once said, "Happiness comes from commitment to a worthy purpose."

I thought about what my own purpose was. What was it that I wanted most from life? It turns out, the list I created was endless, but it started with health, happiness, peace, and contentment. Your list may start with survival; others may have fame and fortune at the top. Some make the pursuit of knowledge their highest priority, and yet others look to religion and philosophy to seek their answers.

A sense of purpose is born of good, positive, constructive, proactive thought and subsequent action. It shows the path to something bigger than the self. As Galileo Galilei (1564–1642), physicist, astronomer, and philosopher, once said, "I cannot believe that God, who has endowed us with sense, reason, and intellect, wants us to forgo their use."

Buddhist thinkers say, "All that we are is the result of what we have thought." As we mature and develop, we will most likely change aspirations, priorities, purpose, and circumstances many times over. By the time we are in our twenties, we begin to make decisions about how to live our lives and which path(s) to take and achievement and ambition move to front and center. With each step, aim, desire, and ambition our purpose becomes further delineated. It is at this point that life often takes on more of a set routine, and we begin to believe we can sit back, secure that we know what's coming down the road.

Unfortunately, this is often just when an unforeseen event or disease can derail us. With a well-defined purpose and determination, however, we can still work toward achieving our goals without losing hope, identity, or direction. Temporary setbacks should not necessarily take us off track, although it's true that they may delay our progression toward the goals we have been pursuing. It may not be an easy task, but a strong, determined mind, a well-looked-after body, and the belief in God, or in something greater than ourselves and in self, can work miracles. On the other hand, the fear of losing what we have can make us afraid to participate fully in life. As Henry Ford said so well, "Whether you think that you can, or that you cannot, you are usually right."

During my cancer treatment I had one solitary purpose in my life, and I worked hard to achieve it. I was determined to live, and live well and long, so I embarked on a plan to follow the protocol I believed would take me in the right direction. I changed my lifestyle for the better and inculcated better habits, which I continue to espouse. I thought positively then and I still think positively now. If I, a simple human being who was only 19 years old, could change my life I know there are plenty more of us out there who are also ready to do the same. Take the plunge. Define your purpose and set out to achieve it.

Interestingly, having a purpose is one of the things that has been found to delay aging. People with defined purposes have actually been found to live longer, happier, and healthier lives. Look around you and see for yourself how people without a sense of direction seem to age much more rapidly. Although our environment and situation influences who we are, we alone are responsible for our own thoughts, lives, and achievements. Having a purpose, whether it is gardening, traveling the world, or teaching yoga, helps us feel in control of our life and situation and provides us with a sense of self-respect and motivation.

Thinking outside the box

The expression "thinking outside the box" is just one way of reminding us to look at things from a different perspective. If we keep thinking the same old way, we will do the same old things we have always done—and get the same old results. We are therefore encouraged to think outside the box to derive better results and solutions and to find new options to our challenges. Thinking outside the box, in other words thinking intelligently and creatively, creates a wider network of thoughts, meaning we have more varied options with higher risk-taking abilities.

When the mind thinks beyond its preconceived limits it can explore new horizons beyond its expected boundaries. For an individual who is told that he or she has cancer and has to undergo a long, arduous treatment process, staying stuck inside the box means negativity and ongoing despair. On the other hand, beyond the box lies a universe of possibilities and approaches. Out-of-the-box thinkers are always ready to explore new ideas and to act upon them to prove them correct; out-of-the-box thinkers explore, innovate, and create, nurturing new methods to combat problems. Thinking outside the box requires us to leave our tried-and-true comfort zones and explore the unknown *without knowing the outcome*. It requires us to take a leap of faith and do the unexpected in order to better ourselves, our health, and our quality of life.

In Figure 5-1 you will find an interesting exercise highlighting the ability we all have to think outside the box.[67] If you take a moment to attempt to complete the challenge, you may find that your problem-solving abilities are greater than you thought. (Directions and exercise on page 344)

When you think you may have figured how to think outside the box, see Addendum 1 at the end of this book for the answer.

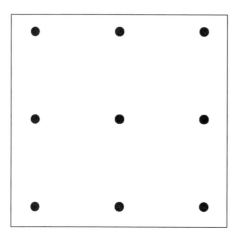

FIGURE 5-1. Thinking outside the box. (Source: San Graal School of Sacred Geometry, Grassy Branch Loop, Sevierville, Tennessee. Reprinted with permission ©1995-2007. *www.sangraal. com*)

DIRECTIONS: Draw this simple box of dots on your own little scrap of paper and begin as follows:

- The idea is to connect the dots with lines, but to use *only four lines* to do it.
- Position your pencil on one of the dots.
- Do not allow the pencil to come off the paper; that is, do not pick up the pencil and start from another place in the box. You must use one continuous flow of writing once you start.

Achieving sound mental health

Albert Einstein once said, "A human being is part of the whole, called by us Universe; a part limited in time and space. He experiences himself, his thoughts and feelings as something separated from the rest: a kind of optical delusion of his consciousness." Einstein went on to explain that this delusion is synonymous with a prison for our mind. "Suffering under delusion" means that many of us human beings go about our lives on autopilot, in the sense that we tend to go about our daily business without really giving much thought to what we are doing and why we are doing it. Most of us have not developed the consciousness to act as witness to our own behavior, or the ability to closely observe what is occurring without reactivity or judgment. If we free ourselves from this prison of the mind we can begin to see things as they really are. If we do break out of our self-imposed bondage, we can embrace humanity and nature in their beauty and splendor and feel liberated in our pursuit of security and happiness.

Just as our physical bodies require homeostasis to stay healthy, so does our mental state. According to Sigmund Freud, we all have three components that work together to produce our behaviors. These three components—the *id*, the *ego*, and the *superego*—need to be balanced for acquiring rational, sound mental health.

The id. The id is that unknown part of the subconscious mind responsible for managing our unconscious thoughts and desires. The id is responsible for the drive to fulfill our basic needs, such as food, drink, warmth, sleep, love, procreation, elimination, and sudden aggressive behavior. In essence, it is that "mindless" part of us that tends to ignore all other components and possibilities in order to immediately gratify what it seeks.

The ego. The word *ego* is derived from the Latin word for "I." It is that part of the personality involved with perception, defensiveness, cognitive, and rationalizing functions. Freud described the relationship between the id and the ego like that of a horse and rider. While the horse, the id, is the energy or driving source, the rider, the ego, controls the destination and achievement of the goal. The ego works on principles, recognizes and respects behaviors and norms, and attempts to balance that approach with the id's attempt at getting what it wants. At times, the "horse" will make impulsive and immature decisions, and it is at this time that the ego will defend itself and our behaviors in order to rationalize or "make things right."

It is the ego that facilitates an understanding of negotiation and comprise between the id and the superego, forming an appropriate bridge between the two and allowing them to express themselves.

The superego. According to Freud, the superego is that manifested balance between ego and id. It is that part of us which drives our need for consciousness, or mindfulness; the part that seeks out right from wrong and dictates that right will rule over wrong. The superego has been likened to the "moral police of the mind." When we enjoy a balanced ego we are in a position to satisfy the needs of the id, yet not upset the superego. Not always an easy task, we only acquire this skill as we mature and become more capable of prioritizing life's objectives. A headstrong id leads to the development of a selfish individual, while an overcompensating superego keeps us from growing beyond a certain limit—keeping us "inside the box"—as each attempt to break out is governed and set by rigid morals and standards.

This interaction of the three components, id, ego, and superego—our conscious and unconscious mental and emotional processes—is called *psychodynamics*. Imbalances among the three lead to disruption in personality, behavior, and attitude.

For example, an overabundance of ego manifesting in self-centeredness can lead to a sense of detachment from the rest of the world. But it is also the ego that provides the "illusion of safety" we all need as a method for understanding the world and our role within it. In this way, anxiety, an integral facet of human nature, is often accompanied by feelings of guilt, embarrassment, and inadequacy. According to Anna Freud, Freud's sixth child who followed up on her father's extensive research, the ego employs the use of a defense mechanism to combat these feelings of anxiety and the accompanying destructive feelings. More recent studies, however, add further delineation to this explanation by pointing out the difference between "defense" mechanisms and "coping" mechanisms. While defense mechanisms are largely unconscious and irrational, coping mechanisms are often based on more conscious and rational thought processes. Typical ego defense mechanisms can involve aggression, compensation, denial, displacement, fantasy, humor, identification, rationalization, regression, sublimation, and withdrawal, all utilized to protect us from anxiety that could be caused by our id's impulses. A healthy superego, on the other hand, removes our inner friction, helps guide us over the naturally occurring hurdles in life, and is the basis for balanced growth and maturity as we age.

From time immemorial, writers have written about the ego from a spiritual point of view. In his book *A New Earth: Awakening to Your Life's Purpose*, Eckhart Tolle says, "Listen to people's stories and they could be entitled 'Why I cannot be at peace now.' The ego doesn't know that your only opportunity for being at peace is now. Or maybe it does know, and it is afraid you may find this out. Peace, after all, is the end of the ego."[68] The ego here points to our deeply ingrained self-referential, self-seeking disposition, the hidden and capable adaptive attitude that revolves around us. Ego, acting as a usurper and a pretender, can cut us off from God, nature, and people—and even more so from our own self. Some religions and spiritual pursuits beseech us to cast the ego aside, to be free of it, in order to evolve as spiritual beings. When that happens the ego joins forces with our deeper selves and we become "one." Generally speaking, to help free ourselves of the ego's efforts at control, we need only become more aware of our thoughts and emotions. As a Hindu proverb says, "There is nothing noble in being superior to some other man. The true nobility is in being superior to your previous self."

Dr. Wayne Dyer, an American self-help advocate, author, and speaker, has spent a lifetime studying similar subjects. Said to bring "humanistic ideas to the masses," Dyer's work reflects wisdom and self-awareness, something he is dedicated to sharing. According to Dyer, Jesus was not teaching Christianity as such, but rather kindness, love, concern, and peace, and this is what Dyer also attempts to do. Dyer talks about ways to change our lives through healing and by overcoming the ego's hold on us through seven simple and doable steps that facilitate freedom from the ego.[69]

Stop being offended. It helps us to understand that the behavior and actions of others need not be of any real consequence for us. What offends us only weakens us. If we go looking for reasons and occasions to be offended, we certainly find them everywhere, but putting energy into being offended only creates negative energy—which is what produced the offense in the first place.

Let go of your need to win. Ego prefers to divide us up into only two groups: winners and losers. But thinking this way is detrimental for our self-esteem—especially if we take into account that "winning" all the time is next to impossible. Competing against oneself and always trying to improve is by far a more constructive approach.

Let go of your need to be right. Avoid conflict and tension, as these lead to hostility and loss of goal. Developing new options to resolve conflict helps make you feel more receptive and free from anger, resentment, and bitterness. When you let go of the need to be right, you are always able to reach closer to your goals.

Let go of your need to be superior. Greatness doesn't come packed with superiority. Staying humble is a great virtue and helps us avoid assessing ourselves and others solely on the basis of appearance and achievements.

Let go of your need to have more. The ego is never satisfied. Although it is good to keep striving for improvement and reaching toward our goals, setting ourselves up to never be satisfied and to always want more in order to be happy does not help us achieve success or contentment.

Identify with yourself, not with your achievements. First and foremost, we are creations of God; we are the tools in His hands. It helps to see ourselves that way and therefore give credit to the power of intention in our own lives. We are much more than our achievements, whether as human beings, parents, friends, or family members. Don't let lack of gratitude and the constant seeking of "more" take you away from—or keep you from—your purpose.

Let go of your reputation. Reputations are real only in the mind of others, and only according to what we do or have done—in other words, our achievements. If we concentrate only on pleasing others, we will be disconnected from our purpose and guided by their opinions. Always listen to your inner voice to guide you and stay connected to your source.

Employing faith and an impartial judgment not only contributes to a sense of tranquility, but helps us stay focused. The next time you find yourself immersed in a tangle of unhappy thoughts, stressors, or problematic behavior, remind yourself that there is something you can do to help yourself. Close your eyes and breathe deeply in and out. Let go of all resentment and ugly thoughts, and hold onto only precious moments. The mind opens to reality and truth when we understand our feelings and do not allow them to overpower us. I remember talking to a former cancer patient who said that the hardest part of dealing with her illness was healing her mind. The response that came to me was, "Your body is forgiving; why not your reasoning?" Eventually, her belief that cancer was not killing her and her faith that she was being cured were the mainstays on her road to recovery, making it less traumatic and more bearable. This woman's experience speaks to the philosophy that healing begins the moment we release our resistance.

It was Rabbi Hillel who once said there are three questions we should all ask ourselves: *If I am not for myself, who will be for me? If I am only for myself, what good am I?* and *If not now, when?* And as Dr. Martin Luther King, Jr. said so succinctly, "Take the first step in faith. You don't have to see the whole staircase, just the first step."

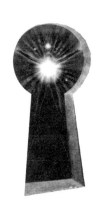

6. Complementary Alternative Medicine (CAM) Therapies

"There is nothing more difficult to take in hand, more perilous to conduct, or more uncertain in its success than to take the lead in the introduction of a new order of things."

- Niccolo Machiavelli (1469-1527)

We've come a long way

I magine our forefathers—and -mothers—coming to live in the 21st century. I wonder how they would react to the changes that have occurred. Would it be a pleasant surprise, an unbelievable experience...or a rude awakening? What we accept as everyday facts of life now would probably appear as dreams, or possibly nightmares, to them. But in general, I suspect they would be proud of how many of their thoughts and ideas have come to fruition, how their insights and ingenuity about everything from home remedies to inventions have burgeoned based on their experience, trial-and-error experiments, and good ol' common sense. And we have come a long way. Coronary bypass surgery, organ transplants, hip and knee replacements, and genetic engineering are now routine and many cures have been discovered for diseases that were fatal just a few years ago.

Medical science has indeed advanced in leaps and bounds. In addition to developments in conventional medical science, whole new avenues have opened up in the field of complementary and alternative medicine as well. Historical evidence reveals many complementary and alternative therapies that date back thousands of years; unfortunately, it is only recently that these modalities have begun to gain the recognition and acceptance they deserve. I believe the healers throughout history would be delighted to see that so many of their thoughts, ideas, and practices are now being researched and implemented.

Defining terms

Today, credible evidence has proven that complementary medicine plays a vital role in the healthcare system and can have a significant positive impact on our health.

Although the terms *complementary* and *alternative* medicine are often used synonymously, they do not mean the same thing. Complementary medicines are supportive therapies that work simultaneously *with* conventional medical care for treatment of specific ailments. The dictionary defines "complementary" as "supplying mutual needs or offsetting mutual lacks." Some examples of complementary therapies include meditation to reduce stress, or massage to assist in alleviating discomfort resulting from a treatment protocol. These are noninvasive, non-pharmacological, nonsurgical, integrated therapies that help the body in the healing process. Complementary therapy incorporates both diagnostic and therapeutic disciplines that are outside the realm of conventional healthcare practices.

Alternative therapy, on the other hand, is used *instead* of conventional medicine for treatment of specific ailments. It is used as a direct replacement for traditional medical practice. The dictionary defines "alternative" as something that "exists outside traditional or established institutions or systems." Examples might be adopting a special diet instead of treating cancer directly with surgery or radiation, or taking megavitamins to fight disease rather than undergoing chemotherapy treatments. While every individual has the right to choose what is best for him or her, this book is solely based on my experience, which resolved itself through the *combination* of conventional therapy, which eliminated my disease, and complementary and alternative therapies, which supported me in healing my body and continue to make sure the disease process has stayed away.

Alternative practices may include, but are not limited to, acupuncture, chiropractic, massage, meditation, Reiki, and osteopathy. Currently, many people utilize healing practices like these in the United States. The National Institutes for Health has a division called the National Center for Complementary and Alternative Medicine (NCAM).[1] This organization conducts and supports research, trains CAM researchers, and provides information about CAM to the general public. In 2007, for example, NCAM conducted a National Health Interview Survey to question Americans regarding their health- and illness-related experiences. The survey gathered information on 23,393 adults, age 18 years or older, and 9,417 children, age 17 years and under. Results of this survey found that in the United States, approximately 38% of adults (about four in 10) and approximately 12% of children (about one in nine) were using some form of CAM.[2] The survey also found that people of all backgrounds use CAM therapies, but that its use among adults is greater among women and those with higher levels of education and higher incomes. The NCAM survey also found that natural products, deep breathing, meditation, chiropractic, osteopathy, massage, and yoga were the most commonly used treatments, and that though people use CAM for an array of diseases and conditions, the most utilized treatment was for musculoskeletal problems, such as back, neck, or joint pain. Other ailments treated by CAM therapies include head or chest colds, anxiety and depression, stomach upset, headaches, recurring pain, and insomnia. CAM modalities are also used by many as preventative measures to protect the nervous system, musculoskeletal system, digestive system, cardiovascular system, endocrine system, lymphatic system, and the immune system. After all, what better way to avoid the experience of illness or disease than to prevent it?

Remember, the use of CAM does not undermine conventional medicine. It does, however, belong right alongside conventional medicine as a viable, necessary, complementary adjunct to the traditional healthcare system's offerings. Patients, therefore, should feel free to discuss CAM therapies with their medical doctor before, during, and after their treatments.

CAM practices

There are a number of practices that form a part of the vast body of CAM services. Common CAM therapies include acupressure, acupuncture, aromatherapy, Ayurveda, chiropractic, herbal medicine, homeopathy, hypnosis, massage, relaxation techniques, meditation, naturopathy, osteopathy, reflexology, Reiki, visualization, yoga, tai chi, and qigong for enhancing, accelerating, and reinforcing the healing process. According to Josephine P. Briggs, M.D., director of the National Center for Complementary and Alternative Medicine, "The public's concept of health is broader than preventing and treating disease. Increasingly, Americans are using strategies that they can employ themselves to improve their health, maintain wellness, and improve quality of life."[3]

In Figure 6-1 (on the next page), we see a graph of a telephone survey undertaken by researchers at the University of Exeter.[4] The purpose of this survey was to research the popularity of CAM therapies in the United Kingdom and worldwide. The graph demonstrates that Germany leads the pack in CAM practices, with almost 65% of the adult population practicing some form of therapy. Canada comes in a close second with close to 60%, followed by France, Australia, the United States, Switzerland, Belgium, Sweden and the United Kingdom. Herbalism, aromatherapy, homeopathy, acupuncture, massage, and reflexology were among the most popular CAM therapies utilized. In Germany and France, a significant number of CAM techniques are practiced by medical doctors, while in the United States CAM practitioners are generally chiropractors and osteopaths. Apart from osteopaths and chiropractors, who are licensed doctors in their specialties, it is not mandatory for complementary and alternative medical practitioners to be licensed before they begin practicing in the United States. However, many practitioners are now members of various accredited organizations that serve to standardize and regulate the various forms of CAM practices.

FIGURE 6-1. The role of Complementary and Alternative Medicine (CAM): One-year prevalence bar graph of CAM in various countries. (Source: *British Medical Journal.* *http://bmj.bmjjournals.com/cgi/reprint/321/7269/1133.pdf*)

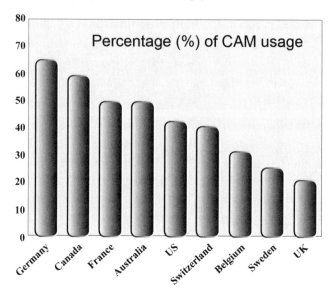

Most complementary practitioners are bound by a particular philosophy as the basis of their treatment and believe that complementary therapeutic intervention restores balance to the body by assisting in the natural healing process, rather than by targeting the individual disease or a troublesome symptom. An example of complementary intervention might be to advise the patient receiving conventional medical treatment about ways to supplement healing by applying lifestyle and dietary modification along with relaxation techniques.

Headquartered in Seattle, Washington, the Academic Consortium for Complementary and Alternative Health Care (ACCAHC) is a good example of how the world of healthcare is changing. This organization is dedicated to shifting medicine toward a more holistic healthcare system. ACCAHC's core membership consists of organizations representing acupuncture, massage therapy, chiropractic, midwifery, oriental medicine, naturopathic medicine, and other traditional world medicines. ACCAHC predicts "a healthcare system that is multidisciplinary and enhances competence, mutual respect, and collaboration across all complementary and alternative medicine and conventional healthcare disciplines. This system will deliver effective care that is patient-centered, focused on health creation and healing, and readily accessible to all populations."[5]

As my interest piqued, I set about investigating the more commonly known CAM therapies, but the subject is so vast that I had a hard time figuring out where to begin. To simplify my research, I started with topics I had vaguely heard about from time to time. I did not attempt to rate these topics or modalities, because all I wanted to do was learn about each one without trying to judge it. In doing so, I was able to view each one as a distinct entity that holds as much weight as any other.

Because the study of CAM is, in effect, endless, with new ideas entering the field all the time, this chapter attempts to cover some of the more common therapies popular in the United States in the 21st century.

Acupuncture

Acupuncture is an ancient form of healing that has been in practice in China for at least 2,000 years (some say as many as 5,000) and is one technique of Traditional Chinese Medicine (TCM). Acupuncture was known and has been used in the West as far back as the 17th century. Its first recognized use was in Paris at the Paris Medical School in 1810 by Dr. Louis Berlioz. In England, John Churchill was the first acupuncturist to publish results relative to acupuncture treatment for rheumatism in 1821. In the United States, acupuncture has grown in popularity over the last 30 years, in part due to President Nixon's trip to China in 1971. It seems that on this trip, a journalist from the President's group fell ill and required medical treatment. The reporter was so impressed by his speedy recovery, which had been aided by the use of acupuncture for his postoperative pain, that he shared his experiences upon returning to the United States.

Traditional Chinese Medicine is based on the theory of *qi*, or "life force." Two symbols, a broken line signifying "the receptive," and an unbroken line to signify "the creative," represent the two major universal life forces which denote the vital energy circulating through the pathways of the body's meridians, or energy pathways. This qi energy needs to be balanced for the individual to achieve optimal health. *Yin*, represented by the broken line, and *yang*, represented by the solid line, are manifestations of qi, dualities which symbolize the philosophy behind all Traditional Chinese Medicine and its application. It is said that yin and yang are opposites which together create the whole, and that in the practice of TCM, yin, the dark, passive, female energy, and yang, the light, active, male energy, are regulated and brought to balance for attainment of spiritual, emotional, mental, and physical wellbeing. The methods of Traditional Chinese Medicine are comprised of both internal and external forces that approach disease as disharmony within the body, or between the body and the environment. The seven internal forces are joy, anger, worry, thought, sadness, fear, and shock; the six external forces are wind, dryness, cold, moisture, fire, and heat. Two other causes of disharmony, which are neither internal nor external, are fatigue and food. Furthermore, in Oriental medicine all organs are considered in the individual's treatment protocol, not only the organ perceived to be affected with the problem. This is because it is believed that one organ's condition affects all the others; as a result, the entire body is affected.

Where conventional medical doctors monitor blood flow through the blood vessels with Doppler ultrasound and electrical activity in the brain with an EEG, acupuncturists appraise the flow of vital energy through the various *meridian* lines in the body to reverse any imbalances.

Acupuncture is widely practiced in this country by thousands of doctors, dentists, acupuncturists, and other practitioners to alleviate many types of pain. In fact, according to a 2002 National Health Interview Survey (NHIS), 1.4% of respondents (representing 3.1 million Americans) said they had used acupuncture in the prior year.[6] In a study at the University of Michigan, for example, 20 women diagnosed with fibromyalgia (a chronic pain disorder) were randomly assigned to receive either traditional acupuncture or simulated acupuncture treatments over four weeks. While both traditional and simulated acupuncture groups showed a reduction of pain, the traditional acupuncture group showed significantly greater reductions in pain levels.[7] Studies like this show us that during the process of diagnosis and treatment, the assistance of acupuncture can not only help manage illness, but promote good health through prevention. And as there are virtually no side effects with acupuncture, more and more people are turning to this treatment for continued health.

With growing understanding of this field, more and more medical practitioners are also advising patients about the benefits of acupuncture, and its popularity continues to rise. The last five years have also seen an increase in the field of *integrative medicine*, a combination of Western and Oriental medicine. Cancer patients, for example, can be found undergoing chemotherapy to destroy cancer by a conventional medical practitioner, while simultaneously undergoing treatment with an acupuncturist to decrease any associated side effects and improve immune system responses through the balancing of qi.

Treatment by acupuncture has been found to provide relief from common addictions like smoking and drug addiction, and studies suggest that acupuncture is helpful in many cases of anxiety, depression, allergies, asthma, arthritis, back pain, colitis, digestive disorders, dizziness, fatigue, headaches and migraines, insomnia, menstrual disorders and menopausal syndrome, indigestion and nausea, and weight management and control. In 1996, acupuncture's growing popularity led the U.S. Food and Drug Administration to reclassify acupuncture needles for use by licensed practitioners for public safety and effectiveness. This requires the administering of sterile, nontoxic needles labeled "for single use" by qualified practitioners only. The needles used are very thin, about the width of a hair, and, unlike hypodermic needles, are solid and do not cut the skin. When inserted properly, the application of these needles is generally not at all painful. Similar to any therapy, however, the response to acupuncture varies from person to person. When performed by a licensed practitioner, acupuncture has been found safe and effective and, as said before, without side effects. Completely non-addictive, people frequently report a sense of wellbeing, revitalized mental clarity, and feelings of serenity and peace during and after treatment.

Preventative acupuncture is utilized for those individuals who are symptom- and disease-free, but are looking for ways to ensure their body maintains its homeostasis and health. Healthcare providers often refer patients to acupuncturists, but acupuncture treatment does not require a medical referral. Naturally, it is advisable to check the practitioner's credentials to ensure he or she is licensed and has met the standards for treating patients. Treatment costs vary depending on the length of treatment and the number of times treatment has been recommended. A problem may be resolved in a few visits, a few weeks, or even longer, depending on the nature of the condition. Acupuncture is one of the CAM therapies now recognized by some insurance carriers, so check with your insurer before beginning treatment to see if acupuncture is part of your insurance plan. Regardless, when it comes to your health, this kind of treatment is money well spent.

Acupressure

Acupressure is similar to acupuncture as it is also an ancient healing therapy developed in China more than 5,000 years ago and based on the same TCM philosophy. Instead of fine needles, however, physical pressure is applied by the hand, elbow, or other device to different acupuncture points along the meridians of the body. Acupressure is said to be excellent in healing for the whole person—mind, body, and spirit. The two most common styles of acupressure are *Shiatsu* and *Jin Shin Do*, therapeutic methods that induce relaxation while balancing the flow of vital energy and promoting health. Shiatsu, the Japanese form of acupressure, is literally translated as finger (*shi*) pressure (*atsu*) therapy and involves the application of vigorous and firm pressure, and Jin Shin Do, or "the way of the compassionate spirit," involves a gentler pressure on the acupuncture points. Both methods stimulate the body to follow its own rhythms and restore the natural flow. Acupressure encourages the body's natural curative abilities and is a safe, effective complement to conventional healing methods.

Aromatherapy

Aromatherapy is yet another therapy under CAM's wide umbrella. In essence (no pun intended), aromatherapy uses the psychological and physiological therapeutic properties of essential, or volatile, plant oils to improve the individual's health and disposition. Aromatic essential oils and compounds are extracted from the leaves, stems, flowers, bark, roots, seeds, twigs, berries, rinds, and bulbs of plants, and then diluted, to be used for various purposes. The benefits of aromatherapy are derived through inhalation of the oils, which restore, relax, and rejuvenate body, mind, and spirit.

The word *aromathérapie* was coined in the 1920s by a French chemist named René-Maurice Gattefossé. After a lifetime of researching the properties of essential oils, Gattefossé was convinced that plant oils and extracts had positive effects on many physical and emotional ailments. For example, the scent of lavender oil is now known for its calming effect, which aids in relaxation and the reduction of anxiety. Peppermint oil is commonly used for nausea, indigestion, and irritable bowel syndrome; patchouli is used for the treatment of headaches; and rosemary oil is often recommended as a mental stimulant to aid memory and concentration.

Tracing its origins back more than 4,000 years, aromatherapy is one of the oldest techniques of holistic healing. For instance, translations of hieroglyphics found in the temple of Edfou have shown that aromatic oils were used by Egyptians and their priests for the purposes of formulating perfumes, cosmetics, medicines, and for embalming. The Greeks, who attained their knowledge of aromatherapy from the Egyptians, then went on to make many of their own new discoveries. Ancient Chinese herbal books dating back to about 2700 B.C. also tell us that aromatherapy was an accepted healing tool in that culture. These works detail information about more than 300 plants and their uses. In India, the traditional medical system of Ayurveda also continues its long-time use of aromatic and herbal massage for various ailments of mind and body.

Aromatherapy is reported to strengthen the self-healing process by stimulating various bodily systems. Inhaled fragrances activate centers in the brain; this encourages relief from stress through the natural alteration of the mental state, the removal of energy blockages, and the facilitation of the flow of blood and oxygen. Today, aromatherapists' comprehensive, in-depth knowledge of essential oils allows them to custom blend different oils for different results.

Circulating essential oils is achieved by evaporation of the aromatic constituents into the atmosphere with different types of devices. Some use direct heat as a means of evaporation, while others prefer candle diffusers or ceramic or brass rings placed on light bulbs. How olfactory aromatic oil works is an interesting process whereby, upon inhalation, the oils affect the body in a variety of ways. When the scent of the oils enters the nasal passages, they stimulate highly specialized olfactory nerve endings. The nerve endings then send messages directly into the limbic system of the brain, the central location of all memory, behavior, and emotion. Here a physiological chain of events occurs in the body to positively affect the nervous, endocrine, and immune systems.

The results of using aromatherapy vary from individual to individual. Most schools of thought agree that essential oils do have an overall positive effect, but no particular oil is known to induce exactly the same effect in everyone. This is because there are many variables that can affect the outcome, such as the nature of the essential oil used, the type of ailment, and/or the individual's general disposition. Today, products for aromatherapy are widely and easily available in the form of wax and soy candles, diffusers, essential oils, and oil burners.

With over 150 essential oils currently available, some known for their chemical properties as natural antibiotics, antifungals, antiseptics, and antivirals, aromatherapy has become a convenient adjunct for use alongside conventional medicine. During cancer treatment as well, the use of aromatherapy is a simple method for reducing stress and anxiety. Aromatherapeutic massage and touch involves the addition of concentrated plant oils to massage lotion, and is yet another method for encouraging patients to connect with others by building and fostering relationships.

With its acknowledged benefits, the popularity of aromatherapy continues to grow. Aromatherapists now publish their own quarterly journal, the *International Journal of Essential Oil Therapeutics*, for individuals and groups with an interest in the bioactivity of aromatic plant applications on both humans and animals.[8]

Reading about the benefits derived from such profound therapies, I couldn't help but think about how much of a difference they might have made for me when I was suffering so much anxiousness during my own cancer treatment. That is why I am dedicated to raising awareness for people undergoing long, arduous treatment by sharing the noninvasive avenues open to them to reduce the stress associated with their own cancer treatment procedures.

Ayurveda

Ayurveda is a form of CAM originating in the Indian subcontinent. The term is a combination of two words, *ayur* and *veda*, where ayur signifies "life," and veda, "science," and can be loosely translated as the "science of life." There is no documented evidence as to the origins of Ayurveda, though the first discovered writings on the subject are thought to have been produced during Vedic times (from the second and first millennia B.C. to the 6th century B.C.). Ayurveda is based on belief in the principle that there are five primary elements in nature: space, air, fire, water, and earth. Ayurveda stresses that these five elements are not only in the environment, but within us; that is, nature's "elements" are found in the form of matter and energy, equivalent to the body and soul; when the five elements of nature (outside) are combined with the matter and energy (inside) we become one. Inside the body, these five elements are represented by three doshas, or energy types, *vata*, *pitta* and *kapha*. These forces are known as *tridoshas*, based on the fact that we are comprised of a combination of all three.

Vata directs the law of movement, the force which is expressed by nerve impulses, circulation, respiration, and elimination. Pitta is expressed through the metabolism, the conversion of food into nutrients absorbed by the body, and intracellular metabolism. The kapha dosha, including the elements of water and earth, embodies growth and protection. Cerebral spinal fluid, which protects the brain, spinal cord, and mucosal lining of the stomach, are examples of how kapha manifests in the body. In the physical world, space and air combine to form the vata dosha, fire and water constitute the pitta dosha, and earth and water comprise the kapha dosha.

Ayurveda believes that each of us is a unique combination of vata, pitta, and kapha, manifestations of the greater universe where all living and non-living things are interconnected and exist in a state of balance. Diseases are said to arise when there is disharmony in us, between us, and with the universe. Ayurvedic practitioners design treatment protocols to address any imbalances that exist to help the body be more adaptable in bringing about physical, psychological, and spiritual change. Various herbs and medicines are also prescribed in Ayurvedic therapy and have been shown to have useful healing properties. For example, the Neem (*Azadirachta indica*) tree has compounds shown to increase immunity by boosting lymphocyte and T-cell counts. *Terminalia arjuna* is a plant which has been shown to reduce angina pain, heart failure, coronary artery disease, and hypercholesterolemia.

Kerala Ayurveda is one of the most popular Ayurvedic treatment modalities, originating in Kerala, India, in which a variety of treatments and rejuvenating therapies, including herbal baths, massage with special oils, dietary recommendations, yoga, and meditation are utilized to treat conditions of the mind, body, and soul. It is the aim of Ayurveda to cure not only the ailment, but to promote longevity through good health.

In the United States, the National Institute of Ayurvedic Medicine (NIAM), established by Dr. Scott Gerson in 1982, is recognized as the most reliable resource for Ayurvedic treatment. At one time, Dr. Gerson was the only doctor in the country who practiced both conventional and Ayurvedic medicine. Though Ayurvedic practitioners do not require licensing in the U.S., certain standards have been created to address treatment protocols and the legalities of practice. As per the 2007 survey by the National Center for Health Statistics, about 200,000 United States adults had used Ayurveda within the 12 months prior to the survey.[9] (If you are undergoing Ayurvedic treatment and conventional medical therapy concurrently, always inform your medical practitioner to confirm there is no contraindication with simultaneous use.)

Chiropractic medicine

Chiropractic is a complementary and alternative healthcare system that focuses on diagnosis, treatment, and prevention of mechanical disorders of the musculoskeletal system in order to control their effects on the nervous system and on overall physical health. Chiropractic systems of CAM influenced me and my life so profoundly that I studied to become a doctor of chiropractic, and have been in private practice now for over 25 years. Chiropractors are licensed physicians, accredited by state and national boards.

The word *chiropractic* is derived from the Greek meaning "done by hand." The foundation of chiropractic therapy lies in the principle that the body can heal itself if the skeletal system is properly aligned to allow the nerve impulses transmitted through the nervous system to flow freely without obstruction. Information from the brain through the spinal cord regulates the functioning of all cells, tissues, and organs in the body by receiving and sending messages through the spinal nerves. Any misalignment, or *subluxation*, in the vertebrae that make up the spinal column housing the spinal cord and where spinal nerves exit, can therefore impede spinal nerve function. A *vertebral subluxation* can alter neurological function, which, in turn, can cause neuromusculoskeletal and visceral disorders. Simply put, when spinal nerve function is blocked, the brain's communication to all the other structures becomes blocked also; this creates a state of *dis*-ease by keeping the body's "innate intelligence" from being expressed, both directly and indirectly, on normal bodily functions.

The exact origin of chiropractic cannot be traced specifically, as many different types of physical manipulation of the spinal column and skeleton have been practiced worldwide for more than 1,000 years, but it has been documented that ancient Greek, Roman, Oriental, and Indian doctors have used this form of therapy to treat many health problems. Hippocrates is known to have explored spinal manipulation and its effect on general health, as is Galen, the well-known 2nd-century physician, who recognized the importance of an aligned spine in the curing of disease. It wasn't until 1895, however, that Daniel David Palmer, healer, scientist, and founder of the first school of chiropractic (in 1897), discovered not only that subluxated vertebrae could cause impeded nerve function and further disease, but that adjusting or correcting these segments back to their normal positions could facilitate healing and have a profound effect on an individual's health and wellbeing. This theory was further developed by many others, including Palmer's son, B. J. Palmer.

Spinal manipulation is the predominate technique utilized in chiropractic treatment. Contrary to some popular belief, chiropractors do not limit themselves to symptoms arising from musculoskeletal problems, such as lower back and neck pain, and misalignments caused by sports, work, or auto accident injuries, but also take an active role in more preventative, or "family," spinal health considerations. At times, manipulation to other osseous structures of the body, as well as physiotherapy, diet and nutrition changes, and exercise regimens are recommended to complement adjustments to the individual for the achievement of overall long-lasting good health. According to the 2007 survey conducted by the National Center for Complementary and Alternative Medicine, about 8% (or 18 million) of all American adults and 3% (or 2 million) of all American children had received chiropractic manipulation in the prior 12 months.[10]

Chiropractic is one of the few CAM therapies that shares some features with other health professions. These elements include stressing a balance between environment, health, and lifestyle, and focusing on the cause of the illness, rather than its symptoms, and the centrality of the nervous system and its close relationship to the body's structural integrity. Chiropractic also distinguishes itself from other modern medicinal techniques with its credible philosophy of healing naturally and effectively through noninvasive methods that emphasize the individual's own recuperative and healing abilities. As one of the most frequently used CAM practices for treatment, chiropractic holds a unique complementary position within the healthcare system of the United States. Today most patients have the benefit of insurance coverage for at least part of the cost of their chiropractic treatment.

Osteopathic medicine

Osteopathy is a unique form of medical practice. The term *osteopathy* comes from the Greek word *osteon*, meaning "bone," and *pathos*, meaning "to suffer." Osteopathic physicians believe that disease is a result of an imbalanced relationship among the body's anatomical structures, organ systems, and physiological functions. This system of healing uses modern medical techniques to diagnose and correct imbalances in the body's structure, including all muscles, bones, ligaments, and organs. Correction is facilitated with a whole-person, hands-on approach.

The origin of osteopathy can be traced back to 1874 when Dr. Andrew Taylor Still finished his tour of duty as an Army doctor during the Civil War. Disillusioned with the traditional practice of medicine, Still began to focus his work on restoring health through more primary manual techniques, those now known as osteopathic manipulations. Still's research led him to the conclusion that the musculoskeletal system plays a vital role in health and disease and that correcting the body's structural imbalances often enables the body to heal itself.

Today the osteopath's work involves restoring the body's natural healing system by gently applying the correct amount of pressure to the body to facilitate proper joint movement, organ correction, and muscle action. This work in turn facilitates healing in the joints, muscles, and organs, eliciting a positive physiological response.

Osteopathy and chiropractic are based on similar principles in that both are holistic methods of healing that target the spine and other bony structures of the body. Both practices share the philosophy that structure affects function, as well as the understanding that mental, dietary, and lifestyle factors have an inseparable relationship with health. The difference between these disciplines can be found in the state laws that govern each profession's scope of practice. Where both chiropractors and osteopaths are trained in manipulation of the musculoskeletal system to facilitate healing, of the two, only chiropractors are trained in correcting vertebral subluxations, and only osteopaths are licensed to prescribe medication and perform surgery. Furthermore, osteopathy is not limited to bone problems, as the name might suggest (although the bony skeleton is considered the foundation of the body, and any disruption in the skeleton is viewed as a possible precursor of illness). Osteopathic physicians in the United States often practice medical specialties, such as radiology, surgery, orthopedics, neurology, and pediatrics, to coincide with their osteopathic training.

Common disorders that may be alleviated with osteopathic treatment include neck and back problems, joint pain, traumatic injury, asthma, gastrointestinal problems, neurological problems, and allergies. According to the American Association of Colleges of Osteopathic Medicine, there are 55,000 licensed osteopathic physicians in the United States, and this number is growing steadily.

Naturopathic medicine

The foundation of naturopathic medicine, like other complementary and alternative medicine practices, is that the human body has the innate ability to heal itself. Naturopathic doctors are practitioners who prefer and utilize natural remedies, such as manual therapy, herbalism, diet, and counseling, as a way to facilitate healing and combat disease, and espouse the minimal use of surgery and drugs. The word *naturopathy* was coined in 1895 by Dr. John Scheel, but it was Dr. Benedict Lust who held its registered name. Lust was a trained hydrotherapist (see page 370) who graduated from the New York Homeopathic Medical College and from the Universal College of Osteopathy. Lust eventually founded the American School of Naturopathy in New York in 1902, but the field remained fairly unpopular at the time due to the major reorganization of the American Medical Association and its influence on medicine during that period. Meanwhile, due to its simplicity, adaptability, and cost effectiveness, naturopathy was popularized in many countries. In India, for example, the practice was made accessible to everyone by Mahatma Gandhi.

In the 1970s, a revival of interest in naturopathy in the United States and Canada in conjunction with the holistic health movement occurred, and naturopathic doctors began incorporating work in nutrition, botanical medicine, homeopathy, hydrotherapy, psychology, and acupuncture into their practices. Naturopaths are trained in conventional medical science and are granted licenses by each state's Naturopathic Board of Medical Examiners.

The six fundamental principles of naturopathic medicine are similar to the Hippocratic Oath: to trust the body's wisdom to heal itself; to look beyond the symptoms to the underlying cause; to utilize the most natural, least invasive, and least toxic therapies; to educate the patient in health; to view the body as a whole; and to focus on overall health, wellness, and disease prevention. Naturopathic medicine seeks to promote the restoration and revival of health by following the simple basic rules of health and by acknowledging that these rules can be found in nature—good eating, a healthy lifestyle, and avoidance of things impure to the body. It is the role of the naturopathic physician to identify and remove obstacles to good health, thereby creating an environment conducive to healing.

Holistic physicians

Physicians who are *holistic* are allopathic doctors with training in natural healing remedies. In addition to their conventional medical training, education often includes holistic and natural approaches to patient treatment, including nutrition, acupuncture, homeopathic medicine, herbs, psychology, and counseling. Holistic doctors advise patients about lifestyle, nutrition, outlook and attitude, prescribe natural remedies, and at times refer patients to other medical specialists. Holistic doctors offer a unique combination of conventional medicine and CAM therapies; this approach provides a balanced approach of the best of Western medicine's advanced technologies and the preventive and natural techniques of complementary medicine. Dr. Ralph Bircher, son of Dr. Maximilian Bircher-Benner, whose influence on the health reform movement in Europe has lasted long past his death in 1939, operates the famous Bircher-Benner clinic in Zurich. Dr. Bircher has said of holistic practice, "The treatment is really a cooperative of a trinity—the patient, the doctor, and the inner doctor." In this sense, practitioners recognize that healing has to occur from the inside out, not only the outside in, and are devoted to treating the whole person—the mind, body, and spirit—in the individual's interest. Chinese medicine, naturopathy, acupuncture, and homeopathic methods are some of the therapies adopted by holistic doctors. In addition to the medical care provided, holistic care offers supportive care for long-term health and wellbeing.

Holistic nursing

Holistic nursing is yet another effective branch of holistic healing. Holistic nursing encompasses all nursing involved in the healing of the whole person. Per the American Holistic Nurses Association, or AHNA, holistic nursing is defined as "all nursing practice that has healing the whole person as its goal." Holistic nursing is a specialty practice that draws on nursing knowledge, theories, expertise, and intuition to guide nurses in becoming therapeutic partners with people in their care. This practice recognizes the totality of the human being— the interconnectedness of body, mind, emotion, spirit, social/cultural relationship, context, and environment."[11]

As the concept of "holism" supports the fact that an individual is an integration of mind, body, spirit, and the environment, holistic nurses become therapeutic partners with individuals, families, and whole communities to aid healing. The well-rounded, complementary care they provide as part of their clinical practice focuses on physiological, psychological, and spiritual needs. Holistic nursing requires a remarkable shift in consciousness and intention, because in addition to the usual knowledge and compassion implemented in conventional medicine, this field adds the critical techniques of massage, therapeutic touch, intuition, and spirituality to education and modes of treatment. In this way, medical, complementary, and alternative modalities are all addressed.

The guiding principle in holistic nursing can be summed up in one word: *care*. These nurses interact with a single-minded thoughtfulness and sensitivity. The individual's positive change in outlook, ever-evolving acceptance, and wellbeing are the healthy by-products of the love and care holistic nurses provide. As Florence Nightingale, believed to be one of the first holistic nurses, once said, nursing puts a patient "in the best conditions for nature to work upon him."

The art of caring for another human being unselfishly to help him feel better and working toward his wellness, healing, and cure demands dedication, devotion, hard work, and strength of character; these are the qualities embodied by holistic nurses.

Registered dieticians

When it comes to knowing what kinds of food to eat, how many calories to consume, and where to find the best sources for our daily requirements of vitamins and minerals, many of us may feel left in the dark. This is where registered dieticians (RDs) are available to help us make healthier choices for ourselves. These experts are devoted to providing education and counseling, preventing disease, and promoting health through food choices.

Qualified registered dietitians fulfill coursework that must be approved by the Commission on Accreditation for Dietetics Education (CADE) of the American Dietetic Association (ADA). Licensure includes completing a bachelor's degree, passing a national examination, and completing a supervised CADE-accredited practice program of six to 12 months under supervision at a healthcare facility, community center, food service management, or other food dietetics facility. The dietitian also has to complete professional continuing education credits to maintain licensure. Many registered dietitians hold additional certifications in specialized areas of practice.

More and more hospitals and other healthcare facilities employ the services of trained dietitians. These are the diet and nutrition professionals who manage the food services of institutions, such as schools, company cafeterias, and prisons, distribute food, and promote healthy eating habits through research and development. RDs work in clinical and community settings as clinical dietitians, community dietitians, food service dietitians, research dietitians, administrative dietitians, consultant dietitians, or business dietitians. Other nutritional workers who assist registered dieticians may include dietary assistants, dietary clerks, and dietary managers and workers.

Clinical dietitians work in hospitals, private practice, or other healthcare facilities and help plan daily food charts to meet the individual's nutritional needs. They also develop and implement highly beneficial nutritional programs for the speedy recovery and wellness of the patient. The American Dietetic Association reports that 47% of its members work in this setting.

Community dietitians coordinate wellness programs directly in communities or through various organizations within the community. They are involved in the application of knowledge of food and nutrition according to lifestyle and geographical areas, and organize their dietary knowledge with public health agencies, day care centers, and recreational camps.

Food service dietitians, as the name suggests, are dietitians specializing in and responsible for large-scale food planning and distribution. Their work involves coordination, assessment, and preparation of food, as well as its storage and distribution. They work with healthcare facilities, cafeterias, restaurants, educational institutions, food service programs, and corporations to manage and direct other service staff to schedule the delivery of nutritious food.

Research dietitians are those involved in the research and development of nutrition and who work around the clinical aspect of nutrition. They study human nutrition for health development and disease prevention, generally in hospitals and research establishments.

Administrative dietitians, also known as managers and directors of dietetics departments or nutrition services, oversee organizational food and nutrition departments. Responsibilities include hiring, training, supervising, and managing all the dietitians on staff.

Consultant dietitians are dietitians who are in private practice and who independently provide nutritional and diet-related services to individuals, groups, or healthcare facilities.

Business dietitians are the resource link for the media. They work as experts on television and radio and in various publications, including daily newspapers, magazines, and journals.

Since registered dietitians have the capacity to formulate types and amounts of food and fluid for their patients, they need to be knowledgeable about each individual's illness, health history, and metabolism, as well as the biochemistry of the nutrients and food components being recommended. For example, for diabetics the dietitian has to design meals in which the carbohydrates, proteins, and fats consumed by the patients encourage healthy blood-sugar levels. In the case of a patient with high cholesterol, recommendations would be made for reducing cholesterol intake through diet, one of its main sources. Likewise, cancer patients undergoing treatment often suffer from a partial or complete loss of appetite. The registered dietitian is trained to formulate meals that will not only be appealing, but also provide the correct caloric and nutritional values required to complement the current treatment. Dieticians designate special diets, recommend nutritional supplements, and counsel patients and their families, with the goal of preventing and treating illness through proper dietary regimens. Dieticians encourage a disciplined approach to eating habits that support long-term health.

The American Dietetic Association is the nation's largest organization of food and nutrition professionals with more than 67,000 members.[12] There are also other organizations committed to public health issues, including the American Society for Nutrition. With a membership of more than 3,600, its members, scientists, and practitioners are involved in improving quality of life through education and research about nutrition.[13]

The British Nutrition Foundation is one of a number of like organizations with a mission of interpreting a variety of nutritional and dietary scientific data to "generate and communicate clear, accurate, accessible information on nutrition, diet and lifestyle…relevant to the needs of diverse audiences. Through active engagement with government, schools, industry, health professionals and journalists, [BNF] also aim[s] to provide advice to help shape and support policy and to facilitate improvement in the diet and physical activity patterns of the population."[14] Their goal is to disseminate reliable information and develop strategic partnerships to create a greater impact on the population in hopes of promoting significant lifestyle changes to improve the health and wellbeing of society at large.

Physical therapy

Physical therapy is a healthcare profession that provides services to individuals to develop, improve, maintain, and restore physical movement and functional ability. Physical therapists treat disorders of the muscles, bones, and joints with physical agents, such as heat, water, light, electric stimulation, manual massage, joint mobilization, and exercise. Because physical therapy is inherently a one-on-one approach, it has been called "the science of healing and the art of caring." A viable addition to the CAM basket of offerings, physical therapists provide another natural, drugless, hands-on approach to recovery and wellness.

Physical therapists often work with orthopedic problems, such as postoperative joints, osteoporosis, joint and soft tissue injuries, fractures, and dislocations. They also treat neurological conditions, such as strokes, brain injuries, spinal cord injury, Alzheimer's disease, and Parkinson's disease. Cardiovascular and pulmonary physical therapists treat a wide variety of patients with heart and lung disorders, such as chronic obstructive pulmonary disease, heart conditions, and those who are post-coronary bypass surgery. Pediatric physical therapists assist in the early detection and treatment of disorders in the pediatric population. This includes improving gross and fine motor skills, balance and coordination, strength, endurance, and sensory processing and integration.

The American Physical Therapy Association (APTA) is the nation's largest organization of physical therapists, with close to 74,000 members.[15] APTA's goal is to foster advancements in the practice of physical therapy, education, and research. APTA defines *physical therapy* as "the prevention, diagnosis, and treatment of movement dysfunctions and the enhancement of physical health and functional abilities of people," and physical therapists as "health care professionals who diagnose and treat people of all ages who have medical problems or other health-related conditions that limit their abilities to move and perform functional activities in their daily lives. They examine the individual and plan treatments based on their problems to restore function, prevent disability, reduce pain, promote wellbeing, and achieve a better lifestyle." Physical therapists require a license to practice in all states. They must have graduate degrees from an accredited physical therapy program, after which they are eligible to take the national licensure examination permitting them to practice. According to the American Physical Therapy Association in 2009, there were 212 physical therapist education programs; of these accredited programs 12 awarded master's degrees and 200 awarded doctoral degrees.

Physical therapists can be found working in hospitals, outpatient clinics, rehabilitation centers, education and research centers, schools, fitness and sports training centers, industrial settings, and other workplaces. Many are in private practice, and patients are referred to them by physicians.

Massage therapy

Whatever school of thought you espouse, no profession can deny the importance of a healthy musculoskeletal system. That is why naturopaths, chiropractors, osteopaths, and medical doctors often recommend massage therapy. Massage therapy is considered one of the oldest and simplest forms of healing. It involves pressing, stroking, kneading, and rubbing different parts of the body to alleviate pain, to relax knotted and tense muscles, improve circulation, remove waste products from muscles, and stimulate overall energy flow. Historic evidence on the benefits of massage is common. Egyptian tomb paintings have been found that depict the art of massage, for example, as do Chinese texts from 2700 B.C. which outline breathing exercises, massage of the skin and flesh, and exercises of the hands and feet for treatment of paralysis and chills. In fact, at one time in Greece and Italy massage was the primary method for relieving pain. About this form of healing, Hippocrates said, "The physician must be experienced in many things, but guaranteed in rubbing because rubbing can bind a joint that is loose and loosen a joint that is rigid."

In India, traditional Ayurveda emphasizes therapeutic massage with medicated or aromatic oils for relaxation and treatment of various ailments. Apart from the relaxation response, the massage works to improve the functioning of the musculoskeletal, neurological, circulatory, organ, and lymphatic systems of the body. Massage has also been found to restore physical, mental, and spiritual equilibrium and is used extensively in intensive care units to provide relief and comfort to the seriously injured.

Massage has also been shown to be an effective complementary modality in patients undergoing cancer treatment relative to pain relief, increased relaxation, management of treatment side effects, and overall improved health. For example, in one study at Memorial Sloan-Kettering Cancer Center, 1,290 cancer patients were evaluated for symptoms over a three-year period. Researchers observed that participants who received massage therapy during their cancer treatment protocols had significantly improved levels of pain, nausea, fatigue, depression, and anxiety.[16] In another study, massage therapy was also shown to be beneficial following lymph node dissection surgery. In this case, the "significant others" (spouse, partner, friend) of the participants were taught how to perform massage, and were asked to perform arm massage as a postoperative support measure on their partners. Results of this study revealed not only that arm massage decreased the participants' pain and discomfort related to surgery, but that it promoted a sense of closeness and support between the subjects and their significant others.[17]

Massage is classified into two groups: Western-influenced massage techniques, such as Swedish, deep tissue, triggerpoint, sports, and chair massage, and Eastern-influenced massage techniques, such as Ayurveda, Shiatsu, Tui na, hot stones, and reflexology. As with other natural cures, massage therapy directs the attention to the body's ability to heal itself. Generally, no specific disease process is treated, though there are times when a specific condition is addressed. For example, overworked muscles can accumulate lactic acid, which can lead to soreness, stiffness, or even cramps in the muscles. In these types of cases, massage can improve circulation and assist in eliminating the waste products, thus speeding recovery and facilitating healing.

Many states in the U.S. require formal training and certification for the practice of massage therapy. Some states require continuing education programs for therapists to keep their knowledge up to date. It is recommended that massage therapy be administered by a trained and licensed individual, and advisable to check the license and certification of the therapist before beginning sessions. It is also a good idea to let your therapist know your past and current health statuses before the massage session begins to avoid any problems you may have. According to the American Massage Therapy Association, it is estimated that there were 265,000 to 300,000 massage therapists and massage school students in the United States as of 2008.[18] This growing rate of therapists is due to the ever more widely accepted use of massage therapy and its recommendation by many clinics, doctors, sports trainers, and physical therapists. Due to its capacity to help individuals both physiologically and emotionally, the American Cancer Society views massage as the most universally beneficial therapy.

Colon hydrotherapy

The more one explores the subject of complementary and alternative therapies, the larger the picture grows. Numerous therapies exist with roots embedded thousands of years back in various civilizations across the globe. One of these therapies is colon hydrotherapy.

The colon consists of four sections: the ascending colon, the transverse colon, the descending colon, and the sigmoid colon. The colon, which winds through the abdominal cavity to end at the anus, serves to store waste, reclaim water, maintain the water balance, and absorb some vitamins. The colon also functions to perform the immense task of eliminating the waste it has stored in the form of feces and nonspecific toxins. Although the colon cleanses itself naturally without assistance to some degree, the benefits of thorough cleansing in the form of hydrotherapy are well documented throughout history.

The use of an enema was seen as far back as 1550 B.C., in an Egyptian medical manuscript known as *Ebers Papyrus*. Hippocrates and Galen also recognized the use of enema therapy for treatment of a number of ailments. In these ancient civilizations, the preferred methodology was to inject fluid via the use of a hollow reed (found in any body of water) to stimulate the flow of water into the rectum. Hydrotherapy is often compared to an enema, but enemas treat only the lower bowel. Colon therapy, on the other hand, cleanses the entire colon to flush out the wedged fecal matter, toxins, residue, and parasites for thorough detoxification.

In his book, *Guide to Better Bowel Care*, Dr. Bernard Jensen states, "The need to detoxify and cleanse the body has never been greater than right now. People are more toxic-ridden today than ever in known history. The widespread existence of toxic substances and the levels at which they are found are becoming a nightmare as illness continues to take its toll. Nearly all the patients I see have some kind of bowel disorder associated with toxicity, even if they are unaware of it."[19] Jensen's findings have been substantiated by others. In her book, *Gut Wisdom: Understanding and Improving Your Intestinal Health*, for example, author Alyce M. Sorokie reveals that her undertaking to help others came from her own experience of losing her father to colon cancer. She asks, "Could we learn something from our symptoms?" and answers, "According to the Royal Society of Medicine in Great Britain, in an article titled 'Death Begins in the Colon,' almost every known chronic disease is due directly or indirectly to the influence of more than 36 bacterial poisons that are absorbed from the intestines into our blood streams. It is no wonder that allergies, obesity, acne, constipation and other digestive problems, fatigue, heartburn, gas, joint pain, and skin problems are some of the health problems that may be caused by a toxic intestinal tract. This accumulation of toxins from an imbalance of the flora lining the intestines occurs due to unhealthy eating habits and poor lifestyle choices and as a result, can ultimately manifest a wide array of physical symptoms."[20]

Very often we do not eat the right foods or get enough fiber in our diets. Many of us do not consume enough fruits and vegetables and/or drink enough water. In other words, we neglect some of the necessary components for healthy digestion. If we continue to neglect to treat our digestive system correctly, we can easily develop a sluggish gastrointestinal system, which in turn creates toxic waste build-up. This fecal residue accumulates until it begins to continuously release toxins into the system. None of us are aware of the true amount of toxins with which our bodies are bombarded each day through the polluted air we breathe, the water we drink, and the processed foods that we eat. The human body is incredibly adaptable to this exposure in that the colon, liver, and kidneys naturally function together to purge toxins from the body to keep it healthy. But there comes a point where the magnitude of toxins becomes too large to detoxify. As a result, vital organ functions become adversely affected, increasing our risk to many diseases, including cancer.

This trend for poor digestive health supports the fact that colon cancer (as mentioned earlier) is the second-most common type of cancer, resulting in close to 20% of all cancer deaths in the United States.

Symptoms of intestinal dysfunction due to poor colon health include, but are not limited to, loss of appetite, asthma, backache, bad breath, eczema, fatigue, gingivitis, indigestion, insomnia, nausea, swelling, and weight problems. One of the most commonly seen symptoms is appendicitis, an inflammation in the appendix, which is often due to fecal toxicity.

Colon hydrotherapy is also called colon irrigation, a procedure where close to 20 to 35 gallons of warm water gently flush the colon. Sessions are performed in clean, sanitary settings, generally lasting 45 minutes. Normally, when a session begins, the individual learns what to expect with regard to physical sensations, instrumentation, and the most comfortable position to assume when lying on the table in order to facilitate the gentle insertion of the rectal tube. The colon is then filled and flushed with the warm water. Participants are generally advised to relax as much as possible during the procedure so that a complete and thorough irrigation is possible. Toward the end of the procedure, the rectal tube is gently withdrawn and the individual is provided with instructions on how to relieve any remaining water. Breathing techniques, massage, pressure points, reflexology, and other methods may be introduced by the therapist during the procedure to aid in the removal of any toxic waste that may be present.

The International Association for Colon Hydrotherapy (I-ACT) provides general information about treatment and the type of results one can expect from this procedure.[21] I-ACT promotes the use of FDA-certified equipment and disposable nozzles to ensure public safety. In the U.S., the growing recognition of and demand for colon cleansing has given rise to a number of clinics specializing in this particular field. Colon hydrotherapists assert that the natural treatment by colon hydrotherapy leads to general overall wellness through detoxification.

Traditional Chinese Medicine

Any discussion about CAM would not be complete without a discussion about Traditional Chinese Medicine (TCM) and doctors of Chinese medicine. TCM is a therapeutic intervention based on principles that have evolved over the past 4,000 years. Chinese medicine treats manifested symptoms that result in illness; these are believed to stem from energy imbalances and disharmony in the different systems of the body. Doctors of Traditional Chinese Medicine assess all bodily systems to locate these energy imbalances between the yin and the yang and adjust them accordingly. We have already discussed two fields of TCM: herbal medicine, the use of natural plant compounds specially formulated to treat symptoms, and acupuncture, the use of needles to balance the body's meridians or energy lines. Other techniques of Chinese Medicine include qigong, the ancient method of working and moving energy throughout the body, and tui na, the art of ancient Chinese massage, which focuses on pushing, pulling, and kneading muscle to bring the body into balance. Dietary approaches to balance qi and wellbeing are also part of the TCM toolbox.

Today, TCM is sought for prevention and treatment of many ailments, such as early cardiovascular disease, hypertension, allergies, respiratory problems, gastrointestinal problems, and neurological disorders. People also turn to TCM as a complementary therapy for healing and wellness during cancer treatment.

Reiki

This Japanese technique for stress reduction, relaxation, and healing is known as *Reiki*, a form of therapy administered by the "laying on of hands." Reiki comes from a combination of two Japanese words, *rei* and *ki*. *Rei* means "universal;" *ki*, as mentioned earlier, signifies the "vital life force energy," the basis for all life. Reiki is said to have originated in Tibet thousands of years ago when seers and prophets developed a system based on sounds and symbols to stimulate healing energies. In the early 1900s, when a Japanese educator named Dr. Mikao Usui rediscovered this system, he set about studying the ancient sounds and symbols extensively and chronicled the ancient *sutras*, or precepts. What he discovered was that the sounds and symbols contained inherent energies that could be used to activate healing processes in the body. Calling this healing modality by the name of Reiki, Dr. Usui began to teach the system to a handful of people throughout Japan and the Western world, where its principles were ultimately adopted in the 1970s.

Reiki practitioners believe that when the life force energy is low or blocked we are more likely to get sick; when it is high, we are more capable of being—and staying—healthy. This unblocked, free-flowing energy is considered the spiritually guided life-force energy in all of us. When this energy is transferred from the practitioner—in other words from the person with a strong energy field to the person with a weaker energy field—healing can occur. Reiki is performed by placing one's hands near or on a particular part of the body of the patient. Since the person requiring healing extracts energy from the person giving it, both the giver and receiver play an active role in this transfer. The energy created balances the body and restores the patient's natural capacity to heal. As the name suggests, Reiki allows the life force to harmonize body, mind, and soul. Although Reiki techniques vary from place to place and instructor to instructor and have been modified over time, the four basic original techniques remain as follows: *Byosen Reikan-ho, Hatsurei-ho, Reiki Mawashi*, and *Shuchu Reiki*.

Byosen Reikan-ho is a description of the energy of disease, something that is detected with the hands. *Byo* means "disease," *sen* means "future," *rei* signifies "energy and soul," and *kan* is "emotion and sensation." This technique can be performed on oneself or others and involves sitting or standing at ease by yourself or next to the recipient. First, calm the mind with auto-suggestions. Then place the hands on or above the body, moving them around until a difference in sensation, such as heat, cold, or, in some cases, the absence of any feeling, has been noted. The longer one holds one's hand(s) over affected and/or various areas, the more these sensations tend to increase. This process signifies one cycle, to be completed with a prayer of thanks.

Hatsurei-ho is a technique for enhancing spiritual growth by cleansing and energizing the body. Hatsurei-ho involves meditation with a particular posture and focus on the mind. Prayer, concentration, and visualization are involved in this technique of Reiki, with an added emphasis on breathing methods.

Reiki Mawashi is the traditional method of what is called the "Reiki circle," a process that helps practitioners feel the flow of energy. A group of practitioners holds hands and forms a circle to start the Reiki flowing, first in one direction and then in the other. Reiki energy transfers from person to person, and the group begins to move with the energy expressed.

Shuchu Reiki is another method of group Reiki. *Shuchu* means "focus" or "center." In this technique, a number of practitioners surround the individual and channel their energy to that individual to improve his health and wellbeing.

Distance Reiki. This method incorporates the sending of Reiki energy from a distance. The simple "law of correspondence," or the "law of similarity," is achieved by way of thoughts and concentration and is done by visualizing and stating (mentally or verbally) the name of the recipient. Distance Reiki allows the Reiki to reach the concerned person, who then receives the energy sent.

The benefits of Reiki are numerous and include relaxation, removal of blockages of energy paths, elimination of toxins, and the generation of wellbeing and spiritual contentment. As a result of this energy transfer, many people experience a general sense of improvement throughout the body due to better metabolic function. One often hears people who undergo Reiki therapy say that they experience a feeling of warmth and a sense that an "inner glow" is flowing through them and radiating throughout the body. A true complementary therapy, Reiki treats the body as a whole and can be incorporated into one's daily life in addition to any other concurrent treatment(s). The last 30 years has seen a steady growth in the number of Reiki practitioners, especially since many hospitals and healthcare centers are now integrating Reiki therapy with conventional medicine to aid in healing.

Tai chi

The central philosophy of tai chi is based on what sage Lao Tsu wrote in the *Tao Te Ching*: "Yield and overcome; bend and be straight. He who stands on tiptoe is not steady and he who strides cannot maintain the pace." Embracing these words, tai chi can be said to be a way of merging this dynamic duality of yin and yang. Here in the West tai chi is considered a moving form of yoga combined with meditation.

While accounts of tai chi's history often differ, the most consistently important figure in its past is a Taoist monk in 12th-century China named Chang San-Feng. It is said that Chang observed the movements of the snake and crane and concluded that their movements made them the most able to overcome strong, unyielding opponents. Chang went on to develop a set of exercises that imitated the movements of various animals in order to encourage the individual's ability to adapt to change by blending the soft with the hard, and strength with yielding. Chang's ideas evolved into a system that affirms the fact that smooth, focused, unhurried, gentle, fluid movements benefit the entire body. General health benefits include:

maintenance of good health, stress management, equilibrium, flexibility, and cardiovascular fitness. Individuals complaining of arthritic symptoms express noticeable relief from this particular art as the postures of tai chi gently work muscles and enhance concentration to improve the flow of vital energy through the body.

Different schools, or styles, of tai chi, exist, that have been named after their founders. The main schools in existence today are the Chen, Wu Shi, Hu Lei, Sun, Yang, and Wu styles. In the United States, the Tai Chi Chuan Federation is an umbrella organization dedicated to the promotion of tai chi for health and self-defense. The Federation brings tai chi practitioners together from all over the United States for support and educates qualified tai chi instructors through its certification programs.

Qigong

Along with tai chi, another form of Eastern restoration is the art of qigong. Qigong is the branch of Chinese medicine that involves coordination of various breathing patterns with specific, learned postures and movements to move and distribute energy through the body. We know qi means energy; *gong* means "effort." Simplified, qigong becomes the practice of cultivating energy. The Qigong Association of America explains qigong as "the skill of attracting vital energy with self-healing properties, combining both movement and breathing techniques." The combination of these techniques guides the energy and supports the body's self-healing capabilities.

Both qigong and Reiki encompass what are known as two types of energy fields: *veritable* and *putative*. Veritable energy is energy that can be measured, such as vibration, or sound, electromagnetic force, and magnetism. Putative energy fields, also called "biofields," are frequencies, which thus far we have not been able to reproduce or measure.

Beginners in qigong start with some basic movements combined with a few breathing methods, while advanced participants enter more detailed study involving a greater number of both. The National Qigong Association USA recommends qigong as another form of alternative and complementary therapy,[22] and the division of the National Center for Complementary and Alternative Medicine at the National Institutes of Health lists the complementary and alternative medical practices of qigong and Reiki as viable therapeutic options.[23]

Yoga

In any discussion about health through movement, breathing, and/or meditation, we must also include yoga. The practice of yoga originated in India and is one of the six schools of Hindu philosophy. The word *yoga* itself originates from the Sanskrit word *yuj* meaning "unite" or "join." It signifies the union of the inner soul with the universal soul, said to be the gradual ascent to the divine. Through the use of yoga methods, one can master the mind by slowing thought and restraining the senses. Yoga goes beyond the physical aspect of wellbeing to delve into the inner divine of being, attempting to achieve balance and harmony between mind and body in the same way many other complementary and alternative therapies do. To continue the quest toward self-enlightenment, yoga stresses simple techniques, including breathing exercises, postures, gentle movements, relaxation and meditation.

In the sixth chapter of the Indian sacred scriptures, or Bhagavad Gita, Lord Sri Krishna explains yoga as a method of deliverance of pain and sorrow, saying, "When the mind, intellect, and self are under control from restless desire, through the practice of yoga, one is in communion with God. One finds fulfillment within him and abides in reality. There is nothing greater than this, and one who achieves it cannot be moved by sorrow. From this, we understand that yoga presents us with the ability to control our mind and gain peace within ourselves. With a peaceful inner self, sorrow would not affect us. This is the real meaning of yoga—a deliverance from contact with pain and sorrow."

While yoga techniques have a universal theme, different schools of thought exist relative to its methods. Some concentrate on the alignment of the body, some on breathing techniques and movement, and still others emphasize the fluid flow of movements. While yoga is still yoga, it is a matter of personal preference which technique you prefer. Preference does not imply that one is better than another, but rather that they are simply different in approach and style. There are so many types of yoga that compilation of an exhaustive list would mean listing the same aspects with very little variation, so instead I have chosen to outline a few types with significant distinguishing methodologies below:

Hatha yoga. This method of yoga stresses postures and breathing techniques and is the most commonly practiced form of yoga in the West. Some forms of Hatha yoga focus on the alignment of the body and coordination of breath and movement; some stress holding each posture for a certain duration of time. Breathing techniques play a very important role in all types of yoga, including Hatha yoga.

Anusara yoga. *Anusara* means "following the heart," or "to move as the will moves." This kind of yoga emphasizes the alignment of the outer and inner bodies to induce spiritual awakening.

Ashtanga yoga. Often referred to as "power yoga," this practice combines aerobic and physically strenuous workouts to tone the muscles and discipline the mind. Its main goal is to build strength, stamina, and flexibility, while detoxifying the body.

Ananda yoga is a combination of affirmations and yoga postures with gentle movement and breathing exercises; its goal is to gain inner awareness and strength by moving through various stages of awakening the body's ability to realize changes in its energy level.

Kundalini yoga. *Kundalini* is considered the vital force that lies dormant within all of us. When it is activated by the practice of yoga, one is led toward spiritual awakening and eventual salvation. This type of yoga emphasizes breathing and aims to stimulate rapid energy flow to bring about pure knowledge, joy, and love. Its practice focuses on raising the "coiled" kundalini energy at the base of the spine upwards through various poses, movements, breathing, and meditation.

Kripalu yoga encourages us to understand the wisdom of the body and to work within its limits. The participant begins with postures in accordance with his or her body's capabilities and restrictions and progresses from there. The second stage involves holding particular postures for extended time to develop concentration. The third stage is considered meditation in motion, and allows for sequential and spontaneous posturing.

Sivananda yoga involves gentle techniques that combine chanting, meditation, and deep relaxation. This style of yoga encourages a healthy lifestyle, vegetarianism, and positive thinking.

Viniyoga. Viniyoga is a form of yoga that requires an understanding of a person's present condition, personal potential, appropriate goals, and the means available to expedite those goals. This type of yoga is often recommended for beginners due to its individualized methods of practice.

Bikram yoga is performed in a room set at a high temperature, where the participants sweat while performing a series of 26 *asanas* (various bodily positions assumed in yogic exercise) to warm the body and stretch the muscles, ligaments, and tendons.

Iyengar yoga focuses in great detail on posture alignment and precise movements of the arms and legs in order to achieve better concentration. It incorporates over 200 classical yoga *asanas* and 14 different types of *pranayamas* with variations.

Yoga has been shown to have numerous benefits. I have personally found that its practice helps to cultivate a mind, intellect, and body free from restlessness, and that this freedom helps bring about peace and fulfillment. Most commonly, participants experience an increase in flexibility through the stretching of muscles and joints, but practicing yoga can also help those who are working through times of fear and sorrow achieve fulfillment. Yoga has been found to strengthen the immune system, offer total detoxification of the body, and stimulate the vital organs. Furthermore, through both breathing and postures, yoga has been shown to reduce heart rate and lower blood pressure. Many who practice yoga find they have a remarkably renewed zest for life as the aging process slows and energy levels are enhanced. For patients undergoing treatment for major illnesses and who may suffer from a sense of disorganization due to ongoing fatigue, yoga can also be an excellent way to begin the reintegration process.

Cancer patients often feel isolated and disillusioned during and even after treatment. Practicing yoga can help us regain our "center," that part of the self that may get lost in the process of curing our physical state of disease. Experiencing this sense of reintegration through the various postures of yoga helps us regain strength and flexibility of both body and mind, and supports the body's capacity for self-healing.

Yoga is by no means a cure for cancer or any other major illness, but it *can* provide relief from the side effects of treatment and can go a long way toward helping us achieve long-lasting health on all levels. Since yoga supports the building of resilience and faith, it can help us develop our inner resources so that we are better able to deal with the changes in our lives and help us see these changes as opportunities for growth. The diagnosis of any life-threatening disease typically sets off a chain reaction of feelings, including shock, denial, anger, fear, guilt, loneliness, depression, despair, and helplessness. Yoga can help us to manage the anxiety, stress, and pain, while at the same time empower us to continue to move in a direction that supports our health.

Herbs

My quest for knowledge soon led me to the world of herbs, where I found no shortage of advertisements, promotional materials, and testimonials praising their exceptional healing power. After doing my own research, I came to the conclusion that herbs indeed contain compounds that can be preventative, restorative, and healing. The word *herb* is derived from the Latin word *herba*, meaning "grass." The definition of the word *herb* is "a plant lacking a permanent woody stem."

Herbs have a variety of uses. Some have medicinal properties and some are aromatic, while others are used for flavor and cooking. Some herbs are even used as pesticides. According to one legend, herbs were said to be "the friend of physicians and the praise of cooks." Chinese history reveals the utilization of herbs for more than 5,000 years for increasing longevity, but it wasn't until the 8th century that the medicinal value of herbs gained acceptance. Since then, we have learned that herbs are safe and beneficial to the body, with relatively few—if any—side effects. Even the Bible has been said to proclaim the health benefits of herbs, as follows: "Their fruit will be for food, and their leaves for medicine." Texts of the ancient Egyptian civilization also contain references to hundreds of herbal remedies, and Hippocrates, the first to practice medicine as an art, teaches us that the power of the cure rests "with nature."

Relative to herbs, our forefathers were way ahead of their time. Many of the remedies used by our grandmothers and great-grandmothers, for example, having been proven effective, are now cast in pharmaceutical form. Millions recognize that nature's herbs are inexpensive and safe and that a main advantage of treating with herbs is their ability to facilitate improvement with the least disruption in the body's natural balance.

In 1933, the Herb Society of America[24] was founded for the purpose of furthering the knowledge and use of herbs by the general public. This organization is "concerned with the cultivation of herbs and with the study of their history and with their role, both past and present, as flavoring agents; as medicinal, fragrant and dye plants; as ornamentals in garden design; as household aids, and as economic plants supplying products for modern industry." Today, the Herb Society continues to broaden its understanding of herbs to meet the challenges associated with a high public interest in herbal information.

If you choose to consider incorporating herbs into your health regimen based on recommendations of friends, family, or health provider, it is advisable to become educated about their properties so you can make informed decisions about their use. Besides accessing information from organizations like the Herb Society, numerous books provide in-depth descriptions of herbs and their uses. Joerg Gruenwald's *PDR for Herbal Medicine*, for example, is written on the template of the original *Physician's Desk Reference*, the yearly publication that compiles manufacturer information pertaining to all prescription drugs currently on the market.[25] The *PDR for Herbal Medicine* also provides comprehensive information, in this case on herb identification, indications, homeopathic indications, side effects, drug/herb interactions, safety, and more.[26]

Herbs are receiving more and more scientific attention of late. A scientific review published in *The Lancet*, for example, has reported that echinacea, a North American flower, can be widely used to reduce the frequency and duration of the common cold. In this study, conducted at the University of Connecticut School of Pharmacy, researchers found that the odds of developing the common cold was reduced 58% by taking supplemental echinacea.[27] Although echinacea is only one among many plants used in hundreds of different health-related products, and there are an estimated 250,000 to 500,000 plants existing on Earth today, only about 6% have been extensively studied for their medicinal properties to date.

A number of anticancer drugs have been developed based on plants as well. Tamoxifen, used for breast cancer treatment, is a product of the yew tree. Vinca alkaloids, anti-cancer medications that inhibit cancer cell growth by stopping cell division, are used to treat childhood leukemia and Hodgkin's disease, and are derived from a variety of periwinkle. Another herb, commonly known in the English language as "foxgloves" and traditionally belonging to the figwort family, is the basis for the drug Digitalis. This pharmacologically active compound is extracted in its pure form to be manufactured as digitoxin, and used for the treatment of heart conditions.

Herbs are generally not known to have side effects, but it is always advisable to consult your doctor to make sure any herb you consider taking is not contraindicated with any medication you may also be taking. For example, hawthorn is known to lower blood pressure and should not be taken with prescription blood pressure medication, as the combination may lower blood pressure too much, and ginkgo biloba, if taken with some diabetic medications, has been found to alter blood levels of medication and directly affect the blood-sugar regulating system of the body.

Herbal teas are commonly consumed for their medicinal properties as well. Herbal "teas" are significantly different from what we might call "regular" teas. Regular tea is derived from the leaves of the *camellia sinensis* bush, also called the tea plant. As mentioned earlier in this book, the leaves are plucked, usually by hand, and then processed to form black tea, oolong tea, green tea, or white tea. Herbal "infusions," on the other hand, do not come from any part of the *camellia sinensis* plant. Instead, they contain extracts of the flowers, leaves, roots, and stems of herbs known for their healthful value and therapeutic qualities. The "tea," or tea bag containing the mixture, is prepared in a prescribed combination to soothe a particular ailment or eliminate a particular problem. There are herbal teas for detoxifying, calming, dieting, and stimulation. You name it, there is an herbal tea for it, whether for settling digestive systems or calming the nerves. Greek Mountain Tea, a popular warm-climate tea in Greece, for example, helps prevent and provide relief from colds, and the *boldo* herb is used in South America to calm upset stomachs and treat liver disease, internal parasites, worms, and malaria.

Chinese medicine attributes benefits of all aromas and flavors to some organ system of the body. The sweet flavor of anise seed, for example, helps the stomach and spleen, while the bitter flavor of dandelion root affects the heart and small intestines. Chamomile, a member of the daisy family, is known to relieve anxiety, hyperactivity, insomnia, and stress, and to help in cases of nausea, colic, flatulence, and irritable bowel. Raspberry leaf, a member of the rose family rich in minerals like calcium, magnesium, and iron, helps in soothing diarrhea, intestinal inflammation, and mouth and throat irritations, and has been found to aid in pregnancy and delivery. Ginger root has been shown to aid circulation and provide relief in cases of colds and lung congestion, and even motion sickness.

Initially popular in China, the science of using plants for medicine dates back to the beginnings of Ayurveda in India. Today, the World Health Organization estimates that 65% of the world's population incorporates the use of plants into the various traditional healthcare systems in some form or another. This use of plants for medicine by humans is called *ethnomedicine*. Research has identified 122 compounds, obtained from only 94 species of plants that are found to be used globally in the form of drugs. It has been discovered that prior to their use as drugs, 80% of these compounds were being used for the same, or similar, ethnomedical purposes. Researchers state, "Because these compounds are derived from only 94 species of plants, and a conservative estimate of the number of flowering plants occurring on the planet is 250,000, there should be an abundance of drugs remaining to be discovered in these plants."[28] For this reason, many different schools of health are now teaching the benefits of herbology as part of their curriculum on alternative therapies.

Homeopathy

Homeopathy is also known as *homeopathic medicine*, a medical system practiced in the United States since the early 19th century. The word "homeopathy" was first used by German physician Christian Friedrich Samuel Hahnemann (1755–1843), considered the founder of this branch of medicine in the United States. The term is a derivation from two Greek words: *homoios*, meaning "similar," and *pathos,* meaning "suffering." In Hahneman's words, "The physician's highest calling, his only calling, is to make sick people healthy, to heal, as it is termed." According to Hahnemann, the principal tenet of homeopathic treatment is that the cause of disease is due to a disturbance of the spiritual, vital force that exists in all of us, and that manifests as specific symptoms. Correcting this underlying disturbance is said to be the only way to cure both the symptoms and the disease. Hahnemann expressed the principle of homeopathy through the Latin phrase *Similia similibus curentur*, which translates to "let likes cure likes," and his system has been successfully utilized for more than two centuries.

Hahnemann's theory that if a particular substance caused symptoms of disease in a healthy person, then small doses of that same substance should be able to cure similar symptoms in a sick person, is based on his work with quinine. Quinine is an alkaloid derived from cinchona bark. Until World War I quinine was the only effective means for the treatment of malaria and its positive effect on fever was well known in Hahnemann's time. Hahnemann tested his theory and described what happened when he consumed two points of a knife of "good cinchona" twice a day: "First the feet, then the tips of my fingers etc. became cold, then my heart started beating, the pulse heavy and fast; then I was possessed by an infinite anxiety, a trembling (but without shiverings of cold), a weakening of all limbs, then beating in the head, reddening cheeks, thirst—in short, all the symptoms of relapsing fever presented themselves successively…." During this experiment on himself, Hahnemann drew the conclusion that quinine was able to cure malaria because it could cause the same symptoms as malaria in healthy people. This is the basic principle of homeopathy.

Homeopathic medicines are made from plants, such as dandelion, plantain, and aconite; from minerals, such as arsenic oxide, iron phosphate, and sodium chloride; and even from animals, such as the venom of poisonous snakes or the ink of the cuttlefish. Homeopathic medicines are made by a process that consists of a series of dilutions and successions, which create potentization. *Succession* is the process of shaking the liquid vigorously to enhance dilution, making the substance fainter, until there is no physical trace of it left. *Potentization* is believed to occur when energy is channeled from the original substance into the final, diluted remedy. In homeopathy, it is believed that the original substance leaves a kind of energy imprint that facilitates the body's ability to heal itself.

Homeopathy arrived in the United States in 1825 with European physicians. By the beginning of the 1900s the U.S. had as many as 22 homeopathic medical colleges and one out of every five doctors was practicing homeopathy. However, by 1910 only 15 colleges remained due to the pull toward the medical model of treating illness, and by the late 1940s homeopathy had lost much of its following. However, the American Foundation for Homeopathy began offering the subject of homeopathy as a post-graduate course for doctors in 1922, and courses on homeopathy continue to be offered by the National Center for Homeopathy today. In the United Kingdom, homeopathy has been available from the National Health Services since its inception in 1948.

Homeopathy is considered extremely cost-effective, especially because it rarely causes adverse reactions, and is readily available to everyone. Laws about the practice of homeopathy vary from state to state, but its practice generally requires licensure and the Food and Drug Administration regulates the production and sale of all homeopathic remedies sold over the counter. In a 2007 National Health Interview Survey done by the National Center for Complementary and Alternative Medicine, an estimated 3.9 million U.S. adults and approximately 900,000 children used some form of homeopathy the previous year of 2006.[29]

Psychotherapy

Psychotherapy is an intentional interpersonal relationship between trained psychotherapists and individuals or groups undertaken to aid in challenges of daily living. It is a behavioral science that involves direct and open interaction with a psychotherapist with the goal of initiating new levels of personal freedom by helping the individual(s) involved gain awareness of the underlying source of current concerns. With the therapist's help, individuals assess how beliefs, attitudes, and past circumstances are influencing their present life, with a goal toward identifying areas in need of change and carrying out appropriate modifications. Many psychotherapists consider themselves instruments in the healing process, understanding that heightened self-awareness leads to the ability to help oneself. Psychotherapy in the United States is performed by a variety of different practitioners, such as licensed clinical social workers, family and marriage therapists, counselors, psychiatrists, and psychologists.

History shows that psychotherapy began in Vienna in the 1880s. During this time, Dr. Sigmund Freud, a trained neurologist, explored mental and physical ailments with the use of what he called "psychoanalytic techniques." These methods incorporated free association, understanding, insight, and the exploration of emotion and fantasy. Freud's work forms the basis for many of the psychoanalytic methods still used today, where thoughts, feelings, ideas, dreams, and emotions of the patient are explored through interpersonal dialogue between the therapist and the individual.

For those undergoing cancer treatment, psychotherapists often act in a combined role of analyst, philosopher, and teacher by providing insight into the choices available. They might also assist in dealing with reactions of fear, anxiety, loneliness, or depression. Broadening one's individual outlook and thought processes is often key to finding increased acceptance of the situation at hand; this means that instead of an ongoing focus on the negativity surrounding an illness like cancer, the individual has a chance to experience feelings of general contentment. As Freud once said, "Look into the depths of your own soul and learn first to know yourself, then you will understand why this illness was bound to come upon you, and perhaps, henceforth, to avoid falling ill." Psychotherapy has long been considered a credible means of expression for working through issues and resolving emotional upheaval, whether from medical or non-medical causes, and cultivating a greater sense of self for the long term.

Biofeedback

Biofeedback is a technique where the individual is trained to control internal bodily processes that normally occur involuntarily to achieve greater health and wellbeing. Biofeedback has been found effective in reducing stress and anxiety, controlling blood pressure and heart rate, mitigating sleep disorders, managing chronic pain, alleviating muscle tension, and affecting skin temperature changes. The four most commonly used measurements of biofeedback are: electromyography (EMG), measuring muscle tension; electrocardiograph (ECG), measuring heart rate; galvanic skin response (GSR), measuring skin temperature; and neurofeedback (EEG), measuring brain wave activity. In a typical biofeedback session, electrodes are attached to the individual's skin. These electrodes feed information into monitoring devices that translate the physiological responses into a tone that varies in pitch, a visual meter that varies in brightness, or a computer screen that shows lines moving across a grid. The biofeedback therapist then leads the individual through appropriate mental exercises. From this feedback, the individual learns which areas could benefit from modification.

The Association for Applied Psychophysiology and Biofeedback (AAPB) is the national association for professionals who treat with the method of biofeedback.[30] The AAPB website is a good place to find qualified practitioners in your area. Practitioners range from nurses to physicians and dentists. Biofeedback is considered a safe procedure that has the ability to improve quality of life through a better understanding of an individual's unique physiology.

Summary

The health practices read about in this chapter constitute an overview of the many offerings available to everyone under the CAM umbrella. Homeopathy, TCM, Ayurveda, and naturopathic medicine constitute one group of the holistic arts. The second group, mind-body medicine, includes yoga, psychotherapy, and biofeedback. The third includes the biologically-based practices, such as herbology, supplementation, and dietary management. Manipulative and body-based practices founded on structure and function comprise the fourth category and include chiropractic, osteopathy, physical therapy, and massage. The last group, the category of energy medicine, encompasses practices like Reiki and qigong. There is no doubt in my mind that disease and death could be significantly reduced with the combined efforts of Western medicine and the various CAM modalities working together to facilitate health and encourage better lifestyle choices.

One ongoing collaborative effort in assessing disease control priorities is the Disease Control Priorities Project. This organization produces evidence-based analysis and resource materials to assist health policy decisions in developing countries with the ultimate goal of improving their health systems and, ultimately, the health of the populations.[31] The Disease Control Priorities Project has identified 19 selected risk factors that increase the chances of developing a disease or disability. These risk factors are associated with millions of deaths each year and include smoking, high blood pressure, high cholesterol, physical inactivity, overweight and obesity, alcohol use, and a low intake of fruits and vegetables. Researchers on this project state that, "Globally, an estimated 45 percent of mortality and 36 percent of the burden of disease were attributable to the joint effects of 19 selected risk factors." From what we now know about CAM interventions, it is easy to see that CAM practices can offer significantly sound support in reducing many of the risk factors that now comprise affliction on a global scale.

The World Health Organization states that Complementary and Alternative Medicine is viewed as "traditional" medicine in many countries and, as such, is considered an integral part of their health systems.[32] *Traditional medicine* is defined by the World Health Organization as "the sum total of knowledge, skills, and practices based on the theories, beliefs, and experiences indigenous to different cultures that are used to maintain health, as well as to prevent, diagnose, improve or treat physical and mental illnesses."[33] In Africa, for example, 80% of the population uses traditional medicine for primary healthcare; in Australia the number is 49%. In China, traditional medicine accounts for 30 to 50% of total healthcare practice, and is fully integrated into the greater healthcare system, where a full 95% of Chinese hospitals incorporate traditional medicine (TM) units. In India, traditional medicine is widely used in its 2,869 hospitals. In Indonesia, 40% of the total population and 70% of the more rural population uses traditional medicine. In Japan, 72% of physicians practice some form of traditional medicine. In Thailand, traditional medicine is fully integrated into its 1,120 health centers as it is in Vietnam, where the healthcare system serves 30% of the population.

Unfortunately, here in the West, CAM and Traditional Medicine has not yet been fully integrated into our healthcare system the way it has in these other countries.[34] As a result, many cancer patients are looking outside the system for help. One recent study, for example, has shown that herbs, vitamins, dietary supplements, and other biochemical products are among the most popular complementary and alternative medicine therapies currently used by pediatric oncology patients.[35] While the researchers of this study stated that more investigation needed to be done with regard to the safety and effectiveness of products and services like these, they also acknowledged that complementary therapies had potential in their role as useful agents in the treatment of pediatric oncology. Furthermore, as conventional medical costs continue to rise, it is important to note that ongoing studies continue to show that CAM therapies are cost-effective modalities of good value.[36]

Admittedly, progress continues to be made, as evidenced by the opening of the National Center for Complementary and Alternative Medicine at the National Institutes of Health in 1998. This significant step was taken due to the growing interest for and utilization of many complementary and alternative medicine methods. Because experience and research have proven that CAM methods provide relief, promote health, are more cost-effective, have so few side effects, and can be instituted alongside any conventional medical treatment, it is not surprising that they have engendered both recognition and trust from much of the general population. I believe, along with many other doctors, that when both supportive care and conventional medical treatment come together, only good manifests, and that the collaboration can only make our healthcare system better. It is like tipping one burning candle to light another—the process doesn't take anything away from the first candle; instead the flame brightens from the joining of the two.

In the late 1970s the concept of holism, specifically CAM, was virtually unknown and unexplored, and the topic was a sensitive one to broach whether in casual conversation or the written word. However, as I researched on my own, learned on my own, and adapted certain CAM therapies into my own life over time, I knew they were vital pieces to an even bigger health puzzle. Health is never based on just one single, solitary factor. It is a culmination of many factors, each having its own unique formula in the health equation. This is probably why more and more people are learning and incorporating holistic healing into their lives.

In recent years CAM therapies have grown by leaps and bounds. Universities are teaching various CAM therapies and the number of professionals qualifying to practice each year is in the thousands. More than one third of the medical schools in the United States now offer courses on CAM, and universities, such as Harvard, Duke, Stanford, and Columbia offer formal programs in mind-body and integrative medicine. Hippocrates' statement, "Cure sometimes, heal often, and support always," is the basis for all CAM practices, which hope to soon see a healthcare system that adopts preventive integrative therapies along with its support for conventional therapies.

In the words of Andrew Weil, M.D., from his book *Health and Healing: The Philosophy of Integrative Medicine and Optimum Health:* "Treatment originates outside you; healing comes from within."[37]

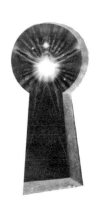

7. Social Wellbeing

"Interdependence is and ought to be as much the ideal of man as self-sufficiency. Man is a social being."

- Mahatma Gandhi

On thriving

nyone who has ever been diagnosed with cancer knows the feeling of separateness and isolation that can occur; it's the feeling of not really fitting in with anyone or anything. Some might experience the feeling daily, others only occasionally. In my case, I was plagued with a feeling of remoteness for over five years before I finally decided to do something about it. One day when I had had all I could take of feeling so disconnected, I decided to pick myself up and go to the bookstore. I didn't really know why I wanted to go; all I knew was that something inside me was telling me to go. When I got there I spotted one of those big club chairs and sat down. Sitting with my arms extended in front of me and my hands on the armrests, I looked around and watched all the people standing in front of bookshelves, quietly thumbing through books. Feeling restless and uncomfortable in my own skin, I knew I had to try something—anything—to make myself feel better. So I got up and began emulating others who were rummaging through books on the shelves for something to read. After picking up and putting back about a dozen books from art to zoology, I still hadn't found anything that appealed to me. Frustrated, I worked my way along the long wall of shelving, continuing to pick up a book here and there. I finally wound up in the self-help section. (Since that day this section continues to be one of my favorites in any book store because I always find that no matter what I'm feeling, I can find something about it on those shelves.) On this particular day, I took down a book and randomly thumbed through the pages. That's when this statement jumped out at me: "The *I* in illness is isolation and the crucial letters in wellness are *we*."[1]

It was at that moment that it dawned on me that I was part of something bigger than myself. That I was part of a collective "we."

Human beings do not fully thrive when isolated from others, and therefore there is much to be gained from one another as members of the biggest race of all—the human race. Not only do we share the common thread of humanity, one mind with access to immeasurable resources, but we are also part of a collective social system in which we can join hands and try to find the meaning in life's boundless questions. It was when I recognized that I was a part of something bigger than myself that I made up my mind to take whatever steps I needed to take to improve the quality of my life. I realized that it would not be possible for me to solve all my life's problems alone; I would need to willingly extend my hand to gain the helping hand of others. When I was sick I had known automatically that I could not cure my illness alone. I knew how much I needed help from others; after all, it was their expertise, kindness, and compassion that saved my life so that I could go on to have a full life. Now, in the same way, it became just as obvious that it was up to me to reach out if I wanted to change my life for the better.

I have come to understand that there are many factors that influence wellbeing—things like access to money, goods, and services and creativity, freedom, health, and education—and that they all affect our mind-sets and how we look at life. In philosophy, the term *wellbeing* is used to express something that is good for the individual, but nowadays it is primarily used as an expression to indicate general good health. Aristotle, the Greek philosopher, once said, "If you are my friend, then my wellbeing is closely bound with yours." This statement refers to the fact that being allies and joining hands is an integral part of each and every person's overall wellbeing. Rudolph Steiner, the Austrian philosopher, literary scholar, artist, and social thinker once said, "A healthy social life is found only when in the mirror of each soul the whole community finds its reflection, and when in the whole community the virtue of each one is living." This reflects the fact that human nature is the sum total of both the social and more personal, or individual, parts.

Having this awareness of the braiding of the two is critical to understanding the need for both individual and social wellbeing. Robert Frost wrote, "To be social is to be forgiving." I believe this means that it is time to let go of whatever individual grudges we may have toward any individual or group and to develop the forgiving part of our natures. When we do this we can engage in all the good society has to offer us—and what we as individuals have to offer society as well. Eventually, there comes a time when we need to simply bury the hatchet. To let go of the past and to forgive, while extremely difficult at times, is an important element in the healing process for each of us.

On "wellbeing"

There are also a number of other definitions of "wellbeing." Economists, for example, define it as the individual's "quality of life." The *Random House Dictionary* defines it as "a state of health, happiness, and prosperity." The World Health Organization defines wellbeing in terms of health, where health is "a complete state of physical, mental, and social wellbeing and not purely the absence of disease or infirmity." All three definitions are a reminder that it is the inalienable right for each of us to have a healthy quality of life and to experience wellbeing throughout our lives.

If I were to ask any number of people what "social wellbeing" means, the answers would certainly differ from person to person. That's because perspectives naturally vary based on ideas, beliefs, and experiences. Some say wellbeing is being healthy. Others say it is having social, spiritual, mental, and physical components in balance. There are some who feel that it is a broader composition of factors, such as feeling a sense of belonging in an environment, and in terms of employment, demographics, and community. No matter what the definition might be, however, there is a collective consensus that the larger concept of social wellbeing is manifested in some way, shape, or form in all of our lives. It is a clear cooperative understanding that in acting as a whole we share an absolute united and impenetrable strength. It takes a compassionate community to create and expand on this ideal, not only by providing opportunity for all in areas of health, education, safety, security, and employment, but by offering a peaceful existence as well.

The idea of including a discussion about social wellbeing in this book strengthened as I talked to people at meetings organized by my office, Cancer Care, and the American Cancer Society. I already knew from my own experience that recovering from a major illness like cancer was generally a lonely and lengthy process. But what I realized as I spoke to these groups was that for those of us who have undergone treatment, socialization was even more critical because we need contact with others to regain our sense of self, of who we are, and of how we fit into the world. In fact, socialization influences every aspect of our health, our work, our life at home, and our leisure time.

Social wellbeing begins with making a personal choice to get involved, choosing a direction, and taking on a sense of social responsibility with optimism. It means making an attempt to create new relationships and embracing existing ones. This choice is born from the desire to be a part of the social fabric that clothes and supports our daily lives. How do we begin to feel a sense of social wellbeing? There are two ways. The first is through something called *concentrated group settings*. These are settings where we interact with other people through a shared medical interest, such as joining a support group or cancer discussion. The other way is through *coordinated leisure settings*, where we join a group to share the same experience, like going to a concert, lecture, art or music class, going to the movies or the mall, or attending a sporting event—in other words, participating in social events in a leisurely, nonmedical setting. In both kinds of settings, age and gender are non-factors. For most people, just being in the presence of others in a social setting is enough to supply a much-needed energy boost. Regardless of the types of choices you make as you live your life, whether you choose to be a part of concentrated or coordinated groups—or both—there is no doubt that you will feel yourself enhanced relative to health, functional abilities, feelings of independence, overall positive changes in lifestyle, and, of course, wellbeing.

Social wellbeing and social work professionals

There are a number of professions that contribute to the social wellbeing of both individuals and society at large, including social work, therapeutic recreational therapy, and home health care. The people who serve in these professions work in conjunction with physicians and other healthcare providers to assist those of us who need help living a better quality life.

Social workers are healthcare professionals concerned with social problems, their causes, and their impact on society as a whole. In the early 20th century two evolving factions were attempting to define the true nature of social work. The first was led by Mary Richmond, who developed teaching materials for charity organizations and societies nationwide. Richmond became director of the Russell Sage Foundation's Charity Organization Department in New York City and was a serious advocate for the establishment of professional schools for the study of casework, and for the need for the creation of formalized social work education. Jane Addams, one of the first women to receive the Nobel Peace Prize in 1931, led the second faction attempting to define the parameters of "social work." Although she did not consider herself a social worker, per se, Addams was a strong advocate for children's and women's rights. Her pursuit of a higher social and civic life for women and children led her to found Hull House, a center dedicated to instituting and maintaining educational and philanthropic enterprises and investigating and improving the condition of the industrial districts of Chicago. To celebrate Addams' achievements, the state of Illinois has named December 10 as Jane Addams Day. The organizations started by Richmond and Addams both advocated for the betterment of men, women, and children of all ages and ethnicities, and their debate over whether social work should be considered a profession continued to be deliberated for many years. Social work as we know it today did not come of age until later in the 20th century, but has the same roots in philanthropy, social reform, charity, and compassion toward others in times of need.

The National Association of Social Workers defines professional social workers as those who "assist individuals, groups, or communities to restore or enhance their capacity for social functioning, while creating societal conditions favorable to their goals." As trained professionals, "social workers help people overcome some of life's most difficult challenges: poverty, discrimination, abuse, addiction, physical illness, divorce, loss, unemployment, educational problems, disability, and mental illness. They help prevent crises and counsel individuals, families, and communities to cope more effectively with the stresses of everyday life."[2] The social worker is defined as "a professionally qualified person employed in the administration of social service, charity, welfare, and poverty agencies." The social workers of today often act as a link between community health agencies and the government to advance the social conditions of the disadvantaged of entire communities by providing services of psychological counseling, guidance, assistance, and support in various forms.

Social workers help people function, help them solve individual and family problems or conflicts, and offer support for ongoing physical and mental health. They help in cases of inadequate housing, unemployment, disability, or even substance abuse. There are social workers working in schools, institutions, hospitals, community centers, and in many rehabilitation centers. There are those who work with children in foster care, in fund-raising, in the production of educational materials, and in counseling services. In hospitals and other medical institutions, social workers offer educational services to patients and their families regarding both the facts around disease and the effects of treatment related to disease.

Social work is currently the largest and most important social service profession in the United States, and encompasses an extensive spectrum of services. A report published by the U.S. Department of Labor reveals that in 2008 there were 642,000 jobs held by social workers in this country, most of them in the healthcare and social assistance industries. This report categorizes the number of social workers employed in various capacities as follows:[3]

- child, family, and school social workers 292,600
- medical and public health social workers 138,700
- mental health/substance abuse social workers 137,300
- all other social workers 73,400

Individuals who have been treated for cancer or who are concerned about cancer sometimes take on a role not unlike the role of social worker, where they become "patient advocates." Today National University, the second-largest, private, nonprofit institution of higher learning in California, has developed a graduate certificate in this new field of patient advocacy. This program defines "patient advocates" as those who "work to protect and enhance patients' rights and become agents of change in the healthcare system." The National Cancer Institute's Specialized Programs of Research Excellence (SPORE) also reflects this approach of advocacy. SPORE does this by means of providing grants that promote interdisciplinary research, and by connecting basic research findings to clinical settings which involve both cancer patients and populations at risk for cancer.[4] SPORE investigators are multidisciplinary teams, including social workers, that work in collaboration with patient advocates to plan, design, and implement research programs that may impact cancer prevention, detection, diagnosis, and treatment. Working closely with patient advocates allows the teams to coordinate the sometimes difficult interactions between patients, doctors, researchers, and institutions. Today it is quite common to see members of the cancer-conscious public asked to join in these discussions to bring a first hand community perspective to the healthcare debate. One such setting occurs when individuals offer to willingly put themselves at risk by participating in clinical trials in order to help find a cure for cancer—in essence, courageously agreeing to be part of an experiment so they might one day be integral in the solution. In these situations, social workers play an active role in establishing the bridge between research and human testing.

The American Cancer Society's National Cancer Information Center (NCIC) is a nationwide 1-800 help line. This phone line is open 24 hours a day, seven days a week to answer calls and emails from anyone with questions about cancer, including cancer patients, family members, and friends.[5] Cancer-information professionals who answer calls are required to have a college degree or equivalent and many are professionally trained social workers who are highly educated in cancer resources. As part of the NCIC team, these warm, sensitive, and service-oriented individuals are considered reputable and dependable in their goal of meeting the needs of individuals and their families who are dealing with cancer. Because the responsibilities of social work intervention are so varied, including, but not limited to the behavioral, social, and support methodologies related to all facets of cancer and its treatment, social work as a profession has become highly recognized in the field. Really, there is no other profession like it—in depth or breadth. As the Association of Oncology Social Workers (AOSW) in 2001 states, the role of social work is to "advance excellence in psychosocial care of persons with cancer, their families, and caregivers through networking, education, advocacy, research, and research development."[6] Currently more than a thousand members of AOSW from around the world are doing their best to provide the best in psychosocial cancer care.

Networking facilities

The concept of networking has transcended into medical facilities throughout the country to provide total health service management under one roof. One of these facilities is the Comprehensive Cancer Center at the University of Michigan. As the name suggests, the Comprehensive Cancer Center provides collaborative, integrated care in one facility, where health professionals from all specialties and researchers in the areas of both basic and clinical science share a building with the patients. This facility offers comprehensive diagnostic treatment, and support services to cancer patients in an environment that reflects their mission: "The conquest of cancer through innovation and collaboration." Along with conventional oncology treatment, this center also provides nutrition counseling, art therapy, social work, psycho-oncology support, and various complementary therapy programs.

One complementary opportunity provided to cancer patients at the Comprehensive Cancer Center is the Voices Art Gallery.[7] The Voices Art Gallery was established in 1999 to offer those living with cancer an opportunity to share their stories through art. By recognizing the influence of art in the healing process and displaying artwork created by people undergoing treatment, the Cancer Center encourages, supports, and guides those diagnosed with the disease and the people close to them. It is my opinion that this center's collaborative methodology is ground breaking and that their initiative will be the cornerstone of cancer care in the future.

Many Voices of Cincinnati, Ohio is another organization that has been a forum for thousands since 1989.[8] Many Voices was created to aid people with Dissociative Disorder, a condition found in people suffering from physical, sexual, or emotional trauma, and uses art as one medium for "reconnecting" and facilitating the process of healing. This organization's philosophy states, "Though our past lives may be troubled, our present lives can be improved, and our futures can be transformed."

Integrated efforts in healing continue to grow in the United States and throughout the world. One of the simplest ways to renew one's sense of self is through social support networks, a natural expression of the ways people come together. This has been proven true for many individuals, including the 98 women with early stage and regionally advanced gynecologic cancers who participated in a study in 2000. When investigators followed the women in this study during their first year of cancer treatment to assess mood, quality of life, and coping strategies, two significant results were noted: not only did those women who sought greater social support develop higher levels of social wellbeing, but they showed improved doctor-patient relationships as well.[9]

In another study at Stanford University's School of Medicine, quality social support was shown to have a direct improvement on mental wellbeing in women with metastatic breast cancer. This result was found to be associated with lower cortisol concentrations; since decreased cortisol indicates healthier neuroendocrine functioning,[10] researchers believe overall outlook on life can indeed affect and be affected by the body's responses.

The opposite has also been found to be true, where having a poor social network can impact survival. In the Nurses' Health Study, for example, an elevated risk of mortality was found among the breast cancer survivors who were socially isolated. This study followed 2,835 women diagnosed with stage 1 to 4 breast cancer between 1992 and 2002, assessing levels of isolation specifically related to a lack of close friends, relatives, and adult children.

This research further reported that those women who tended to be poorly socially integrated prior to their breast cancer diagnosis also had a 66% higher risk of mortality from any cause, and a two-fold increased risk of mortality from breast cancer.[11]

In the book, *Psycho-Oncology*, coauthor Jimmie C. Holland states that social support provides three important elements to support health.[12] The first is element is "cognitive." This means the individual has access to information and feels good about the social support she receives through the social network in place. This kind of social support helps the individual feel positively about herself, to have positive expectations about the future, and to feel confident about her ability to exercise personal control. The second element supporting health, Holland says, is "affective benefits," or increased positive emotions and reduced negative emotions. The third element, "behavioral benefits," is revealed through decreased risk behaviors, increased behaviors that promote health, and the seeking-out of appropriate treatment for symptoms. It is Holland's belief that "the cognitive, affective, and behavioral benefits (which are likely to be interconnected) of social ties and social support [can] impact cancer incidence, mortality, and survival by altering biological pathways. Biological pathways include cardiovascular, neuroendocrine, and immune function, [and] research has linked social support to better functioning in all three domains." American poet Maya Angelou agrees. "I've learned that every day you should reach out and touch someone," she says. "People love a warm hug, or just a friendly pat on the back."

The profound relevance and impact of social support networks also makes them powerful safeguards against the tendency to experience low levels of optimism when confronted with cancer and its treatment. "Low optimism," a not atypical perspective for those who find themselves in this kind of situation, can be viewed as a generalized belief and expectation that negative outcomes are more likely than positive ones. Supporting this theory is a study of 77 African American women who were being treated for non-metastatic breast cancer and assessed based on their levels of social interaction. Researchers in this case found that those women with high levels of social support were shown to experience improvement in their coping skills, a mechanism which acted as a cushion in their defense against feelings of low optimism relative to treatment.[13]

Social "not so wellbeing"

While collaborative social consciousness has been shown to help patients in many studies like these, individuals who have or have had cancer know that cancer takes a toll on one's social surroundings. So, here I would like to explore the social "not-so-wellbeing" side of cancer.

We know that before we had cancer things were different. That's why it is extremely common to feel that before we had cancer we also had *something*—whether that was a routine, a day-to-day familiarity, or simply a sort of regularity to our lives. Many of us woke up, ate breakfast, went to work, came home, and got ready for bed...only to do the same thing again the next day. This was our life, whether good, bad, boring, mundane, or exciting in its execution. This was the normal, everyday life to which we had become accustomed. Then, one day, cancer came. Suddenly everything we knew to be real, ordinary, and habitual was gone.

Getting that feeling back where we have an expectation of normalcy may be easier said than done, what with the ordeal of cancer treatment and its residual physical and psychological adjustments, including coping with depression, fears of recurrence, anxiety about what the future will bring, and any number of other aspects related to assimilating back into the social setting from which we've been separated. Furthermore, a return to "normalcy" is not only about healing ourselves, but about healing the family unit after its experience with cancer as well as our relationships outside the home. Reintegrating into the workplace, feeling comfortable enough to interact with the world at large, keeping abreast of insurance-related issues associated with the treatment of disease, making decisions about future medical care—these are just some of the concerns with which we are faced when finding our path back to society. Everything might have seemed "the same" before cancer appeared, but returning to living our lives the way we lived them in the past only serves to remind us that, somehow, after cancer, things are very different.

This type of experience is supported by a survey undertaken by the Lance Armstrong Foundation, which revealed that people who have experienced cancer also experience many challenges in other areas of their lives. In the area of relationships, for example, the survey revealed that 58% of cancer survivors reported dealing with sexual changes and 25% reported having dating problems. In the area of finances, 43% reported facing decreased income and 25% went into debt. With regard to cancer's impact in the workplace and insurance, 32% reported lack of advancement, and 34% felt trapped due to health insurance considerations.[14] Furthermore, the addition of practical problems, such as the resultant lack of money and/or loss of health insurance may contribute to worse outcomes for medical treatment and put the survivor at higher risk for illness, disability, and death.[15]

For many survivors, there is a longing to get back to living as normal a life as possible. For someone like me, this meant the way of life I had before cancer. For others it may mean trying to find a new way of "being normal." As many of us know, however, this can be a difficult process. It's time to face the fact that no matter how hard we try, we are not the same and we will never be the same again. Finally recognizing this "after-cancer-treatment period" is an important and distinct phase of the cancer experience. With this in mind, a committee at the Institute of Medicine (IOM) of the National Academies was established to examine the range of medical and psychosocial issues faced by cancer survivors and to make recommendations to improve their health care and quality of life. In 2005 the Institute published *From Cancer*

Patient to Cancer Survivor: Lost in Transition specifically for the purpose of helping cancer survivors move through this after-cancer stage and move forward in their lives.[16] In this report's executive summary, the committee admits freely that this particular phase of cancer care has been "relatively neglected in advocacy, education, clinical practice, and research," and thus discusses strategies for improving the quality of care and life for cancer survivors and their families. The report also recommends that a "survivorship plan" be designed to meet the new challenges that lie ahead once the individual's needs have been addressed. A "survivorship care-plan" records the individual's cancer history, makes recommendations for follow-up care, and strategizes actions that promote health. This approach can be an opportunity for the individual with cancer to find meaning in the experience, to learn new things about himself, and to learn how to live a life with a sense of optimism for the future. Often times, just having an outline of where you are and where you need to go can be a great start on the road to permanent health.

Making a difference

Learning about new approaches and trends in the realm of cancer work has continued to confirm my belief that greater strides can be accomplished with a group collective action than by a single individual trying to do it alone. For instance, it has made me realize that when I was ill, I was unaware of any society, organization, group, club, or alliance available to answer the multitude of questions I wanted to ask. Feeling alone and ashamed at the time, it's possible I would have been reluctant to join any group at first. But once I had learned more about the benefits, I probably would have jumped at the chance. In fact, I know I would gladly have participated in an organized program where people were dedicated to answering my questions and providing emotional support, just as I know that that kind of encouragement would have increased both my understanding and my self-confidence. Now, with the Internet at our fingertips, libraries packed with research journals, and book stores stocked with resources, the magnitude of information is as comforting as it is overwhelming. Not only has the wealth of information spread by way of inventory, but so have the organizations available to support people with virtually all types of disease.

These support organizations not only define illness, but focus on much broader themes. They are dedicated to servicing and promoting good health by informing the public about everything from treatment and cure to prevention. From these expanded sentiments about health, treatment today has become much more than tests, hospitalizations, drugs, and follow-up care. This means that for those individuals who are tired of being in the typical medicinal group-health setting, such as a hospital or clinic, there are alternatives available where they can receive similar health benefits but in nonmedical settings. Patients today seek outside support from family members, friends, religious groups, organizations, support groups, and even fellow patients. Expanding our views, educating ourselves, and heightening our awareness in as many areas as possible helps direct our energy to receiving the good that comes from being a part of something larger than ourselves. That's why support groups that are filled with people who know what you have been through—or are still going through—and who want to help in every way they can, are so vital.

In the United States we are incredibly fortunate to have numerous support organizations at our disposal. Some of these organizations are committed to specific diseases and provide vast social support networks. The American Heart Association, the American Diabetes Association, the Multiple Sclerosis Foundation, the National Association of People with AIDS, the Alzheimer's Association, and the American Parkinson's Disease Association are only some of the many organizations where we can get the help we need.

Cancer support

Numerous organizations exist specifically to assist individuals with cancer and provide support for their families. One of the oldest of these organizations is the American Cancer Society, founded in 1913 by 15 prominent doctors and business leaders in New York City.[17] At that time, the ACS was known as the American Society for Control of Cancer. Today, the American Cancer Society is one of the best resources for cancer information in the world along with the National Cancer Institute, the organization referenced many times in this book and the United States' federal government's principal agency for cancer research.[18] The NCI conducts, coordinates, and funds research about cancer, explores the causes of cancer, classifies diagnoses, evaluates treatment, and assesses prevention issues. The common denominator of most of the societies, organizations, groups, and alliances associated with cancer support is their widespread approach to reduce cancer mortality, decrease incidence, reduce suffering associated with either cancer or its treatment, provide family assistance, and contribute to a better quality of life. Through ongoing efforts, researchers hope to see cancer reduced to a treatable condition within a few years. As highlighted in Chapter Three of this book, statistics and research about cancer are shared by many agencies and accessible to all of us, helping us to stay informed on where we are and where we need to go relative to the war on cancer.

"Concentrated" support groups

Most support groups for people with cancer or who have had cancer promote encouragement and assistance by improving cancer awareness through education. Support groups often help reduce an individual's sense of alienation by giving him/her the opportunity to talk with and be heard by others in the same or similar situation. Consistent, ongoing support is the key to helping individuals who are physically and emotionally dealing with the diagnosis of cancer. Quality medical care combined with fundamental emotional support makes the journey through diagnosis and treatment considerably less daunting. Just about anyone going through this process, or who has just ended the process, needs support to at least validate the often overwhelming multitude of feelings that come up while dealing with the disease. Support groups help reestablish—or instill—confidence so we can naturally regain feelings of wellbeing, the feelings that can become lost as we progress. Groups help reduce anxiety levels and encourage participants to make use of the personal resources and activities available to them through the group. This is the time when "social wellbeing" means a team effort, one which can consist of psychologists, social workers, survivors, psychotherapists, educators, religious groups, recreational therapists, friends, and family—all working together for the wellbeing of the individual.

Cancer support groups are available for everyone who has any type of cancer, in any stage. A support group is not about sitting around a room rehashing the misery of the disease and discussing survival rates, however. Many cancer groups organize outings, plan events, and invite speakers to share insights about coping with day-to-day-life issues. Community cancer support groups are easy to access and offer a convenient way to get actively involved. Meetings are held at various locations, such as hospitals, churches, community centers, and even at private homes.

One support program dedicated to educating people about cancer is I Can Cope. Sponsored by the American Cancer Society, this organization provides classes both online and in areas nationwide.[19] For those individuals unable to be in the company of others or simply not ready to be, many online support groups are accessible at the click of a mouse. One of these is Oncochat (*www.oncochat.org*), a group providing casual peer support to people with cancer, family, and friends.[20] Another online support group called the Cancer Support Community provides support 24 hours a day, seven days a week and is the world's largest employer of psychosocial oncology mental health professionals in the United States with a network of personalized services and education for all those affected by cancer.[21]

The American Cancer Society sponsors an online support community as well, called the Cancer Survivors Network. This social community was created by and for cancer survivors and their families and friends. It is designed to allow members to connect with others via personal home pages, chats, personal stories, and moderated discussions.[22] One of the many areas where the Cancer Survivors Network offers support is for people who are coping with cancer while working at their jobs. Again, as anyone with cancer knows, the reaction and behavior of coworkers and colleagues can be challenging at best. People often react in unexpected ways when confronted with someone dealing with cancer. They can surprise us with their generosity—or their inability to relate. It's not uncommon to experience feelings of sadness, uneasiness, and shock, as well as understanding, encouragement, and compassion coming from people in the workplace. Awkward, ambiguous comments might be due to an individual's own sense of fears around illness, or simply a discomfort based on not knowing what to say. To be honest, sometimes people who have the best intentions can still be downright clueless about what someone with cancer is feeling. Frankly, some people would be better off not saying anything at all—but that doesn't necessarily keep them from trying. I remember thinking, *We're the same people we were* before *we had cancer, aren't we? When did I become "contagious" to the point where people have difficulty approaching me, saying something supportive?* What I learned is that people can feel overwhelmed by simply not knowing what to do, what to say, or how to say it. That's why support organizations offer opportunities to discuss and prepare in advance for situations when they arise.

Gilda's Club is another well-known organization, founded in honor of the late, great comedian Gilda Radner, who died of ovarian cancer. It was Gilda Radner's dream that all people affected by cancer have access to the same kind of emotional and social support that she received during her illness, and her vision has materialized to clubs of this type worldwide.[23]

With the incidence of cancer on the rise, more and more support groups are evolving to provide practical assistance, guidance, spiritual and mental support, and consistent encouragement. Most strive to educate through wellness programs and outings by encouraging free thinking and dialogue. Some even provide assistance with transportation, medical equipment, and food. In general, there is no charge for these services and most are funded by charitable donations from individuals, corporate gifts, grants, and sponsorships.

The National Cancer Institute and the National Institutes of Health have compiled a "who's who" list of some of the non-profit organizations throughout the country that provide full-time cancer support. Although the list is not comprehensive, it offers a very good start by providing information about these organizations on a national scale. It includes phone numbers, addresses, and websites, so individuals can contact them directly. This list includes groups like the American Cancer Society, the American Brain Tumor Association,[24] Man to Man (a prostate cancer support group),[25] and Look Good, Feel Better, a group developed by the Personal Care Products Council.[26] Sponsored by the American Cancer Society, this particular group focuses on helping women offset appearance-related changes from cancer treatment, with the ultimate goal of improving self-esteem, self-image, and quality of life. Reach to Recovery, a rehabilitation program for both women and men who have had breast cancer,[27] is a program striving to help patients cope with the physical, emotional, and cosmetic needs arising from both cancer and its treatment. C3, or the Colorectal Cancer Coalition, as the name suggests, is an association dedicated to supporting those diagnosed with colorectal cancer.[28] Cancer Care, Inc. is another national nonprofit agency that provides counseling and support groups, education, financial assistance, and other practical help to people with cancer and their families.[29] The Candlelighters Childhood Cancer Foundation, a nonprofit organization dedicated to children,[30] is the largest publisher and distributor of free childhood cancer books in the country and provides information and awareness for children, adolescents, and advocates. The Cancer Hope Network is another group that provides free and confidential one-on-one support to cancer patients and their families. This organization matches cancer patients and/or family members with trained volunteers who have themselves undergone and recovered from similar cancer experiences.[31]

There are also organizations that focus solely on the various aspects of breast cancer. I was surprised and pleased, for example, when I came across an organization that provides support for men with spouses who have breast cancer, so that these husbands may be better able to support their wives during their experience. The group, called Network of Strength, also has a Partner Match Program, which provides education and support for any caregiver who is supporting a wife, partner, or loved one.[32] Susan G. Komen For The Cure is another committed organization. One of the most high-profile branches of the cancer awareness crusade, this pink-ribbon program is highly recognized for promoting cancer awareness and raising millions of dollars each year for breast cancer research.[33]

LIVESTRONG (the Lance Armstrong Foundation) is another non-profit organization committed to strengthening and inspiring people with cancer.[34] Founded in 1997 by champion cyclist and cancer survivor Lance Armstrong, LIVESTRONG focuses on prevention, access to screening and care, improvement in the quality of life of cancer survivors, and investment in cancer research. The Lung Cancer Alliance is another such nonprofit organization, dedicated solely to providing patient support and advocacy for people living with or at risk of lung cancer.[35] The Lung Cancer Alliance provides free peer-to-peer mentoring support, a matching service for clinical trials, an online survivors' community, and a quarterly newsletter on a wide variety of topics.

I have also learned about a number of organizations involved in "grass roots" movements as well. The National Coalition for Cancer Survivorship, for example, is the oldest survivor-led cancer advocacy organization in the country, championing quality cancer care for all Americans and empowering cancer survivors. NCCS believes in evidence-based advocacy for systemic changes at the federal level in how the nation researches, regulates, finances, and delivers quality cancer care.[36] Pink-Link, an online cancer organization comments on its website, "Cancer is a club that you didn't ask to join," and hosts a free membership which offers immediate access to fellow survivors, family members, medical professionals, and others who, in essence, become "pen pals" via the Pink-Link website.[37]

R. A. Bloch Cancer Foundation focuses on support and education as well. This organization was cofounded by the honorary chairman of the board of H & R Block, Inc.[38] The goal of the R.

A. Bloch Cancer Foundation "is limited to projects that help people who are diagnosed with cancer to have the best chance of beating it as easily as possible." The foundation offers a cancer hotline to answer all questions, sponsors an annual Cancer Survivors Rally, and invites physicians to discuss new treatment options.

With the number of support groups continuing to grow and the variety of choices being offered, cancer is no longer the isolating experience it once was. Today candid, open discussions with doctors, patients, family, friends, caregivers, social workers, and therapists take place everyday. These dialogues help stimulate an array of feelings, often helping individuals to find newfound courage and generate improved attitudes with positive expectations and outcomes.

Once discussions get underway, where everyone freely participates, anything goes. Because discussions don't have to be limited topically, they often run the gamut from general health, fitness, exercise, diet, and family to environmental issues and even politics. Some cancer survivors clubs invite others who have gone through treatment to share their own experiences and to inspire others who are still undergoing treatment. Forums like these allow delicate and sensitive issues to be shared in a nurturing, cooperative environment. In this safe place, individuals can share common ground around tough topics and begin restoring shaky confidence and rebuilding self-respect. Groups like these also advocate a foundation for healthy living, which includes regular screenings, checkups, exercise regimens, dietary considerations, and prevention.

What I have found is that while all share the watermark of cancer, each group has its own unique approach in how it goes about supporting each person's individual needs. Some put more emphasis on social and recreational therapies, some on legislation, others on fundraising, and still others on logistical support and the distribution of educational materials. There is no doubt, however, that whatever the focus, participating in support groups can vastly improve quality of life for cancer patients and caregivers alike.

There are too many support groups, networks, organizations, clubs, societies, and other groups to list them all here and new ones are being conceived all the time. I don't think anyone could have imagined the overwhelming outpouring of support that has been generated for people who are struggling with cancer. As American feminist, activist, and writer Sonia Johnson once said, "We must remember that one determined person can make a significant difference, and that a small group of determined people can change the course of history."

Therapeutic recreation

The American Therapeutic Recreation Association (ATRA) defines therapeutic recreation as "a treatment service designed to restore, remediate, and rehabilitate a person's level of functioning and independence in life activities, [and] to promote health and wellness as well as reduce or eliminate the activity limitations and restrictions to participation in life situations caused by an illness or disabling condition."[39] ATRA was established in Washington, D.C. in 1984 as a nonprofit organization representing the interests and needs of recreational therapists. Its primary objective is to promote maximum functional benefit through therapeutic recreation. In 2008, recreational therapists held about 23,300 jobs in the United States, with 24% in nursing care facilities and others working in hospitals, residential care facilities, and state and local government agencies.[40] Recreational therapists are certified by the National Council for Therapeutic Recreation and are required to recertify every five years.

Therapeutic recreational therapists help people cope with various ailments, addictions, and illnesses. They focus on developing ways to perform meaningful leisure activities for those who find themselves limited. They utilize a wide range of techniques to accomplish the individual's goal regardless of age, disease, disability, or financial or social standing. Therapeutic recreational therapists work with people with various medical problems, such as stroke, spinal cord injuries, cardiovascular disease, cancer, multiple sclerosis, and chronic pain. They provide treatment though techniques that include arts and crafts, sports, games, dance, drama, music, and community outings. These activities are meant to develop and nurture the mental, physical, and social wellbeing of their patients. For individuals requiring long-term care, recreational therapists provide leisure activities either privately or in group settings.

One of the main objectives for the therapeutic recreational therapist is to prevent further medical problems and complications for each individual. Research has shown the following physical, psychosocial, and cognitive benefits from undergoing therapeutic recreational therapy:

Physical benefits:

- increased immune system activity
- reduced pain and stiffness
- better flexibility, agility, and balance
- improved cardiovascular functioning
- improved muscular strength and endurance
- reduced dependency on medication and healthcare services
- reduced secondary disability and related higher care costs

Psychosocial benefits:

- increased self-efficacy and self-confidence
- increased, better-developed and better-controlled motor movements
- better handling and control of stress
- increased skills of conversation and cooperation
- reduction in depression, loneliness, and self-pity
- improved morale and general satisfaction
- improved overall competence
- better acceptance of disability or disease

Cognitive benefits:

- reduced confusion and disorientation
- heightened alertness
- improved problem-solving skills, attention span, memory, and perception

According to the Centers for Disease Control and Prevention, "People with disabilities are less likely to engage in regular moderate physical activity than people without disabilities, yet they have similar needs to promote their health and prevent unnecessary disease."[41] The reasons for not exercising can be anything from not feeling able to participate or not knowing where to start. Overall, collaboration with a therapist or a program can be a good way to start to bring about considerable, but gradual changes, by enhancing motor development, social skills development, social interaction skills, communication, and behavior, all while improving the intellectual, emotional, mental, and physical aspects of health. (See Tables 7-1 through 7-5 for listings of the many benefits of recreational therapy.)

TABLE 7-1. Benefits of recreational therapy for individuals with physical disabilities.

Psychosocial benefits	Physical benefits
Enhanced body image perceptions	Enhanced immune system
Attitudinal changes toward disability	Reduced pain
Increased self-confidence	Increased muscular strength
Controlled stress levels	Improved flexibility and balance
Increased efficiency	Better cardiovascular functioning

TABLE 7-2. Benefits of recreational therapy for individuals with developmental disabilities.

Physical benefits	Cognitive benefits
Improved motor skills	Improved attention span
Improved athletic skills	Enhanced decision-making skills
Better agility	Increased independence of choice

TABLE 7-3. Benefits of recreational therapy for individuals with psychiatric disabilities.

Reduction of symptom	Social impact
Reduced anxiety	Improved social skills
Reduced depression	Better socialization techniques
Reduced tension	Better cooperation
Reduced negative thoughts	Improved communication skills

TABLE 7-4. Benefits of recreational therapy for the elderly.

Physical health	Health benefits
Decreased blood pressure	Enhanced cardiovascular fitness
Increased muscular strength	Better bone strength
Increased mobility	Decreased body weight and fat

TABLE 7-5. Benefits of recreational therapy for children.

Psychosocial benefits	Physical benefits
Enhanced body image perceptions	Enhanced immune system
Attitudinal changes toward disability	Reduced pain
Increased self-confidence	Increased muscular strength
Controlled stress levels	Improved flexibility and balance
Increased efficiency	Better cardiovascular functioning

Home care

Home care, also called domiciliary care, is personal care service that is provided in a patient's home by healthcare aides. Qualified home-health aides help perform both medical and non-medical care, offer mental and physical support, and provide emotional strength and compassion for those who require assistance with activities of daily living. As a profession, the career of home-health aide is expected to be one of the fastest growing through the next

10 years due to society's aging population. Employment in nursing, residential care facilities, hospitals, and home healthcare services are all expected to rise.

In most cases a high-school diploma or equivalent educational background is a prerequisite for this job. However, in some states the only requirement for employment is on-the-job training. The National Association for Home Care and Hospice (NAHC) offers national certification for personal and home-care aides. Certification is a voluntary demonstration to show that the individual meets industry standards. In 2008, about 1.7 million jobs were held in the home-health-aide arena. The majority of jobs were in home-healthcare services, individual and family services, residential care facilities, and private households.[42]

Home-health aides provide an indispensable service to the community at large. They typically work under medical supervision to help the elderly, convalescent, disabled, and those needing support while recovering from an illness. Their duties vary, but can include personal care, medication administration, basic housekeeping tasks, and the accompaniment of individuals to doctor's appointments and exams. They may help with advised exercise regimens, provide assistance with crutches, wheelchairs, or artificial limbs for the disabled, and file reports regarding patient progress and changes to healthcare providers and family.

With such a large number of diverse responsibilities, home-health aides typically need to be the personification of patience and perseverance as well as have the capacity for common sense and knowledge. Working familiarity of the home environment relative to patient safety, the ability to safely deliver personal care, and the knowledge of proper use of assistive equipment (such as wheelchairs and mechanical lifts) are all prerequisites in this profession. Because home-health aides do anything and everything that a family member might do to look after sick or convalescing individuals, and because smaller nuclear families are on the rise, aides are in great demand for people living alone and/or who are alone for the better part of the day.

Caregiving

We've talked a lot about how disease not only affects the person with cancer, but all of those in connection with that person as well. Cancer affects *everyone*. In fact, a disease like cancer involves so many people in the process of treatment and recovery that it would be difficult to name them all. Even the person who accompanies the patient to the hospital for treatment deserves distinction for being there at the right time and doing the right thing for the individual's welfare. And while the lives of patients undergoing treatment change—often radically—so do the lives of the people around them.

Caregivers are integral to the patient's life and crucial to the patient's recovery and wellbeing. They are the people who do whatever it is that needs doing—from medicating, bathing, cleaning, and transporting to being good company, and all without compensation or salary. Most primary caregivers are spouses, partners, or adult children. In the absence of family, close friends, neighbors, relatives, and even coworkers may take on some of these responsibilities. As medical care is constantly changing, with many patients given the choice to spend time at home as opposed to in the hospital while undergoing treatment, this shift has reduced the need for hospital confinement. As a result, the patient's ability to create his or her own healing environment has taken a giant step to the forefront. This trend has also shifted a good deal of the responsibilities from trained health professionals to caregivers.

Most people find personal satisfaction in looking after their loved ones, feeling that no one else can look after them as well as they can. However, caregiving is extremely demanding and requires a great deal of energy, patience, and emotional flexibility because patients have different personalities, capabilities, and needs. It is not unusual for caregivers to feel that the job of giving care has been thrust upon them. It can feel overwhelming and burdensome—something we wouldn't mind giving to someone else with seemingly more skill, knowledge, and patience than we feel we have to offer. Mixed feelings can easily turn into frustration and anger unless we are able to channel our feelings appropriately. That is why, if at all possible, sharing and delegating caregiving responsibilities to reduce the load can help prevent these feelings from surfacing.

Caregivers are notorious for not taking enough time for themselves. Because we tend to spend so much time and effort on the one for whom we are caring, it's important to remember how much care *we* need in order to keep up our efforts. We need to be emotionally and physically sound in order to keep the care going to the degree required and we need to take the time to pay attention to our own needs in order to pay attention to the needs of others. Our roles may differ from day to day, but we can't forget that our priority must be to take care of ourselves first.

A good caregiver is a positive influence and instrumental in an individual's recovery. Encouragement, kindness, and understanding go a long way toward aiding recovery and healing. Therefore, caregivers need to be strong enough to make decisions, handle potential emergencies, and understand medical situations should they arise. If there is a setback due to complications from treatment, the caregiver can be the one to guide the patient to understand the problem and assist in solving it. In essence, caregivers help the patient lead as normal a life as possible; that can mean becoming involved with the treatment process and trying to keep the individual from feeling alone or alienated. It can be a real challenge for a caregiver to make his/her availability known without being overbearing and controlling, to give the patient his or her personal space, but always be on hand in case a need arises. The caregiver's multifaceted role makes him or her an integral part of a caring team, a team player with the common objective of improving the patient's life as much as possible.

Needless to say, the life of a caregiver can be difficult at times. Unfortunately, most of us will find that there are no guidelines or classes in "caregiving" available when we find ourselves suddenly propelled into the role. Here are a few of the things it helps to remember if we find ourselves in the position of helping someone else who is coping with an illness:

Try not to press issues. It's okay to be the one to step back, to be willing to listen to the individual's concerns. It generally does not help to push or pressure anyone to do anything, but rather to remember that only when an individual is ready to make a change will the change occur.

Try to be gentle. When an individual shows resistance to an exercise program, for example, it can be difficult to convince him otherwise. Start with simple things, allowing the person space to find his own motivation. Offering options such as, "Would you like to go for a walk or would you prefer to stretch a little at home?" can provide enough of a bridge for the person to take the initiative to get started. Remember, the mere act of planting a mental seed can manifest huge results.

Look after your own health. Coping with a sick person and attending to his or her needs is no easy task. Concern coupled with strain can impede our own health and wellbeing to the point where we can no longer handle the immense responsibility of caring for another. Eating, sleeping, exercising, and socializing are all important for our own care. We need to set time aside for ourselves to do the things we like to do, making sure not to limit ourselves to the company of the person needing our care. We need to remember that we are human beings with our own needs and capabilities, dislikes, difficulties, and challenges.

Get support. Research has shown that support of friends and family is vital to both the person with cancer as well as the caregiver. It's not uncommon to feel isolated and overwhelmed in the day-to-day care of another. So don't be afraid to ask for help. Reach out to family, friends, and other caregivers; you'll be glad you did.

Accept feelings of negativity and then move on. It would be all but impossible to continue in the role of caregiving without experiencing occasional bouts of negativity, frustration, and even anger. Thoughts of failure, depression, fear of the unknown, and the monotony of an ongoing routine can bring us down. As caregivers, we need to remember that we are working in the individual's best interest and for his wellbeing. We are doing the best we can even when we feel we could be doing better. Under the circumstances we must try not to feel guilty or blame ourselves. Remember, each of us is only one person, and we can only do what we can do.

Religious and spiritual groups

When we go through the anguish of illness, it is common to turn to our faith to find solace. But it is also common to question our faith during these trying times as well. Illness, especially long-term illness, can be painful, isolating, and unpredictable, raising questions as we go through the process. Religious groups can be and often are the basis for support for people struggling in their daily lives by providing guidance, compassion, prayer, conversation, and companionship. While spirituality comes from within, expressing this divine spirit within a religious context can expand on that conviction. According to George Bernard Shaw, "There is only one religion, though there are a hundred versions of it." Religion is that unwavering devotion to faith and observance that allows the sensitivity of one's spiritual values to be expressed. The practice of religion can become the bridge to spirituality within us; that spirituality can then express itself through our religion and religious beliefs.

The practice of religion and the expression of spirituality are very personal choices, and the decisions to practice them are based on what we as individuals feel and believe. Doctors and caregivers need to respect individual religious and spiritual practices, understanding that we are all different in the way we express our preferences. Some of us seek to draw inner strength by receiving something as simple as a hug from another human being. Others find solace in reading a religious text upon awakening or when getting ready for bed, and there are those who find comfort wearing and touching a religious artifact. But, whatever we choose, we need to allow ourselves the time and place to receive with our spirit.

William Ellery Channing, Unitarian theologian, once said, "Difficulties are meant to rouse, not discourage. The human spirit is to grow strong by conflict." In Matthew 7:7-8, it is said, "Ask and it will be given to you, seek and you will find, knock and the door will be opened to you. For everyone who asks receives, he who seeks finds, and to him who knocks the door will be opened." Joining and being a part of a religious or spiritual group can aid in the flowering of the spirit anytime, but especially during times of need. It has been rightly said that anger is natural, grief appropriate, healing mandatory, and restoration possible. In this way, group efforts often support healing and ultimately revitalize our life and reinforce our will to live.

Various programs organized by religious groups, ranging from prayer meetings to healing music projects where soothing, uplifting music is performed, are offered almost everywhere and in many settings. Some groups offer crafts and conversation, where art supplies are provided and enriching conversation is invited. Chaplains, rabbis, priests, ministers, and pastors are available for spiritual guidance in their denominations, and even hospitals are becoming more conscious of the need for religious and spiritual support due to the realization that the combination of medical care and spiritual support goes much further to aid and bolster wellbeing.

Studies have been undertaken to establish that religious faith does in fact have positive physiological effects on those struggling with illness. In one large study of cancer patients, for example, the possession of a religious faith was identified as a significant factor in determining a range of psychosocial needs. When 354 participants responded to the Comprehensive Psychosocial Needs Questionnaire, it was found that 83% said they had some sort of religious faith. It was also revealed that overall these participants were less reliant on health professionals, had less need for information, attached less importance to the maintenance of independence, and had less need for help with feelings of guilt, issues around sexuality, and certain practical matters than those participants who said they had no religious faith. In addition, significantly, researchers found those respondents in the religious faith group had fewer unmet needs overall.[43]

In another study, 33 women, age 65, of Protestant, Catholic, Jewish, and other faiths, were recruited within six months of their diagnosis of breast cancer to look at the relationship between religious faith and the ability to cope with cancer. In this case, researchers found that religious and spiritual faith provided a full 91% of respondents with the emotional support necessary to deal with their breast cancer, 70% with the necessary social support, and 64% with the ability to make meaning in their everyday life, particularly during their cancer experience.[44] As the Indian spiritual leader Sri Sathya Sai Baba once wrote, "Where there is faith there is love; where there is love there is peace; where there is peace there is God; and where there is God there is bliss." With this universal understanding, it is safe to say that when we surrender to a "higher power," or an invisible force, we can heal in a way that is truly miraculous.

Coordinated socializing

Now that we've talked about all the different types of concentrated group socializing through organized support groups, let's look at other ways to experience a social setting. Coordinated leisure settings offer the chance to socialize with people you enjoy in places unrelated to any kind of instruction or medical setting. Picnicking, going on outings to the movies or to a museum, going for a drive, taking a walk in a garden, visiting a historic site, going fishing or shopping or taking a nature hike, going to the beach, attending a concert, taking a trip, joining a sport, or going dancing—all are good examples. If you are not the type of person generally inspired to participate in these types of activities, it helps to know that you can receive some social benefit by merely being in a random setting in the presence of others. Just strolling through the mall, sitting in a park, walking down a city street, or watching a softball game are indirect ways of being "social," allowing us to receive some positive social connection.

Conversing over a cup of tea. As Bernard-Paul Heroux said, *"There is no trouble so great or grave that cannot be much diminished by a nice cup of tea."* I remember many times I've spent with family and friends over a cup of tea, talking, listening, and just being together. Talking is a great way to share feelings, bond with laughter, and feel a sense of understanding. Listening to one another, asking questions, and losing oneself in the process gives each of us the chance to move toward a healthier self.

We've talked about the health benefits of tea earlier in this book, so it should come as no surprise that I'm an advocate for combining the health benefits of tea with its social benefits. Regular or herbal, drinking tea is a wonderful way to take advantage of what they offer and relax during the process.

Hobbies. Hobbies are a great way to pass the time; not only do they keep you busy, but they bring pleasure at the same time. As Dale Carnegie said, "Today is life—the only life you are sure of. Make the most of today. Get interested in something. Shake yourself awake. Develop a hobby. Let the winds of enthusiasm sweep through you. Live today with gusto." Hobbies are activities that can be a lot of fun within a group setting. Regardless of the venue you choose, hobbies can bring out the best in you when dormant, unforeseen, creative forces are given the opportunity to come alive. Creativity often stimulates feelings of achievement and contentment, welcome requisites on the road to recovery from a major illness.

People who have a hobby are also generally found to be healthier emotionally. "When people do things that make them feel good, like a hobby, it activates an area of the brain called the nucleus accumbens that controls how we feel about life," says Dr. S. Ausim Azizi, Chairman of the Department of Neurology at Temple University's School of Medicine in Philadelphia, who studies brain activity and cell signaling. "Activities you enjoy also stimulate the brain's septal zone—its 'feel good' area—and that makes you feel happy."[45] Hobbies can enhance your creativity, help you think more clearly, and sharpen your focus," agrees Carol Kauffman, Assistant Clinical Professor at Harvard Medical School. "When you're really engaged in a hobby you love, you lose your sense of time and enter what's called a flow state, and that restores your mind and energy. In a flow state, you are completely submerged in an experience, requiring a high level of concentration." Dr. Kaufmann's research has also shown that there is a strong correlation between flow states and peak performance.[45]

Museums. Visiting museums to admire and discuss great works of art through the ages is an enriching experience. Henry Moore, the great sculptor, said, "The creative habit is like a drug. The particular obsession changes, but the excitement, the thrill of the creation lasts." Whether we visit alone or go in a group, spending time in an environment where we are inspired by great art promotes a sense of participation and belonging, and broadens our education and understanding of the human expression.

Imagination used in the creation of art is at the core of the same kind of inspiration we have at our disposal to conceive our own health. The beauty of imagination is that it has absolutely no boundaries or restrictions. It is as a result of this limitless understanding that mind-body medicine has evolved. The field of mind-body medicine is based on a growing area called *psychoneuroimmunology*, or PNI. Psychoneuroimmunology is the study of how the mind influences the body, where "psycho" refers to mood, thoughts, and emotions, "neuro" refers to the neurological and neuroendocrine systems in the body, and "immunology" refers to the immune system. In other words, techniques that use the mind can be applied to change neurological, endocrine, and immunological outcomes. In his book, *Creating Health: How to Wake up the Body's Intelligence*, author Deepak Chopra states, "We have already seen that cancer cells in their mindless, useless multiplication have lost touch with their basic intelligence, the know-how at the genetic level that should regulate proper cell division. Somehow these mental techniques restore intelligence by operating from the mind's awareness. It is one intelligence in our bodies speaking to another and bringing it back to normal. What seems so promising is that the cure grows from within the patient, taking advantage of the mind-body connection."[46]

History. Mahatma Gandhi has said, "The history of the world is full of men who rose to leadership by sheer force of self-confidence, bravery, and tenacity!" I feel we can all learn something from the tough times, the times faced by us as well as by others. History is swathed in wars fought, won, and lost, in glory and fame, and in good and evil. Stories of bravery and valor can be appreciated by reading history and visiting great historical sites. Looking at imposing structures with motifs, engravings, paintings, and sculptures has a tendency to help put situations and time into perspective.

Fishing. As Herbert Hoover once said, "To go fishing is the chance to wash one's soul with pure air, with the rush of the brook, or with the shimmer of sun on blue water. It brings meekness and inspiration from the decency of nature, charity toward tackle-makers, patience toward fish, a mockery of profits and egos, a quieting of hate, a rejoicing that you do not have to decide a darned thing until next week. And it is discipline in the equality of men—for all men are equal before fish." When the body is incapable of undertaking strenuous exercise, fishing provides a good way to pass the time and has gained recognition and importance lately as a contribution to the healing process. For example, over the past few years our armed forces have begun looking at fishing to aid injured and disabled military personnel in their physical and emotional recovery. Project Healing Waters Fly Fishing, Inc., one of these initiatives, was started at Walter Reed

Hospital in 2005 and incorporated two years later to support emotional and physical rehabilitation programs at hospitals throughout the country.[47] In it, soldiers learn about fly fishing and then practice their skills on the surrounding rivers. Due to the soldiers' tremendous response and the benefits derived, 70 other programs have been established so far throughout the United States and Canada.

Theatre. Arthur Miller, renowned playwright, once said, "A theater is so endlessly fascinating because it's so accidental. It's so much like life." There is such joy in watching a play or experiencing the thunderous dance of musical theater. To be part of a group enjoying live theatre can be exhilarating, too...waiting expectantly for the curtain to rise, seeing the beautiful sets which form the backdrop for the actors and actresses, and watching a story come to life. Theatre productions utilize personal stories, mythology, fairy-tale comedy, music, dance, and drama as a means of bringing people closer together by expressing human nature through artistic endeavor. Theatre has been called a therapy of optimism because it often brings out our great hidden potential. It is also a here-and-now experience, something which encourages a forward outlook and sense of optimism.

Movies. As Jedi Master Obi-Wan Kenobi said, "May the force be with you." Any movie buff can relate to this quote from *Star Wars*. And when it comes to life's problems, I admit I can use all the help I can get, and that force is more than welcome! I find nothing takes you away from life's complexities more than a good movie. There are all kinds of movies, for all times; ones that make you cry, laugh, or really think. Of course there are always a few that make you wish you could get your money back! There are characters who inspire empathy and emotional connection, and others who bring on the adrenaline of the thrill of action. There are also characters to whom we can relate by watching their life stories unfold on the screen. Being entertained can help us feel less down in the dumps, help us forget about our problems for awhile, and help us feel rejuvenated. If you can afford it, going out to a movie is always preferable to staying in. It gets you out of the house and into the mix of the community where you can share a common experience. Not only can a movie act as a catalyst for great physical release by getting you to laugh or cry, but it can serve as a distraction or change your perspective about life's problems as well.

Shopping. Shopping is another potential antidote for what ails us—if not taken to the extreme, of course. This brief dialog from the TV series *Sex and the City* says it all: "Honey, if it hurts so much, why are we going shopping?" asks one friend of the other. "I have a broken toe, not a broken spirit," says the second. Going through a major illness can be both lengthy and painful. This means you may have the time but not the inclination to do anything for yourself—for *you*. When you are well enough to go outside, shopping can be great way to give something to yourself. And shopping is not limited to buying; experiencing the process itself is just as important. Browsing, admiring a window dressing, or simply strolling to take your mind off your problems for a while, are all valued elements we tend to overlook. But looking at clothing, going through supermarkets to see what new products are available, comparing products and prices—these can all be ways to treat ourselves to a day outside the house and serve as a welcome change from our day-to-day routine.

Arts and crafts fairs. Millard Sheets (1907–1969), American painter and architect, said, "Good design is a great combination of common sense, unusual imagination, clarity of purpose, aesthetic insight, and a deep reverence for the love of life." Going to an arts and crafts show or a flea market can be a great way to restore this reverence for life. The great thing about arts and crafts fairs is that you can stroll and look to your heart's content and never be obligated to make a purchase. These markets can be found all year round, usually with hundreds of vendors selling weekly. Clothes, crafts, jewelry, furniture, and baked goods are just a few of the things found there. We all love a good bargain, and flea markets offer just that, in addition to entertainment and just plain fun. It helps to enjoy the feeling of a close-knit community in a bustling setting, too. If you're in the mood and have the time, pick up a do-it-yourself art project, bring it home, put on your smock, and have some fun.

Gardening. Hanna Rion, landscape artist and illustrator, says, "The greatest gift of the garden is the restoration of the five senses." Imagine planting flowers or a vegetable garden and watching nature take its course as a bud blooms into a flower or a seed grows into a vegetable. Mother Nature has a wisdom all of her own. Anyone who gardens will surely tell you the joy and pleasure from gardening outweighs the sweat of hard work. As philosopher and Cardinal-Deacon John Henry Newman said in the early 1800s, "...so by a garden is meant mystically a place of spiritual repose, stillness, peace, refreshment, and delight."[48] We can overcome adversity through learning to garden, and understand patience as we wait for the byproducts of our labor to bear fruit. Gardening can relieve depression, idleness, and promote relaxation though the meditative quality associated with the process. We don't necessarily have to garden alone either. Many community gardens have sprung up in recent years, allowing the opportunity to share in a group gardening effort. Gardening can keep you in good spirits by way of connecting with the earth and is the quintessential example of reaping what you sow.

Driving. Taking a drive has always been a source of great pleasure for me. Driving can be the perfect solution when you feel the need to get away. Andrew H. Malcolm of the *New York Times* once said, "The car trip can draw the family together, as it was in the days before television when parents and children actually talked to each other." Driving can be a vehicle to self-realization, self-enhancement, and development. When we drive simply for the pleasure of driving, our mind is open, our thoughts are at peace, and we can allow our mind to wander randomly. When we drive there are no doorbells, phone calls, emails, or other "must-do" projects to detract from our ability to admire our natural surroundings.

Picnicking. Jim Fowler, zoologist and host of Mutual of Omaha's *Wild Kingdom*, once said that the single most important thing is quality of life. "If you have a place where you can go and have a picnic with your family, it doesn't matter if it's a recession or not, you can include that in your quality of life!" Picnicking with family or friends can be a great way to relax. When we think of a picnic, we picture lush green grass, a beautiful landscape, and meals packed in baskets and eaten under a blue sky. Outdoor games or basking in the sun with a book are great ways to be together. The beauty and enthusiasm the day brings can go a long way toward our wellbeing. If health permits, play a sport or spend the day enjoying nature. Based on the premise that outdoor activities are so rejuvenating, most children's hospitals are currently introducing family-centered care policies that are "environmentally based." This means that the hospital offers young patients, their families, and caregivers the chance to experience fun, theme-based gardens and other outdoor facilities: activities that provide welcome relief from an often grueling schedule of treatment and help bring back some normalcy into family life.

Pets. Loving an animal seems to bring out the best in all of us. François-Anatole Thibault (1824–1944), a French poet, journalist, and novelist once said, "Until one has loved an animal, a part of one's soul remains unawakened." Pets bring unconditional love, trust, and companionship, contributing enormous health benefits in the process. Pet owners often say interacting with their pets helps reduce their stress and anxiety, offers distraction, and generally provides them with feelings of happiness and an increased sense of wellbeing. According to a study conducted at the Baker Medical Research Institute in Melbourne, Australia, research confirms that pets have a number of positive influences on human health.[49] In this study it was found that pet owners had significantly lower levels of systolic blood pressure, plasma triglycerides, and plasma cholesterol than non-owners and, as a result, showed reduced risk factors for developing cardiovascular disease. The reasons for these positive responses have not been clearly identified, but it is apparent that attachment to a pet often brings about important physiological effects, and researchers further speculate that the social companionship of a pet may bring about positive psychological effects as well. Today, dogs and other animals are used in "animal-assisted therapy" programs in various institutions and hospitals to help to improve many patient treatment outcomes.

Dancing. Dancing is another form of socializing that has direct health benefits. Martha Graham, American dancer and choreographer, once said that dance was the "hidden language of the soul." Dancing is a great alternative to aerobic exercise, jogging, or very brisk walking, and provides the opportunity for socialization, meeting new people, and making new friends...all of which can contribute to a higher sense of self. With as many types of dance as there are ice cream flavors, simply choose one that is right for you. Ballet, jazz, tap, hip-hop, swing, Latin, country and western, folk, and belly dancing are just some of the styles to get you moving. In order to test the theory that dance might improve the lives of breast cancer survivors, a pilot research study was conducted at two cancer centers in Connecticut. In this study, 35 women treated within a five-year period were studied to determine the effect of a dance and movement program on both overall quality of life and shoulder function. For the study's purposes, all the participants completed a trial using a therapeutic movement program founded by Dr. Marc Lebed. Lebed's technique, called The Lebed Method, Focus on Healing through Movement and Dance, was designed to reduce swelling, improve range of motion, and promote wellbeing. When the women finished their 12-week intervention, which addressed both their physical and emotional needs following their treatment programs, researchers found that the dance movement initiative substantially improved a "breast-cancer-specific quality-of-life assessment."[50] Moreover, not only did dancing assist in the women's physical and emotional health, but it became for many an expression of joy and celebration. As someone once said, "Anyone who says sunshine brings happiness has never danced in the rain." For me, the expression of dance can be summed up in this quote: "We dance for laughter, we dance for tears. We dance for madness, we dance for fears. We dance for hopes, we dance for screams; we are the dancers, we create the dreams."

Music. I couldn't agree more with Shakespeare, the great playwright, who said that music is the "food of life," or John "Juke" Logan, musician and composer, who said that music is the "medicine of the mind." Music can be helpful in enhancing motor skills, social/interpersonal development, and spiritual growth. Whether you create your own music or listen more passively, music serves as a personal and spiritual balm in whatever form it takes. Rhythm and blues, jazz, country, classical, rock or rap—whatever the style, music has been found to soothe the soul and connect the world. Playing music in the background, going to a concert, or playing an instrument are all great ways to get back into the rhythm of life.

Recovery

Recovery from an illness is a very personal process involving changes in attitudes, values, feelings, and moods. Improving our social interactions at any age can contribute to that recovery process by significantly improving our ability to bond with others and encouraging our cultural sensitivities.

Socializing most often brings out the good in people, but it's always a good idea to choose carefully the types of people with whom you socialize. There are those for whom the misery-loves-company program is the driving force. These are the people who are miserable and want you to be miserable as well. These are the people who always seem to focus on the bad news of the day, for whom the glass is always half empty instead of half full, and for whom impending doom is always right around the corner. I prefer to see life's glass as half full. I prefer to see the brighter, sunnier side of life, not to adopt the doom-and-gloom attitude that some people have. We would be best served to sidestep pessimists wherever they are—in school, at a party, at work, or in the neighborhood—because their energy can have a less than positive effect on our own. I have often looked back and asked myself, *Would my outcome have been different if the love, affection, support, and understanding I received had been grumbling, complaining, and criticism instead?* I am fairly certain the answer to that question would be yes. Admittedly, it is only natural to respond to feeling sick with some negativity and fear, especially during a seemingly never-ending process of treatment. That is why no price can be placed on those family and friends who stand by and give their unwavering positive support during all the highs and lows, as mine did.

Surrounding yourself with social optimism is the single, most critical thing that can keep you centered and on the right track to health. I firmly believe that love begets love, happiness begets happiness, and positivism begets an attitude of general wellbeing. It might take time, but the universe will always respond in kind.

Seeking out the personal experiences of others. There are so many websites, blogs, and message boards on the Internet where inspirational and thought-provoking insights can be accessed. I read about one particular case recently where a woman diagnosed with breast cancer at the age of 35 decided to make a change in her life. She wrote about how after treatment she made it her business to go about her life "as usual." In her words, she "raised her children, sent them to college, and planned their weddings." Twenty years later she was diagnosed with breast cancer for the second time. After the initial shock and time spent in personal introspection, she realized there was no better way to help herself than to help others. She came to understand that she needed to assist others suffering with the disease because in doing so she would be restoring herself.

This woman's unselfish efforts helped many other women in her situation, women who were also scared, skeptical, and doubtful. The experience of giving back helped this woman in her own recovery as well. Her personal affliction became the catalyst for healing, and her limitless comfort and support enriched her life and the lives of the people she touched.

"Then said a rich man, 'Speak to us of Giving.' And he answered: 'You give but little when you give of your possessions. It is when you give of yourself that you truly give.'"

- *The Prophet*, by Kahlil Gibran

Summary

The idea of social wellbeing is based on simple, solid, fundamental principles. With this humanitarian awareness, it is no wonder that so many organizations have evolved for the betterment of all. Medical care is no longer confined to medicine and hospitals, but now encompasses a much broader domain inclusive of personal interaction and group participation. The long-term goal is the achievement of something greater than the general cure of disease; it is the restoration of a person back to wholeness. Developed nations throughout the world are recognizing more and more the need for the continued advancement of political, medical, and social benefits for the population as a whole, understanding that this core vision will be instrumental in bringing about change. It is this kind of change that will allow for profound long-term benefits for us all. To quote a Maori proverb, *"Enhara takutoa, he takitahi, he toa taki tini,"* which translated means, "My success should not be bestowed onto me alone, as it was not individual success, but success of the collective."

On the next page I have compiled a list of organizations dedicated to the people living with and fighting against cancer (see Table 7-6). Although this list is by no means comprehensive, it stands as a humble salute to all those who are doing great work and a humble offering to those who need a helping hand.

And the work goes on...

TABLE 7-6. Organizations (and their websites) participating in the fight against cancer.

Name of organization	Web site
American Cancer Society (ACS)	*www.cancer.org*
• Programs supported by ACS	*www.acscsn.org*
• I Can Cope	*www.cancer.org*
• Cancer Survivors Network	*www.cancer.org*
• Look Good...Feel Better	*www.lookgoodfeelbetter.org*
Other Organizations	
• Man to Man	*www.cancer.org*
• Reach to Recovery	*www.cancer.org*
• American Institute for Cancer Research (AICR)	*www.aicr.org*
• Bladder Cancer Advocacy Network (BCAN)	*www.bcan.org*
• Brain Tumor Society	*www.tbts.org*
• C3 Colorectal Cancer Coalition	*www.fightcolorectalcancer.org*
• Cancer Care Inc.	*www.cancercare.org*
• Cancer Hope Network	*www.cancerhopenetwork.org*
• The Cancer Project	*www.cancerproject.org*
• Cancer Information Network	*www.thecancer.net*
• Cancer Research and Prevention Foundation	*www.preventcancer.org*
• Candlelighters Childhood Cancer Foundation	*www.candlelighters.org*
• Colon Cancer Alliance (CCA)	*www.ccalliance.org*
• Cure Search	*www.curesearch.org*
• ENCORE	*www.ywca.org*
• Fertile Hope	*www.fertilehope.org*
• Gilda's Club Worldwide	*www.gildasclub.org*
• International Association of Laryngectomees	*wwwlarynxlink.com*
• International Myeloma Foundation	*www.myeloma.org*
• Kidney Cancer Association	*www.curekidneycancer.org*
• Leukemia and Lymphoma Society	*www.leukemia-lymphoma.org*
• Lung Cancer Alliance	*www.lungcanceralliance.org*
• Livestrong, Lance Armstrong Foundation	*www.livestrong.org*
• Lymphoma Foundation of America	*www.lymphomahelp.org*
• National Brain Tumor Foundation	*www.braintumor.org*
• National Breast Cancer Coalition	*www.stopbreastcancer.org*
• National Cancer Institute	*www.cancer.gov*
• National Marrow Donor Program	*www.marrow.org*
• National Children's Cancer Society	*www.children-cancer.com*
• Marie Curie Cancer Care	*www.mariecurie.org.uk*
• Macmillan Cancer Support	*www.macmillan.org.uk*
• Patient's Advocate	*www. patientadvocate.org*
• Spousal Caregiver Support	*www.wellspouse.org*

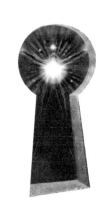

8. Lifestyle

"Your lifestyle—how you live, eat, emote, and think—determines your health. To prevent disease, you may have to change how you live."

- Brian Carter

Conscious living

There are two great days in our lives: one is the day of our birth and the other is the day we decide how we want to live our life. Our life is a reflection of our beliefs, values, ideas, and the decisions we make every day. Lifestyle, therefore, is a choice. We are all born with the ability to make choices, and we can use this ability to find our way to good health, happiness, and wellbeing.

Lifestyle, according to the Random House dictionary definition, consists of "the habits, attitudes, tasks, moral standards, economic level, etc., that together constitute the mode of living of an individual or group." Lifestyle has also been explained as "an individual's expression of life," and sociologists define lifestyle as the way an individual or a group lives, including such elements as consumption, entertainment, dress, and social relations—all of which reflect both our attitudes and our values.

Take a moment to reflect on how you live on a daily basis. What kinds of activities and attitudes make up your daily routine? Is there a possibility for modifications in your lifestyle that will positively impact your health and wellbeing? I personally believe that most of the time people want to make changes for the better, but don't always know where, or how, to begin.

For example, it is all too easy to become habituated to leaving things the way they are; that is, to become accustomed to doing things a certain way as we quietly go about our daily lives. As we live day to day we often unknowingly develop routines and habits; some of these habits may seem to make our lives simpler to negotiate, but they aren't always the best ones to maintain—in other words, they can do more harm than good. I know from my own experience that changing the less constructive aspects of one's lifestyle can be difficult. I also know that with conscious effort and perseverance it is certainly possible to exchange poor habits for better ones and to feel better as a result. As we continue to feel better and better, we build the cornerstones for a healthier lifestyle, and this modified lifestyle naturally breeds confidence for even more productive changes. Simple practices, such as buying the right foods at the supermarket, scheduling the day, preparing meals with thought and care, practicing good hygiene, allowing time for recreation and relaxation, and maintaining an optimistic outlook all make for a healthy, balanced lifestyle.

But no one can force us to make these changes. No one likes to be pressured or put in a position where they have to defend their actions—or inactions. In fact, constant badgering often has the *opposite* effect on the individual receiving the lecture on doing something different. It seems an all-too-common aspect of human nature that nagging only serves to make us automatically rebel, even when it's in our best interest to comply. And the reality is that when we feel pushed to do something we consciously—or unconsciously—do not want to do, it's unlikely anything will change. We may do nothing, dig in our heels further, or even take a turn in the opposite direction out of spite.

I have come to understand that the best kind of change comes from within and happens only when we are ready. This readiness comes in our own way and in our own time. It occurs when we finally realize that making some sort of change will not only enhance our own welfare and happiness, but positively affect our loved ones as well. We have to *want* to change in order to receive what this change for the better has to offer.

With this in mind, let's look at the six major categories of a healthy lifestyle: diet, exercise, mental attitude, socialization, spirituality, and rest.

Diet: the habit of eating

A healthy, balanced diet is composed of fruits and vegetables, complex carbohydrates, such as whole-grain bread, cereal, and pasta, and protein-rich foods such as fish, eggs, lentils, dairy products, and some meat. Foods low in saturated fat, salt, additives, and sugar are far better choices for achieving health. Let's look at each category and its role in a healthy lifestyle.

Carbohydrates. In recent years low-carbohydrate diets have gained popularity as the way to good health. But, in actuality, a healthy diet is one that combines all the food groups—in the right proportions and consumed in moderation.

Carbohydrates should constitute about 60% of all the food consumed on a daily basis. Carbohydrates are an excellent source of energy and supply nutrients, such as minerals, fiber, and vitamins. Meals may be complemented with carbohydrate-rich foods, such as vegetables, pasta, rice, and potatoes, as long as the quantities consumed are within generally accepted guidelines.

Carbohydrates may be perceived as "fattening" foods; however, gram for gram, the calorie content of carbohydrates is less than that of fat. That is why *how* we cook a food becomes as important as the type of food we eat. Smothering a complex-carbohydrate food in butter or a cream sauce can defeat the purpose of attempting to eat healthfully.

Complex carbohydrates are plant-based foods, such as grains, nuts, seeds, fruits, and vegetables, which contain high-nutrient value per calorie and are the predominant sources of fiber in most diets.

Whole-grain foods containing complex carbohydrates are definitely a better choice than foods made of refined grains. Whole-grain breakfast cereals, whole-wheat bread, whole-grain couscous and pasta, and brown rice are excellent additions to any meal of the day. With a high fiber, vitamin, and mineral content, these foods help protect us against many diseases.

Dietary fats and cancer. Heart disease is not the only condition that has been linked with fat intake. Researchers suspect a significant association between dietary fat and certain cancers. For example (though more research is needed to continue to establish causal relationships), researchers at the Harvard School for Public Health suggest that there is credible evidence that diets high in animal fat and saturated fat increase the risk for prostate cancer in men and breast cancer in postmenopausal women, and that a high intake of trans fats is associated with the risk of non-Hodgkin's lymphoma.

Here again, the type of fat—and not the total amount—appears to be the critical factor. Over the last 25 years researchers have produced dietary guidelines for reducing the risk of cancer.

> **Reduce your intake of unhealthy dietary fat.** Every major health organization from the Centers for Disease Control, the American Heart Association, and the National Cancer Institute to the World Health Organization has concluded that Americans must continue to reduce their saturated fat intake for better health and prevention of disease.
>
> **Remove known carcinogens from your diet.** Studies have confirmed the presence of cancer-causing substances, or carcinogens, in many food ingredients, including pesticides, acrylamides (found in fried foods), and synthetic food additives.
>
> **Reduce your intake of red meats.** If you make the decision to include red meat in your diet, baking, broiling, and poaching is preferable to frying or charbroiling to avoid the formation of carcinogenic compounds in the cooking process.

Eat nutritious food. Eat foods that are high in cancer-inhibiting nutrients, such as phytochemicals and antioxidants, which reduce the damaging effects of free radicals.

Limit or eliminate alcoholic beverages. While there is considerable conflicting evidence about the benefits of the occasional, or even daily, glass of wine, many studies suggest that the constant consumption of alcohol can increase the risk for cancer of the liver, breast, prostate, colon, and rectum.

Restrict sodium intake. To effectively cut back on sodium, restrict your usage of table salt and read food labels to look for "no added salt" or "reduced sodium" versions of your favorite foods.

Fruits and vegetables. Research shows that eating at least five portions of a variety of fruits and vegetables every day contributes to protecting us from a whole host of diseases, including heart disease and cancer. About 80 gm of fruit represents one portion; that means each day we should be consuming at least 400 gm of fruits and vegetables. Fruits can easily be eaten with breakfast, as a snack after lunch, or as dessert after dinner. The amount we need to eat to get this daily portion varies with the fruit, as illustrated by Table 8-1.

TABLE 8-1. Daily fruit portions.

One portion of 80 gm (2.82 oz) of fruit:	
1	Apple, banana, orange, pear, or similarly sized fruit
2	Plums, or other similarly sized fruit
½	Avocado or grapefruit
1	Slice of a large fruit, like melon
3	Tablespoons of fresh fruit salad or stewed fruit
1	Handful of cherries, berries, or grapes
1	Glass of fruit juice (without additives)

A portion of fruit with breakfast, a salad at lunch, and a portion of fruit or some juice in the evening (recommended by experts to be limited to one to two cups a day) are all good ways to ensure that we meet our body's daily requirement of five servings of fruits and vegetables. If your digestive system has difficulty consuming certain fruits or vegetables, eat only the ones you are able to tolerate. Sometimes individuals will experience a problem with digestion due to medical treatment or surgical intervention. If this is the case and you are unable to tolerate certain fruits and vegetables in their raw form, I recommend the use of a juicer, which allows you to get the nutrient value without the fiber.

There is a wide variety of vegetables from which to choose that can be found in most supermarkets. Table 8-2 supplies examples of one 80-gm portion of various common vegetables.

TABLE 8-2. Daily vegetable portions.

One portion of 80 gms (2.82 oz):	
3 heaping tablespoons	Cooked carrots
3 heaping tablespoons	Cooked peas
3 heaping tablespoons	Cooked sweet corn
4 heaping tablespoons	Cooked green beans
4 heaping tablespoons	Cooked cabbage
4 heaping tablespoons	Cooked spinach
2 spears	Cooked broccoli
8 florets	Cooked cauliflower

Fish. Fish is an excellent source of protein and contains many vitamins and minerals. Oily fish in general is a rich source of omega-3 fatty acids, which have been shown to reduce the risk of some cancers and to help maintain a healthy heart. Some oily fish that are conveniently available at supermarkets are salmon, mackerel, trout, herring, fresh tuna, and sardines. Consuming 4-oz portions twice a week is recommended for both men and women. Low-oil fish, such as mahi mahi, canned tuna, haddock, and hake, are also good sources of protein, although these are somewhat lower in omega-3 fatty acid content. Fish like shark, swordfish, and marlin, while good sources of protein, contain high levels of mercury, a known toxin, and should be eaten in moderation. Shellfish like lobster, shrimp, crab, mussels, and scallops are high in minerals, protein, and cholesterol. Because of their high cholesterol content, however, it may be prudent to consume them less frequently than other sources of protein.

Poultry. Poultry is a category of domestic fowl raised for food, such as chicken, turkey, duck, and geese. Poultry has less fat and fewer calories (especially when the skin is removed) than red meat. Poultry contains less saturated fat than red meat as well; however, it is still not considered a "good fat" (as mentioned previously). Salmonella and campylobacter are two potentially deadly strains of bacteria that are sometimes found in raw chicken and are responsible for millions of reported cases of food poisoning each year. That's why it is so important to cook poultry thoroughly, never allow raw poultry juices to come in contact with other food, and always use soap and warm water to wash all surfaces and utensils that come in contact with it.

Fats. Fats and oils are part of a healthy diet, so the type and amount of fat makes a difference in our overall health. Fats supply energy, and essential fatty acids serve as carriers for the absorption of the fat-soluble vitamins. Fats serve as building blocks of membranes and play a key regulatory role in various metabolic functions throughout the body. To maintain a healthy lifestyle, consume less than 10% of your calories from saturated fatty acids, consume fewer than 300 mg per day of cholesterol, and keep trans-fatty-acid consumption as low as possible. Limit your intake of fats and oils high in saturated and/or trans fatty acids by choosing foods low in these products. Keep your total fat intake low, with most fats coming from sources of polyunsaturated and monounsaturated fatty acids, such as fish, nuts, and vegetable oils.

Milk and dairy products. The foods in this group are important sources of protein, vitamins, and minerals, and are particularly rich in calcium for maintaining strong bones and teeth. Common milk and dairy sources found on the supermarket shelves are milk, cheese, and yogurt. It is not necessarily true that everyone "needs" milk or needs to consume milk products. What is important is getting adequate sources of calcium and protein in your diet, whether it comes from milk or other sources, to ensure a healthy, balanced diet. If you make the decision to include milk in your diet, the following comparison of the types of milk generally seen on supermarket shelves, including their caloric content and fat content per 8-oz serving, may be useful (see Table 8-3).

TABLE 8-3. Milk content per 8-oz serving.

Milk	Caloric content	Grams of fat
Whole milk	150 calories	8.0 gm fat
2% milk	120 calories	4.5 gm fat
1% milk	100 calories	2.5 gm fat
Skim milk	80 calories	0 gm fat

Portion size. Eaten out lately? If you have, it's hard to miss the fact that portion sizes have gotten larger. While this may seem as if we are getting more for our money, increased food portions may not be the best thing for our health. This "super-sized" eating can mean significant excess calorie intake, especially when consuming high-calorie foods. According to the Centers for Disease Control and Prevention research studies, people naturally consume more calories when faced with larger portions. The important thing to remember is that more does not necessarily mean better. Too many calories in a single meal can significantly burden your digestive system; as a result, excessive weight gain can occur, which increases the risk for chronic health problems. Portion control, therefore, becomes a critical element of health management. Since none of us carry scales, spoons, or measuring cups with us when we dine out, we can simplify our choices by equating common everyday objects with portion size, as illustrated in Table 8-4.

TABLE 8-4. Serving sizes. (Source: *www.aarp.org.*)

One portion, or serving, is equal to…	
Grain products	What one serving looks like
1 cup cereal flakes	size of a fist
1 pancake	a compact disc
1/2 cup cooked rice, pasta, or potato	1/2 a baseball
1 slice of bread	a cassette tape
Fruits and veggies	
1 cup salad greens	a baseball
1 medium fruit	a baseball
1/2 cup raisins	a large egg
Dairy and cheese	
1-1/2 oz cheese	4 stacked dice
1/2 cup ice cream	1/2 baseball
1 cup milk, yogurt, or fresh greens	size of a fist
Meats and alternatives	
3 oz meat, fish, and poultry	deck of cards
3 oz grilled/baked fish	checkbook
2 Tbsp peanut butter	ping pong ball
Fats	
1 tsp oil	size of your thumb tip

Body weight. Weight is a never-ending battle for many people today. While it is certainly true that some weight gain may be based on genetics or due to some metabolic imbalance in the body, I have found that the majority of weight issues are due to the fact that people do not know how to eat healthfully and do not know the best ways to be comfortably physically active. In January 2009, the National Center of Health Statistics, a division of the Centers for Disease Control, reported that maintaining a healthy body weight has been shown to reduce the incidence of many diseases, including cancer; however, more than 34% of Americans are considered obese, and 32.5% are considered overweight. Calculating your Body Mass Index, based on height in relation to weight, is a quick and easy way to determine if you are the correct body weight (see Chapter Four for details and chart). You can also get more information about your BMI on the support pages of the National Institutes of Health's website.[1]

Fluids. Water is the ideal drink for staying hydrated throughout the day, with the added benefit of being calorie-free and sugar-free. Water plays an important role in every single bodily function—from regulating temperature, to energy production, to removing toxins.

When we want a change from water, fruit juice is a healthy alternative to get the hydration we need with the taste we want. Orange, apple, pear juice, and so on; the list of what's available is virtually endless. Fruit juice is not only a good source of water, but of carbohydrates and vitamins as well. When purchasing juice in a supermarket, it's better to buy juice that is 100% fruit juice with no added sugar.

Other popular beverages that contribute to daily fluid intake are vegetable juice, herbal teas, lemonade (from squeezing your own lemons), soy milk, and rice milk. Regular tea and coffee are beneficial due to their antioxidant properties, but are often disparaged by some for their caffeine content. Beverages that contain alcohol, while not my preferred recommendation, also deserve to be mentioned, especially since alcohol has been an accepted social drink for centuries. Limiting intake to no more than two drinks per day for men and one drink per day for women is recommended.

Exercise. Along with the previous benefits mentioned earlier in this book, it is believed that exercise may reduce serum insulin and Insulin Growth Factor 1 (IGF-1) levels in the body. IGF-1 is a polypeptide that is secreted by the liver and acts as an important mediator between the growth hormone and growth throughout fetal and childhood development. IGF-1 is important for normal physiology; however, it has also been implicated in a number of disease processes, including cancer, and studies of men and women have raised the possibility that an abundance of this protein may contribute to certain types of cancer.

In one such study, it has been found that women with breast cancer show higher plasma levels of the hormone IGF-1, which may be an indicator of increased breast cancer before the age of 50.[2] Other studies in this area have revealed that estrogen enhances IGF signaling at multiple levels. This is influential because IGF signaling has been reported to enhance receptor activation in human breast cancer cells.[3] The risk for prostate cancer has also been found to be increased in men with elevated plasma IGF-1, with a particularly strong association relative to younger men.[4] In a study at Harvard Medical School, for example, researchers examined blood specimens of 32,826 women who participated in the Physicians' Health Study. Findings in this case indicated that a high blood level of IGF-1 combined with a low level of IGFBP-3 (a growth factor binding protein involved in apotosis and antiproliferative actions) posed a noticeable increased risk factor for the development of colorectal cancer and adenomas.[5] Not only has IGF-I been implicated in these cancers, but insulin-like growth factor-1 has been found to influence the development and progression of ovarian cancer.[6] Currently, researchers continue to examine the role of IGF-1; as a result, chemotherapeutic agents are being developed to block the activity of insulin-like growth factor-1 to slow cancer progression and stimulate apoptosis.[7]

Caloric restriction, or CR, is a dietary approach that involves limiting the amount of daily calories consumed per day. Applied in a variety of different ways, caloric restriction attempts to limit the number of calories an individual consumes, while still maintaining the individual's excellent health and acceptable body weight. Studies have shown that restricting caloric intake may lower breast cancer incidence[8] and that glucose restriction may impair precancerous cell growth.[9]

The factors that can cause variations in IGF-1 levels are genetic profile, age, and sex—in other words, factors over which we have no control. Lifestyle changes, such as exercise, calorie intake, and BMI, however, can influence the potentially altering effect that IGF-1 has on the cells in our bodies, thus impacting our risk for cancer. The factors that *are* within our control and can be managed through changes in our daily living, therefore, are well worth our due consideration.

Again, through exercise and reasonable caloric intake we can maintain a normal BMI—thereby lowering our concentrations of circulating IGF-1. In other words, exercise has huge benefits.

After deciding on an activity that you enjoy (see Table 8-5 for some alternatives), find a time for it in your schedule. Have appropriate clothes and accessories available so you feel comfortable in whatever type of exercise you choose. Do only as much as you can; never do more than you feel you are able to do. Stick with the routine and before you know it that routine will become a habit. Healthy habits can have a significant and amazing impact on lifestyle and one's overall sense of wellbeing. Regular exercise is a crucial part of staying healthy because it improves moods, combats chronic disease, boosts energy, promotes better sleep, and helps manage weight.

TABLE 8-5. Exercise alternatives.

Exercise alternatives
Take the stairs instead of the elevator
Go for a morning walk before your day gets going
Avoid traveling by car as much as possible
Walk to nearby places
Do housework, garden, or rake leaves
Play active games you like and join a group to play them

Rabindranath Tagore, the Nobel Peace Prize essayist, has said, "You can't cross the sea by merely standing and staring at the water." This is true with exercising as well, where a good place to start is by beginning. It keeps us fit and active, helps us live longer lives, and reduces the risk of many diseases, including cancer. Brisk walking, jogging, running, bicycling, lifting weights, aerobic dancing, belly dancing, yoga, tai chi, or kick-boxing...they're all great ways to get moving. Make sure you choose something you like to do. As I've said before, I am an avid believer that doing *something*, no matter how little, especially with respect to exercise, is better than doing nothing at all. The wonderful thing is that you can exercise in so many different ways that your regimen need never become boring or monotonous. Turn it up with music, smart clothes, and friends with whom you can share the experience. It is not an exaggeration to say that these things can provide the motivation we need to get going—and keep going. With physical exercise even a small step can make a big difference. Remember to consult your doctor before undertaking an exercise program.

Mental attitude. Having an optimistic outlook organizes and directs the mind toward wellness. As we have seen in Chapter Five, the power of the mind can be instrumental in overcoming obstacles in our lives. Adopting the practices of affirmations, meditation, and visual imagery helps keep our mind focused on health. Finding a few minutes every day to meditate allows and encourages both the body and the mind to relax. Think about designing and reciting an affirmation each day that encourages and empowers you. Remember that applying your faith daily is the impetus for true miracles to happen and that even the smallest of seeds can become the biggest of trees. And always, *always*, find the time to daydream, because what you vividly imagine can ultimately become your new reality.

Planning. Planning paves the path to achieving our goals. Planning lays down the guidelines, clears the cobwebs in our mind, and gets us to target what we need to do. If we want to attain a healthy lifestyle, it's always good to begin with a plan. Think about your day, the changes that you can make, and the aspects that you can control. In Table

8-6 you will find a list of fast-track behaviors that can help us achieve a healthy lifestyle and a better tomorrow for ourselves and our families.

TABLE 8-6. Fast track to healthy living.

Healthy behaviors	
Eat sensibly	Stay optimistic
Keep hydrated	Don't smoke
Get enough rest	Be in spirit
Move your body	Get out and socialize

Don't smoke. Forewarned, they say, is forearmed. Knowing that cancer is the second leading cause of death in the United States is, for me, enough of an incentive to forever be on the lookout for ways to reduce that risk. One of those ways is to stop smoking. Time and time again, research has shown that smoking causes cancer, specifically lung cancer, which is a greater cause of death than any other type of cancer in both men and women. So, the best advice I can give you is that if you are thinking about starting smoking, don't. And if you do smoke, think about quitting.

Cigarettes, cigars, and pipe tobacco are made from dried tobacco leaves to which flavor-enhancers are added. Four thousand or more chemicals are found in tobacco and tobacco smoke, out of which more than 60 are known carcinogens. According to the American Cancer Society, harmful compounds, such as ammonia, tar, and carbon monoxide, have all been identified in tobacco smoke. Furthermore, smoking has been shown to be a chief risk factor of atherothrombosis, a disease process characterized by atherosclerotic lesion disruption with superimposed thrombus formation, a major cause of acute coronary syndromes and cardiovascular death.

If you are now smoking and decide to stop, here again a little effort is better than none, as indicated in a study in the *Journal of the American College of Cardiology* in 2005. In their findings, researchers from the Kurume University School of Medicine in Japan undertook an experiment with 27 men who were long-term smokers.[10] During the study, some of these men refrained from smoking for a period of two weeks, while others refrained for four weeks. What researchers found was that the blood of the study's participants underwent changes within only two weeks of abstinence in the form of reduced platelet aggregation, most likely due to reduced oxidative stress. Once the participants began smoking again, their risk status returned to pre-study levels. While larger studies are needed, these researchers deduced that quitting smoking can change blood characteristics within as little as two weeks.

According to the National Cancer Institute, tobacco is considered one of the strongest cancer-causing agents. Cigarette smoking remains the leading preventable cause of death in the United States, causing an estimated 438,000 deaths, or about one out of every five, each year. In the United States, it is reported that approximately 38,000 deaths each year are caused by exposure to second-hand smoke. Lung cancer is the leading cause of cancer death among both men and women in the United States, with 90% of lung cancer deaths among men and approximately 80% of lung cancer deaths among women attributed to smoking. Smoking also increases the risk of many other types of cancer, including cancers of the throat, mouth, pancreas, kidney, bladder, and cervix. In 2007, approximately 19.8% of United States adults were cigarette smokers. Twenty-three percent of high-school students and 8% of middle-school students in this country are current cigarette smokers.[11]

Most of us are aware that regular daily exposure to certain environmental carcinogens can lead to cancer because carcinogens have the potential to damage cellular DNA. We must, therefore, take all the preventive measures we can, which includes reducing our exposure to second-hand cigarette smoke, pesticides, and many common household and garden products. In this regard, again remember: when in doubt about the products you use, *go green*. This means looking for environmentally friendly household and garden products that contain naturally occurring compounds that are safe to use because they have no known carcinogenic effects.

Cancer as virus

Viruses can facilitate the onset of some cancers and, according to the American Cancer Society, "Worldwide, infections are linked to about 15 to 20% of cancers. In the United States and other developed countries, it is thought that fewer than 10% of all cancers are linked to infectious agents. In developing countries, infections can account for as much as 20% of all cancers."[12] As early as 1911, Peyton Rous began researching the link between viruses and cancer, but it wasn't until 1966 that his investigative work in the role of viruses in the transmission of certain types of cancer awarded him the Nobel Peace Prize in Physiology or Medicine.

Viruses are organisms so small that they cannot be seen with the naked eye. They are made up of a small group of genes in the form of DNA or RNA and are surrounded by a layer of protein. Because viruses cannot reproduce on their own, they need to break through a living cell and virtually "hijack" the mechanism of the cell machinery in order to produce more viruses. Some viruses insert their own DNA (or RNA) into that of the host cell, affecting the host cell's genes. When this occurs, the cell can be "pushed" toward becoming cancerous.

Several viruses are now known or suspected of being linked to cancer in humans. Research has shown that the principal virus associated with human cancer is the human papilloma virus, known as HPV. The National Institutes of Health estimates the existence of more than 100 strains of HPV; though most are considered harmless, others are considered carcinogenic.[13] HPV is classified as either "low-risk" or "high-risk." Low-risk viruses might cause harmless warts on the skin or benign (non-cancerous) papillomas tumors. High-risk HPVs can lead to oropharyngeal cancer and cervical cancer. Sexually transmitted, high-risk HPVs include types 16, 18, 31, 33, 35, 39, 45, 51, 52, 56, 58, 59, 66, 68, and 73. HPV types 16 and 18 together cause about 70% of all cervical cancers.[13] There has been a noticeable increase in cervical cancer believed to be due to the trend for intercourse at earlier ages, unprotected sex at any age, and multiple sexual partners. The use of latex condoms has been found to be highly effective in reducing exposure to HPV, and currently two vaccines are available for the prevention of cervical cancer caused by HPV, Gardasil and Cervarix. Gardasil protects against HPV types 16 and 18, the two main types of HPVs that cause cervical cancer and against two types that cause 90% of genital warts in both females and males. Cervarix protects against HPV types 16 and 18 only.

Hepatitis, or inflammation of the liver, refers to a group of viral infections that may affect the health of the liver. The most common types are hepatitis A (HAV), hepatitis B (HBV), and hepatitis C virus (HCV). Hepatitis A appears as an acute infection, does not have a chronic stage, and is not progressive. Hepatitis B and C, on the other hand, may also begin as acute infections, but can remain in the body and result in chronic liver problems and disease. Hepatitis B and C are considered oncogenic (cancer causing) based on research that shows that chronic hepatitis B and hepatitis C virus infection is the most common risk factor for liver cancer. Over 1 million people in the United States are chronically infected with HBV, which can be transmitted by unprotected sex, intravenous drug use, the sharing of razors or toothbrushes of infected persons, and when mothers pass the virus on to their babies.[14] Each year an estimated 25,000 persons become infected with hepatitis A, 43,000 with hepatitis B, and 17,000 with hepatitis C. There are other viruses that have also been found to be cancer-causing, such as the polyomavirus, which has been extensively studied for its role in inducing tumors. The polyomavirus has also been found to induce Merkel cell carcinoma, a rare but aggressive form of skin cancer.[15]

Lifestyle has also been shown to have an effect on other cancers, such as cancer of the prostate. This type of cancer is more common in the United States than other countries; for example, as compared to Asia. Interestingly, it has been found that Asian men who migrate to the United States and adopt a Western lifestyle show a higher risk of developing prostate cancer. Diet in combination with physical activity appears to have a direct correlation to the risk of prostate cancer, where men on high-fat diets combined with a sedentary lifestyle appear to be at a higher risk and men with low-fat diets and regular exercise are at a lower risk. Recent studies have revealed that lifestyle changes not only prevent the risk of prostate cancer, but may in fact reverse it in men already affected with the disease.

For example, in 2005, researchers from the University of California studied prostate cancer patients who made changes in their diet and lifestyle. In this study, a total of 93 volunteers with serum PSAs (prostate specific antigen tests) of 4 to 10 ng/ml and cancer Gleason scores of less than seven, were randomly assigned either to an experimental group which was asked to make comprehensive lifestyle changes or to a conventional care control group where no changes were requested. Findings showed that in the experimental group, where comprehensive lifestyle changes occurred, PSAs decreased by 4%, while in the conventional care group PSAs increased by 6%. Researchers concluded that intensive lifestyle changes may affect the progression of early, low-grade prostate cancer in men.[16]

Some families show higher trends for cancer than others. Having the same type of cancers, having rare cancers, or developing cancer before the age of 50 are some, but not all, of the indicators that show that cancer may be inherited. There are many different causes of cancer, however, so know that having a certain gene does not mean in any definitive way that you will develop cancer. In fact, only about 5 to 10% of all cancers are thought to be caused by inherited genes. If you do have a family history of cancer, there are numerous agencies, clinics, and hospitals that provide information and perform screenings and risk assessment. If you are adopted or don't have a detailed family history, try not to worry. Remember that changes to your lifestyle may have more of an effect on your cancer risk than your genes.

Obesity. Obesity has become epidemic in this country. Studies have shown that obese children develop more diseases than children who are at their ideal weight. Many kids are spending less time exercising and more time on the computer, watching TV, or videogaming. It seems every family is busy, and as a result, there are few free moments to prepare nutritious, home-cooked meals. Unhealthy lifestyles begun at a young age have a direct impact on health later in life. If we instill good habits in our children, they will certainly enjoy healthier tomorrows. Table 8-7 provides a good overall list of the things we can do that will best help us get started on the path to healthy living.

TABLE 8-7. Positive lifestyle changes.

Changing your lifestyle
Define your goal
Identify the factors needing change
Introduce the factors that are absent
Eliminate the factors that are undesirable
Begin a schedule to implement these changes

Living healthy starts with making conscious choices about the food we eat. This begins with what kinds of food we purchase in the supermarket. Most of us consider shopping for food as simply *shopping for food.* But the more thought you put into the process beforehand, the better your choices will be. Good health begins with fundamentally sound food shopping. If you buy junk you will feel like junk. If you buy good food you will feel good. It is that simple. Table 8-8 lists some of my own "Dos and Don'ts" for food shopping.

TABLE 8-8. Dr. Doug's "dos and don'ts" shopping guide.

Do...	Don't...
Make a shopping list and stick to it	Buy in a hurry
Read labels and nutrition facts	Skip reading labels and contents
Buy whole-grain breads and cereals	Buy foods with added preservatives and additives
Shop the outside aisle first, where the fresh fruits and vegetables are	Buy instant food
Look for low-fat or non-fat dairy products	Buy breads and cereal made with refined flour
Buy healthy snacks	Buy over-processed food
Make interesting, healthy recipe choices	Shop when hungry

Not only is eating the right food important, but having a kitchen equipped with the correct utensils to process the food is also essential. What good would having the right paint be without the proper canvas, easel, palette, and brushes? Table 8-9 outlines my suggestions for a well-stocked kitchen.

TABLE 8-9. Dr. Doug's well-stocked kitchen.

Kitchen helpers
Steamer
Wok
Sharpened knives
Clean cutting board
Food processor
Peeler
Stainless steel pots and pans; no aluminum or non-stick
Juicer

Cooking safety and hygiene are other areas where we can make improvements (see Table 8-10). Eliminate the use of anodized aluminum cookware and Teflon-coated cookware. Trace amounts of aluminum have been detected in foods where aluminum cookware is used to cook the food, and there is unsubstantiated, but ongoing, research that high-aluminum content has been found in the brains of people with Alzheimer's disease. Non-stick pans are coated with Teflon, a product accidentally invented by a Dupont chemist more than 65 years ago. A chemical present in Teflon known as perfluorooctanoic acid, or PFOA, has been shown to cause cancer in laboratory animals and is estimated to be found in the blood of 90% of all Americans.[17] This chemical, now being classified as similar to mercury and lead, is a toxin that remains in the body for indefinite periods of time. To correct this situation, in a voluntary pact undertaken in 2006, the United States Environmental Protection Agency and eight major companies launched the 2010/15 PFOA Stewardship Program which is committed to the total elimination of PFOAs from emissions and products by 2015.[18]

TABLE 8-10. Cooking safety and hygiene.

Eating Well
Use cookware with non-reactive surfaces
Avoid toxic aluminum and non-stick cookware
Microwave only as a last resort; microwaves cause destructive chemical and structural changes in food
Check your knives for wear and rust; dry before storing and store separately from silverware
Use a clean cutting board without food residue
Use a food processor and juicer; keep clean and dry
Use a heavy-bottomed and steel wok
A good freezer is a must; thaw in a refrigerator only those foods you intend to use that day
Do not re-freeze thawed food
Stock up your refrigerator on a frequent basis to maintain produce freshness and prevent fruits and vegetables from going bad
Maximize the use of your steamer
Bag your produce separately
Wash fruits and vegetables thoroughly before using
Keep garbage bins clean and empty them regularly
Keep refrigerator clean of spills and residue

Cooking at home. Many people these days spend more time at work or in traffic then they do in the kitchen. As a result, busier lives can contribute to the majority of the population's bigger waistlines. This is why the more we can eat at, or from, home, the more control we have as to what goes on the plate. Home-cooking is just not a matter of eating the right foods, but also knowing how to prepare these foods in ways that will ensure they maintain their nutritional benefits. Careful decision-making about cooking techniques has an enormous impact on the nutrient content of the foods we prepare. Planning ahead, therefore, prevents last minute, impulsive fast-food purchases on the run. Most people would like to move in this direction, but don't know where to start. Here are some general suggestions.

Here are some general suggestions. For example, let's say you'd like to plan your breakfast for tomorrow, maybe an egg white on toast with some green tea. After dinner the night before, separate the egg white from the yolk and properly store the egg white in the refrigerator. Put a green tea bag into a travel mug. Put a cooking pan on the stove with the vegetable spray, spatula, and foil (for wrapping the egg in the morning), alongside the pan on the counter. This way, when you wake up, you simply spray the pan, take the egg white out of the refrigerator, pour the egg white into the pan, cook until done, and add the bread. Voilà! Your healthy breakfast is made in less than three minutes. If you cook your egg at the same time you bring your water to a boil, you're ready to fill your travel mug with the green tea bag. In a few short minutes you're all set. Quick, easy, healthy, and ready to go!

The same applies to lunch, if you can muster up enough energy at the end of your day to create something healthy and appealing. Make a lean turkey, lettuce, and tomato wrap, for example, which stores well and stays fresh in food wrap in the refrigerator overnight. In the morning you can add a couple of pieces of fruit. As for dinner, the same applies. If your pots and lids are already out on the stove, non-refrigerated ingredients are on the counter, and the table is already set from the night before (or from that morning, if you have time), you'll be giving yourself the gift of one less thing to do after your busy day. Planning, organizing, and expediting ensure that you can eat healthfully every single day.

The American Institute for Cancer Research, an organization that focuses on nutrition and cancer, understands the need for home cooking strategies. To help people make conscious choices, AICR has published a "how to" guide filled with ideas. The guide is called *Recipe Makeovers—Homemade for Health*. This brochure is one of a series that explains how to prepare foods that give you the most health protection from cancer and other diseases. It contains everything from choosing the right foods to recipes for their preparation. For those who are ready to go to the next level in learning and trying more ideas, AICR's *New American Plate Cookbook* contains 200 recipes, complete with color photographs of many healthy dishes. All the recipes illustrated are delicious, appealing, and, most importantly, cancer-fighting.

Some general rules for cooking at home are listed in Table 8-11.

TABLE 8-11. Rules for cooking at home.

Cooking at home
Use low-fat cooking methods
Steam vegetables
Serve nutrient-rich low-calorie foods first
Broil or bake meat and fish
Serve nutrient-rich snacks
Limit sweet juices
Go easy on toppings and sauces
Substitute spices for salt

Eating in restaurants. Healthy eating need not be something we do solely at home. In fact, more and more choices are being made available in restaurants so that we can eat more healthfully in those settings as well. Since restaurants offer a wider variety of items from which to choose, however, we may have to work harder to avoid temptation. The best way to stay on course is to plan the same way you do at home and to look for the healthiest alternatives available on the restaurant's menu. If healthy alternatives are not readily available, here are some basic guidelines to follow (see Table 8-12):

TABLE 8-12. Making good eating choices.

The right choices
Read detailed descriptions in menu
Check ingredients
Inquire about cooking methods
Concentrate on salads, grains, and vegetables
Ask for sauces and dressings on the side and use sparingly
Order low-fat desserts

Spirituality

Part of any lifestyle is embracing spirituality in daily living. As with the topics of faith and prayer, spirituality can mean different things to different people, and appreciating that fact is important to any discussion on the subject. For some it may be a process of self-discovery; in other words, learning who you are and who you want to be. For some it might be the process of connecting to ourselves and the world. Spirituality can be seen as a call to reach beyond current limitations and beliefs, to get to that next level of growth, or to find meaning, purpose, and direction. It might also be seen as the basis for building a bridge between our essence and a higher power. For some, spirituality might be the pursuit of being one with God or understanding oneself; for others, it is the dawning of enlightenment to guide humanity toward the right and better-organized path. Whatever you believe, however, the incorporation of some type of spirituality in one's life can be a critical component for leading a healthy life.

Incorporating a healthy lifestyle can in and of itself be considered a spiritual way of living. Spirituality can mean discovering inner peace in your life and sharing it with those around you. For me, spirituality entails a general attitude of caring and taking responsibility for my own and others' wellbeing. It is that component which provides direction to life in tough times as well as in all other times. It has been said that there is no mantra higher than meditation, and no worship higher than inner pursuit...and that with these two factors as the driving force, contentment soon follows. I tend to agree in that the pursuit of a spiritually-based existence allows for an ever greater awareness, and heightening awareness enables us to connect with an element which is bigger than self to define our own meaning and purpose. Spirituality establishes a dynamic, progressive, integrative process, which can only encourage and lead us to improved health and wellness.

Below are some simple steps to incorporate spirituality into one's daily life.

Have a forgiving nature. Grudges are like toxins that need to be flushed out of the body to enjoy healthy living. Holding a grudge does nothing but build discontent and anger, an attitude that eventually affects our health and wellbeing—sometimes irrevocably. Forgiveness can liberate the other individual as well as oneself. Both forgiving someone and asking for forgiveness are the hallmark traits of a person of strong spiritual character.

Show gratitude. Being grateful for all that we have by appreciating the gifts of God goes a long way toward increasing our sense of wellbeing. Whether you consider yourself a religious person or not, whether you are a believer in God or not, practicing gratitude washes away feelings of negativity and brings good into your life. A feeling of gratitude can change the way you look at the world and can awaken your senses. Something as simple as thanking God (or the universe at large) for being able to rise in the morning, to go about our daily chores, and eat our meals—in essence, to live our lives—inevitably inculcates a sense of wellbeing and peace.

The act of giving and receiving. I ask myself if my nature is one that gives selflessly and receives with grace. If I can answer yes, then I know my nature is one that can live with contentment. Offering of yourself to someone else, whether it is your love, understanding, time, or material aid, means giving a part of yourself, and giving of yourself increases your own wellbeing, whether you know it or not at the time. Helping an ailing neighbor or sharing a cup of tea with a friend to offer an empathetic shoulder is an act of reciprocity that helps us feel good in a way that buying something never can. Having a friend with whom you share time and energy can engender feelings of gratitude and happiness, but practicing the art of giving and receiving can help us achieve ultimate contentment even in solitude.

Have the ability to appreciate. Appreciation is as much about appreciating our lives and other people as it is about appreciating ourselves. Appreciation acts as a tremendous source of inspiration and energy booster for the person being acknowledged, but giving appreciation also has a positive impact on those who supply the praise. Giving and receiving appreciation is an art in itself, and being generous in our words of appreciation always furthers feelings of creative goodwill.

Have a compassionate nature. Compassion is an emotion that inspires empathy. When we feel compassion, our heart echoes the pain felt by others, and as a result, we can understand their feelings with heartfelt sensitivity. This can help us provide better assistance to those in need and instill feelings of fulfillment for having taken a step to help them.

Respect the inviolability of life. When we approach life with a high level of respect and appreciation, we seem to move toward a greater sense of spirituality as well. As we proceed, we often find our energy gains momentum and we effortlessly move in a more fruitful direction. As a result, the foundation of our thoughts can become blessings that bestow goodness and faith.

Be "social." As discussed, when we talk about socialization we usually mean the way we learn to live within our culture and community and the benefits derived from that way of life. When it is positive, pleasurable and motivational, socializing furthers our education, broadens our horizons, brings happiness, and introduces feelings of wellbeing. Recognizing that we all have something to offer, the act of socializing can be just what we need to transform our attitudes and outlook.

Getting out of the house and being in the presence of others is a great start to receiving the benefits of being social. Exploring your environs is one way to experience the social aspects of your community, so even if you don't talk to anyone, just being "out" helps you stay in contact with the world. It is too easy to hang out at home with remote in hand or computer on…so get out and about, experience the weather, your community, events, and so on. Most towns have great places to eat, intimate places to hear music, and fun seasonal events, and being part of something bigger than yourself increases your odds of climbing out of a rut and meeting new people.

Rest. A good night's sleep, just like proper diet and exercise, is an essential component to our physical, mental, and emotional health. We know that we spend almost a third of our life sleeping and that sleeping enough and sleeping well are key elements for staying healthy and achieving a sense of wellbeing. Therefore, it naturally follows that a sleep-deprived body means a decreased quality of life and negatively impacted health. Inadequate sleep not only disrupts mental health, but also leads to physiological imbalances as well. An Irish proverb sums it up very well: "A good laugh and a long sleep are the best cures in the doctor's book." In Table 8-13 you will find some suggestions for a healthy night's sleep.

TABLE 8-13. Sleeping well.

Getting a good night's sleep
Adhere to a routine for sleeping and waking to facilitate repair and recovery of body functions
Avoid eating just prior to bedtime, as digesting at night requires energy and can make you feel more tired the next day
Eat fruit
Avoid caffeine
Avoid alcohol
Get to bed on time
Use the bathroom right before bedtime
Avoid drugs or reduce intake of drugs just prior to sleep
Maintain correct body weight, as obesity may increase the risk of sleep apnea
Avoid TV in the bedroom, as it stimulates the brain and makes it difficult to fall asleep
Sleep in complete darkness or as close to darkness as possible
Use an eye mask if complete darkness is not possible
Listen to relaxation CDs

(continued on next page)

Avoid electromagnetic fields, such as radio frequencies, in the bedroom
Use an alarm with a soothing sound as opposed to a harsh, jolting sound
Keep bedroom temperature between 60 to 70° F.
Take a warm bath to relax the body and induce sleep
Avoid working in the bedroom and on the bed
Try listening to soothing music which has a relaxing affect
Keep alarm clocks and other electrical devices a minimum of 3 feet away from the bed
Exercise regularly to get better sleep, but don't exercise just prior to bedtime
Try wearing socks to bed; cold feet can keep you up
Read something spiritual or religious before sleep
If your mind is still working, jot your thoughts down and try to sleep again
Try melatonin, an over-the-counter hormone supplement, to improve sleep if behavioral changes don't help
Try eating a snack rich in protein several hours before bed; this can improve the production of melatonin and serotonin essential for good sleep
Avoid foods that cause allergies and sensitivities
Wind up work well before bedtime

Health begins at birth and has to be maintained to the best of our abilities all through life. To that end, making lifestyle changes as outlined in this chapter results in positive changes in mind, body, and spirit. But changes do not just happen; you and you alone must be and live the change. So, imagine, investigate, and implement. Your health will thank you for it. As Ronnie Kaye, author of *Spinning Straw into Gold: Your Emotional Recovery from Breast Cancer*, says, "Learn to make your recovery your first priority."[19]

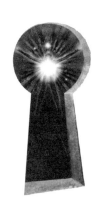

9. Food for Thought

Quotations are fragments of human expression that we use as evidence or illustrations of our own ideas and thoughts. They can serve as support in our daily lives and offer fresh voices of inspiration to invoke introspective thought. I have always enjoyed reading quotes to help me gain a new perspective on life and to help lift me out of the doldrums into which I occasionally fall. Quotes are simple ways to remind me that other people have been through similar situations and have responded in ways that can put me back on my continued journey toward health.

Short notes of wisdom, proverbs, idioms, and phrases can be great sources for awakening. The quotes in the following section relate to daily living, health, wellbeing, physical and mental fitness, friendship, and serenity. They have all been a great source of encouragement and inspiration to me on my journey. I hope they will be the same for you.

Living a king-sized life

Life is just a chance to grow a soul. (A. Powell Davies, 1902–1957, minister)

And in the end, it's not the years in your life that count, it's the life in your years. (Abraham Lincoln, 1809–1865, former president of the United States)

If one could see the miracle of a single flower, one's whole life would change. (Buddha, 563 B.C.–483 B.C., spiritual teacher)

Happiness is the meaning and the purpose of life, the whole aim and end of human existence. (Aristotle, 384–322 B.C., Greek philosopher)

There are two ways to live your life. One is as though nothing is a miracle, and the other is as though everything is a miracle. (Albert Einstein, 1879–1955, physicist)

Laughter: The best medicine

Nobody ever dies of laughter. (Sir Max Beerbohm, 1872–1956, English parodist and caricaturist)

Humor is mankind's greatest blessing. Against the assault of laughter nothing can stand. (Mark Twain, 1835–1910, author)

Cheerfulness is the best promoter of health and is as friendly to the mind as to the body. (Joseph Addison, 1672–1719, English essayist and poet)

Hearty laughter is a good way to jog internally without having to go outdoors. (Norman Cousins, 1915–1990, prominent political journalist, author, professor, and world-peace advocate)

Cheers to health

A wise man should consider that health is the greatest of human blessings, and learn how by his own thought to derive benefit from his illnesses." (Hippocrates, 460–77 B.C., Greek physician)

Nothing will benefit human health and increase the chances for survival of life on earth as much as the evolution to a vegetarian diet. (Albert Einstein)

True enjoyment comes from activity of the mind and exercise of the body; the two are ever united. (Karl Wilhelm von Humboldt, 1769–1859, German naturalist and explorer)

While we may not be able to control all that happens to us, we can control what happens inside us. (Benjamin Franklin, 1706–1770, satirist and politician)

If we could give every individual the right amount of nourishment and exercise, not too little and not too much, we would have found the safest way to health; and

Walking is man's best medicine. (Hippocrates)

Do something everyday that you don't want to do; this is the golden rule for acquiring the habit of doing your duty without pain. (Mark Twain)

When it comes to eating right and exercising there is no "I'll start tomorrow." Tomorrow is disease. (V. L. Allineare, dates unknown)

Those who think they have no time for bodily exercise will sooner or later have to find time for illness. (Edward Stanley, 1799–1869, English statesman and three-time prime minister of the UK)

Hopeful always

We must accept finite disappointment but never lose infinite hope. (Martin Luther King, Jr., 1929–1968, clergyman and civil rights activist)

Most of the important things in the world have been accomplished by people who have kept on trying when there seemed to be no hope at all. (Dale Carnegie, 1988–1955, American writer and lecturer)

The pessimist sees difficulty in every opportunity. The optimist sees the opportunity in every difficulty. (Winston Churchill, 1874–1965, English politician, statesman, and Nobel Peace Prize winner)

Learn from yesterday, live for today and hope for tomorrow. (Albert Einstein)

Hope is both the earliest and the most indispensable virtue inherent in the state of being alive. If life is to be sustained hope must remain even where confidence is wounded, trust impaired. (Eric H. Erikson, 1902–1994, developmental psychologist)

Dynamic faith

Faith has to do with things that are not seen and hope with things that are not at hand. (Saint Thomas Aquinas, 1225–1274, Italian philosopher and theologian)

He who has faith…has an inward reservoir of courage, hope, confidence, calmness and assuring trust that all will come out well —even though to the world it may appear to come out most badly. (B. C. Forbes, 1880–1954, reporter and writer)

Faith in one's self is the best and safest course. (Michelangelo, 1475–1564, Italian Renaissance painter, sculptor,architect, poet, and engineer)

Faith is a living, daring confidence in God's grace so sure and certain that a man could stake his life on it a thousand times. (Martin Luther, 1483–1546, German monk, theologian, and university professor)

There is nothing that wastes the body like worry, and one who has any faith in God should be ashamed to worry about anything whatsoever. (Mahatma Gandhi, 1869–1948, political and spiritual leader)

Wellbeing forever

Wellbeing is attained by little and little, and nevertheless is no little thing itself. (Zeno of Citium, 333 B.C.–264 B.C., founder of the Stoic school of philosophy)

The simplification of life is one of the steps to inner peace. A persistent simplification will create an inner and outer well-being…. (Peace Pilgrim. From 1953 to 1981 a silver-haired woman, calling herself only "Peace Pilgrim," walked more than 25,000 miles on a personal pilgrimage for peace.)

Everyday, in every way, I am getting better and better. (Émile Coué, 1857–1926, French psychologist and pharmacist)

It is now well understood that humans ultimately depend on the health of the planet for their well-being. (Peter Garret, 1953–, Australian politician and musician)

I define joy as a sustained sense of well being and internal peace—a connection to what matters. (Oprah Winfrey, 1954–, actress and talk-show host)

Winning over disease

He who cures a disease may be the skillfullest, but he that prevents it is the safest physician. (Thomas Fuller, 1608–1661, English churchman and historian)

Every human being is the author of his own health or disease. (Buddha)

Natural forces within us are the true healers of disease. (Hippocrates, 460–370 B.C., Greek physician)

Your lifestyle—how you live, eat, emote and think—determine your health. To prevent disease you may have to change how you live. (Brian Carter, dates unknown, singer and songwriter)

The good physician treats the disease; the great physician treats the patient who has the disease. (William Osler, 1849–1919, Canadian physician)

Our way is not soft grass, it's a mountain path with lots of rocks. But it goes upward, forward, towards the sun. (Ruth "Dr. Ruth" Westheimer, 1928–, author and psychologist)

If you want to know if your brain is flabby, feel your legs. (Bruce Barton, 1886–1967, author, advertising executive, and politician)

One step at a time is good walking. (Chinese proverb)

If I am walking with two other men, each of them I will serve as my teacher. I will pick out the good points of the one and imitate them and the bad points of the other and correct them in myself. (Confucius, 551 B.C.–479 B.C., Chinese philosopher)

Connecting with spirituality

The great awareness comes slowly, piece by piece; the path of spiritual growth is a path of lifelong learning. The experience of spiritual power is a joyful one. (M. Scott Peck, 1936–2005, author and psychiatrist)

There are no accidents...there is only some purpose that we haven't yet understood. (Deepak Chopra, 1946–, author)

Happiness cannot be traveled to, owned, earned, worn or consumed. Happiness is a spiritual experience of living every minute with love, grace and gratitude. (Denis Waitley, 1933–, writer and motivational speaker)

To keep a lamp burning, we must keep putting oil in it. (Mother Teresa, 1910–1997, missionary)

The spirit of man is the candle of the Lord. (Proverbs 20:27)

God is great. (Unknown)

God has entrusted me with myself. (Epictetus, ca. 55–ca. 135, Greek Stoic philosopher)

God is at home, it's we who have gone out for a walk. (Meister Eckhart, 1260–1328, German theologian, philosopher, and mystic)

In his will is our peace. (Dante Alighieri, 1265–1321, Italian author of The Divine Comedy)

God can only do for you what he can do through you. (Eric Butterworth, 1916–2003, author, theologian, and philosopher)

I found thee not, O Lord, without, because I erred in seeking thee without that wert within. (Saint Augustine, 354–430, philosopher and theologian)

Secrets of success

We were born to succeed, not to fail. (Henry David Thoreau, 1817–1862, naturalist, philosopher, and author)

The greatest weakness lies in giving up. The most certain way to succeed is to try just one more time. (Thomas Edison, 1847–1931, inventor)

The key to success is to focus our conscious mind on things we desire, not things we fear. (Brian Tracy, 1944–, Canadian author and speaker)

Eighty percent of success is showing up. (Woody Allen, 1935–, actor and director)

Success is more a function of consistent common sense than it is of genius. (An Wang, 1920–1990, inventor and cofounder of Wang Laboratories)

Motivation marches ahead

People often say that motivation does not last. Well, neither does bathing—that's why it is recommended daily. (Zig Ziglar, 1926–, motivational speaker)

All we are is the result of what we have thought. (Buddha)

Do not go where the path may lead, go instead where there is no path and leave a trail. (Ralph Waldo Emerson, 1803–1882, American lecturer, essayist, and poet)

Twenty years from now you will be more disappointed by the things that you didn't do than by the ones you did do. So throw off the bowlines. Sail away from the safe harbor. Catch the trade winds in your sails. Explore. Dream. Discover. (Mark Twain)

You see things; and you say, "Why?" But I dream things that never were; and I say, "Why not?" (George Bernard Shaw, 1856–1950, Irish playwright)

Lifestyle tips

A man too busy to take care of his health is like a mechanic too busy to take care of his tools. (Spanish proverb)

Fresh air impoverishes the doctor. (Danish proverb)

He who takes medicines and neglects to diet wastes the skill of his doctors. (Chinese proverb)

The more severe the pain or illness, the more severe will be the necessary changes. These may involve breaking bad habits, or acquiring some new better ones. (Peter McWilliams, 1949–2000, writer, activist)

Lifestyle intervention requires discipline with a tangible end result that is within reach. It requires personal resolve and a life-long commitment. (Tim Holden, 1957–, American politician)

Destined to fate

If you can't change your fate, change your attitude. (Amy Tan, 1952–, author)

When one door of happiness closes, another opens. (Helen Keller, 1880–1968, author and activist)

Our deeds determine us, as much as we determine our deeds. (George Eliot, 1819–1880, English novelist)

Our fate, whatever it is to be, will be overcome by patience under it. (Virgil, 70 B.C.–19 B.C., Classical Roman poet)

A good head and a good heart are always a formidable combination. (Nelson Mandela, 1918–, former president of South Africa and winner of 1993 Nobel Peace Prize)

Meditation for peace

Plant the seed of meditation and reap the fruit of peace of mind. (Remez Sasson, dates unknown, author and teacher)

Meditation brings wisdom and lack of it leaves ignorance. Know well what leads you forward and what hold you back and choose the path that leads to wisdom. (Buddha)

Empty your mind, be formless, shapeless—like water. Now you put water into a cup, it becomes a cup, you put water into a bottle, it becomes a bottle, you put it in a teapot, it becomes the teapot. Now water can flow or it can crash. Be water, my friend. (Bruce Lee, 1940–1973, actor and martial arts expert)

Prayer is when you talk to God. Meditation is when you listen to God. (Diana Robinson, dates unknown, musician)

Meditation is the tongue of the soul and the language of our spirit. (Jeremy Taylor, 1613–1667, English clergyman and author)

Valuable friendship

Don't walk in front of me, I may not follow. Don't walk behind me, I may not lead. Walk beside me and be my friend. (Albert Camus, 1913–1960, French author, philosopher, and journalist)

The only way to have a friend is to be one. (Ralph Waldo Emerson, 1803–1882, poet)

Friendship with oneself is all important because without it one cannot be friends with anyone else in the world. (Eleanor Roosevelt, 1884–1962, former First Lady of the United States)

What is a friend? A single soul in two bodies. (Aristotle, 384–322 B.C., Greek philosopher)

I find friendship is like wine, raw when new, ripened with age, the true old man's milk and restorative cordial. (Thomas Jefferson, 1743–1826, third president of the United States)

Serenity for the soul

Serenity is not freedom from the storm, but peace amid the storm. (Unknown)

Cheerfulness keeps up a kind of daylight in the mind, filling it with a steady and perpetual serenity. (Joseph Addison, 1672–1719, English essayist and poet)

Boredom is the feeling that everything is a waste of time, serenity that nothing is. (Thomas Szasz, 1920–, psychiatrist and academic)

Nothing can bring you peace but yourself. (Ralph Waldo Emerson)

God grant me the serenity to accept the things I cannot change; the courage to change the things I can, and the wisdom to know the difference. (Reinhold Niebuhr, 1892–1971, theologian)

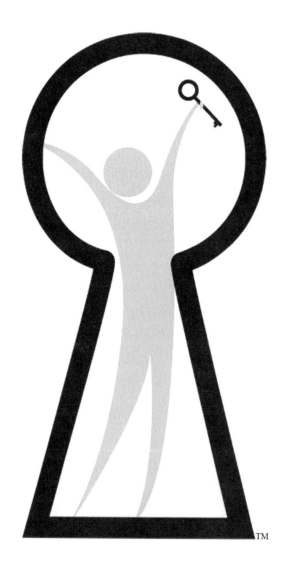

™

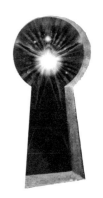

Epilogue

Whether you are recovering from cancer, looking to avert a recurrence, or have the full intention of preventing it altogether, it helps to understand that health is never just one thing. "Health," as conveyed throughout this book, is brought about through a combination of physical, mental, social, and spiritual elements and efforts, and it is this total approach that lowers the risk of getting cancer. How? By increasing one of the body's key capabilities for staying healthy: *the ability of the body to defend itself.*

The body defends itself by having the ability to fight. It defends itself by having the innate resourcefulness to recognize when something is wrong, so that immediate, sustained action can be taken to resolve it. And it is when the body is strong enough to fight that you are in a better position to win.

Building better defenses means making better choices in our daily living—in all areas of life—in our food choices, physical activity levels, social settings, mental attitudes, and spiritual awareness. You can know with certainty from everything you've learned in this book that it is by taking these responsible steps, rather than by leaving things to chance, that you will be led towards a healthier self. Remember, not only do you have a say in what happens, but you have the ability to act and to change what happens as well.

While it is true that making these kinds of lifestyle changes could very well make you feel different from those around you, it is also true that these changes will only continue to evolve a healthier union between you, your inner self, and the universe of which you are a part.

Above all, you will know that you now have the answer—*the answer to cancer.*

References

INTRODUCTION

1. Haylock, P. J. et al. 2006. The Shifting Paradigm of Cancer Care, American Journal of Nursing 106(3):16–19.

CHAPTER 1: The Story Behind the Story (no references)

CHAPTER 2: Health Now and Forever

1. http://www.cancer.org/Healthy/EatHealthyGetActive/ACSGuidelinesonNutritionPhysicalActivityfor CancerPrevention/acs-guidelines-on-nutrition-and-physical-activity-for-cancer-prevention-intro. Retrieved 12/10.
2. http://www.cancer.org/acs/groups/cid/documents/webcontent/002577-pdf.pdf. Retrieved 12/10.
3. http://www.nhlbi.nih.gov/guidelines/obesity/prctgd_c.pdf. Retrieved 12/10.
4. http://www.cancer.gov/cancertopics/factsheet/Risk/obesity. Retrieved 12/10.
5. Petrelli, J. M., et al. 2002. Body mass index, height, and postmenopausal breast cancer mortality in a prospective cohort of U.S. women. Cancer Causes and Control 13(4):325–332.
6. Calle, E. et al. 2003. Overweight, obesity, and mortality from cancer in a prospectively studied cohort of U.S. adults. NEJM, Volume 348(17):1625–1638.
7. Li, A. et al. 2006. Effect of obesity on survival in epithelial ovarian cancer, Cancer 107:1520–1524.
8. Strom, S. et al. 2005. Obesity, weight gain, and risk of biochemical failure among prostate cancer patients following prostatectomy. Clinical Cancer Research. 11:6889.
9. Astin, J. A. et al. 2004. Mind-body therapies for the management of pain. Clin J Pain 20(1):27–32.
10. Zsombok, T. et al. 2003. Effect of autogenic training on drug consumption in patients with primary headache: An 8-month follow-up study. Headache 43(3):251–7.
11. Walker, L. G. et al. 1999. Psychological, clinical and pathological effects of relaxation, training, and guided imagery during primary chemotherapy. British Journal of Cancer 80:262–268.
12. World Federation of Chiropractic. http://www.wfc.org.
13. Toy, J. 2005. Cancer Research UK, BBC. News. http://news.bB.C..co.uk/1/hi/health/4490271.stm
14. Journal of the National Cancer Institute. 2008 100(23):1672–1694.
15. American Association for Cancer Research. http://www.aacr.org/home/public--media/science-policy-- government-affairs/aacr-cancer-policy-monitor/aacr-cancer-policy-monitor-january/cancer-to-become- worlds-deadliest-disease.aspx. Retrieved 12/09.
16. Rosen, E. et al. 2006. BRCA1 and BRCA2 as molecular targets for phytochemicals indole-3-carbinol and genistein in breast and prostate cancer cells. British Journal of Cancer 94, 407–426.
17. Liu, R. H., et al. 2004. Potential synergy of phytochemicals in cancer prevention: Mechanism of action. Journal of Nutrition 134:3479S–3485S.
18. Byers, T., et al. 2002. Reducing the risk of cancer with healthy food choices and physical activity. CA Cancer J Clin 52:92.
19. Johnson, F. M., et al. 2002. How many food additives are rodent carcinogens? Environ Mol Mutagen 39(1):69–80.
20. McCann, D., et al. 2007. Food additives and hyperactive behaviour in 3-year-old and 8/9-year-old children in the community: a randomised, double-blinded, placebo-controlled trial. The Lancet 370(9598):1560–7.
21. Beating the Food Giants, Paul Stitt, Natural Press, 1993.
22. http://www.extension.umn.edu/distribution/nutrition/DJ0974.html. Retrieved 12/09.
23. World Health Organization. Health implications of acrylamide in food. Joint FAO/WHO consultation, Geneva, Switzerland, 25–27 June 2002. ISBN: 02 4 156218 8. http://www.who.int/foodsafety/ publications/chem/acrylamide_june2002/en/.
24. Cornell University, Northeast Regional Food Guide Newsletter, October, 2004.

25. Alavanja, M., et al. 2003. use of agricultural pesticides and prostate cancer risk in the agricultural health study cohort. American J of Epidem 157(9).
26. Zahm, S. H., et al. 1998. Pesticides and childhood cancer. Environ Health Perspect 106(Suppl 3):893–908.

CHAPTER 3: The Truth about Cancer

1. World Cancer Report, 2003. World Health Organization (http://www.who,int/mediacentre/news/releases/2003/pr27/en/.) Retrieved 12/10.
2. CRS Report for Congress. Life Expectancy in the United States. Congressional Research Service, The Library of Congress. Updated August 16, 2006.
3. U.S. National Center for Health Statistics, National Vital Statistics Reports (NVSR), Deaths: Final Data for 2006, Vol. 57, No. 14, April 17, 2000.
4. Centers for Disease Control and Prevention (http://www.cdc.gov/nchs/FASTATS/lcod.htm). Retrieved 08/10.
5. Area Socioeconomic Variations in U.S. Cancer Incidence, Mortality, Stage, Treatment, and Survival, 1975–1999. 2003. Journal of the National Cancer Institute 95(19):1431–1433.
6. American Cancer Society. Cancer Facts & Figures for African Americans 2009–2010.
7. American Cancer Society. Surveillance and Health Policy Research, 2010. Retrieved 08/10.
8. SEER Program, Division of Cancer Control and Population Sciences, National Cancer Institute, 2005, at http://www.caonline.amcancersoc.org/cgi/content/full/56/2/106I.
9. National Cancer Institute SEER Program. http://seer.cancer.gov/statfacts/html/all.html Retrieved 08/10.
10. SEER Program, Division of Cancer Control and Population Sciences, National Cancer Institute. http://www.naaccr.org/index.asp?Col_SectionKey=11&Col_ContentID=50. Retrieved 08/10.
11. Cancer Research UK. http://info.cancerresearchuk.org/cancerstats/world/. Retrieved 08/10.
12. World Health Organization Tobacco Health Toll. http://www.emro.who.int/TFI/PDF/TobaccoHealthToll.pdf. 08/10.
13. Meyerhardt, J. et al. 2007. Association of dietary patterns with cancer recurrence and survival in patients with stage III colon cancer . JAMA 298:754–64.
14. Lewin, M. H. et al. 2006. Red meat enhances the colonic formation of the DNA adduct O6-carboxymethyl guanine: Implications for colorectal cancer risk. Cancer Res 66:1859–1865.
15. Chao, A. et al. 2005. Meat consumption and risk of colorectal cancer. JAMA 293:172–182.
16. Cho, E. et al. 2006. Red meat intake and risk of breast cancer among premenopausal women. Arch Intern Med 166:2253–2259.
17. 10th Report on Carcinogens. NIH. http://www.ntp-server.niehs.nih.gov. Retrieved 08/10.
18. International Agency for Research on Cancer. World Health Organization. http://monographs.iarc.fr/. Retrieved 07/10.
19. Green This! Volume I: Greening Your Cleaning, Diedre Imus. Simon and Schuster, 2007.
20. Susan G. Komen For The Cure. http://ww5.komen.org/BreastCancer/BreastCancerRiskFactorsTable.htmlnce. Retrieved 12/09.
21. BMI Calculator, NHLBI Obesity Education Initiative, 1998. National Institutes of Health, at http://www.nhlbi.nih.gov, Retrieved 12/08.
22. Sprague, B. L. et al. 2007. Lifetime recreational and occupational physical activity and risk of in situ and invasive breast cancer. Cancer Epid Bio & Prev 16:236–243.
23. Leitzmann, M. F. et al. 2008. Prospective study of physical activity and risk of postmenopausal breast cancer. Breast Cancer Research 10:R92.
24. National Cancer Institute. http://www.cancer.gov/cancertopics/factsheet/prevention/physicalactivity. Retrieved 12/09.
25. SEER Cancer Statistics Review, Surveillance Epidemiology and End Results program (NCI SEER). 2003–2007. National Cancer Institute, Cancer Stat Fact Sheets. http://seer.cancer.gov/statfacts. Retrieved 08/10.
26. American Cancer Society. Cancer Facts & Figures, 2010.
27. Hansen, J. 1998. Common cancers in the elderly. Drugs Aging 13(6):467–78.
28. http://www.ncbi.nlm.nih.gov/pubmed/9883401. Retrieved 12/10.
29. U.S. Census Bureau. www.census.gov. Retrieved 08/10.
30. Erikson, C., et al. 2007. Future supply and demand for oncologists : Challenges to assuring access to oncology services. Journal of Oncology Practice 3(2):79–86.

31. Katikireddi, V. et al. 2004. 100,000 children die needlessly from cancer every year. BMJ 328;422.
32. Colditz, G. A. (Editor) and Hunter, D. J. (Editor). *Cancer Prevention: The causes and prevention of cancer, Volume 1*, Kwuler Academic Publishers, 2000.
33. OECD (Organization for Economic Co-Operation and Development). http://www.oecd.org. Retrieved 08/10.
34. PhRMA. Report on 750 new medicines in development for cancer. PhRMA 2008. http://www.phrma.org/files/attachments/09-046PhRMACancer09_0331.pdf. Retrieved 08/10.
35. National Institutes of Health. http://www.cancer.gov. Retrieved 08/10.
36. Office of the Budget. http://obj.cancer.gov/financial/financial.htm. Retrieved 12/10.

CHAPTER 4: Physical Facets of Health

1. American Cancer Society, Physical Activity and Cancer Handbook. http://www.cancer.org. Retrieved 12/10.
2. Centers for Disease Control and Prevention, National Center for Chronic Disease Prevention and Health Promotion. http://www.cdc.gov/nccdphp/dnpa/physical/stats/definitions.htm. Retrieved 1/10.
3. USDHHS, 1996, as adapted from Corbin and Lindsey, 1994.
4. Wilmore, J., Costill, D., Kenney, W. 2007. Physiology of Sport and Exercise. Human Kenetics.
5. Assistant Secretary for Planning and Education. http://aspe.hhs.gov/health/reports/physicalactivity. Retrieved 1/10.
6. U.S. Department of Health and Human Services. Physical activity and health: a report of the Surgeon General. Atlanta: U.S. Department of Health and Human Services, Centers for Disease Control and Prevention, National Center for Chronic Disease Prevention and Health Promotion; 1996.
7. American Cancer Society. http://www.acs.org. Retrieved 01/09.
8. Torti, D. C., et al. 2004. Exercise and prostate cancer. Sports Med 34(6):363–9.
9. Antonelli, J., et al. 2009. Exercise and prostate cancer risk in a cohort of veterans undergoing prostate needle biopsy. J Urology 82(5):2226–31.
10. Giovannucci, E. L., et al. 2005. A prospective study of physical activity and incident and fatal prostate cancer. Arch Intern Med 165(9):1005–10.
11. Lee, I., et al. 1991. Physical Activity and Risk of Developing Colorectal Cancer Among College Alumni. J National Cancer Institute 8(18):1324–29.
12. Harish, K. et al. 2007. Study Protocol: Insulin and its role in cancer. BMC Endocrine Disorders 7:10.
13. Meyerhardt, J. et al. 2006. Impact of physical activity on cancer recurrence and survival in patients with stage III colon cancer. Journal of Clinical Oncology 24(22):3517.
14. Centers for Disease Control. http://www.cdc.gov/nccdphp/publications/AAG/pdf/obesity.pdf. Retrieved 1/10.
15. The Breast Cancer Survivor's Fitness Plan: A Doctor-Approved Workout Plan For A Strong Body and Lifesaving Results, Carolyn M. Kaelin, Francesca Coltrera, Josie Gardiner, and Joy Prouty, McGraw-Hill, 2006.
16. Kerry, S. et al. 2007. Six-month follow-up of patient-rated outcomes in a randomized controlled trial of exercise training during breast cancer chemotherapy. Cancer Epidemiology Biomarkers Prev 16:2572–2578.
17. Holick, C., et al., 2008. Physical activity and survival after diagnosis of invasive breast cancer. Epidemiology, Biomarkers & Prevention 17;379.
18. Drouin, J. S. et al. 2006. Random control clinical trial on the effects of aerobic exercise training on erythrocyte levels during radiation treatment for breast cancer. Cancer 107(10):2490–2495.
19. Dallal, C. M. et al. 2007. Long-term recreational physical activity and risk of invasive and in situ breast cancer: The California Teachers Study. Arch Intern Med 167:408–415.
20. Florin, T., et al. 2007. Physical Inactivity in Adult Survivors of Childhood Acute Lymphoblastic Leukemia: A Report from the Childhood Cancer Survivor Study. Cancer Epidemiology, Biomarkers & Prevention 16;1356.
21. Janiszewski, P., et al. 2007. Abdominal obesity, liver fat, and muscle composition in survivors of childhood acute lymphoblastic leukemia. J Clin Endocrin & Metab 92(10):3816–21.

22. Oeffinger, K. C. et al. 2003. Obesity in Adult Survivors of Childhood Acute Lymphoblastic Leukemia: A report from the Childhood Cancer Survivor Study J of Clin Oncol 21(7):1359–1365.
23. Marchese, V. G. et al. 2004. Effects of physical therapy intervention for children with acute lymphoblastic leukemia. Ped Blood & Cancer 42(2):127–133.
24. Kushi, L., et al. 2006. American Cancer Society Guidelines on Nutrition and Physical Activity for Cancer Prevention: Reducing the Risk of Cancer With Healthy Food Choices and Physical Activity. http://caonline. amcancersoc.org/cgi/reprint/56/5/254. Retrieved 1/10.
25. Blair, Steven, et al., 1989. Physical fitness and all-cause mortality: a prospective study of healthy men and women. JAMA 262(17):2395–2401. http://www.faqs.org/abstracts/Health/Physical-fitness-and-all-cause-mortality-a-prospective-study-of-healthy-men-and-women.html. Retrieved 1/10.
26. Canadian Lifestyle and Lifestyle Research Institute 1997; Physical Activity Benchmarks report 1998.
27. Zumba® Fitness. http://http://www.zumba.com. Retrieved 02/09.
28. National Emergency Medical Association. http://www.nemahealth.org.
29. The New Aerobics, Alan Cooper, M. Evans and Co., 1970.
30. Fairey, A. S., et al. 2002. Physical exercise and immune system function in cancer survivors: a comprehensive review and future directions. Cancer 94(2):539–51.
31. Senchina, D., et al., 2007. Immunological outcomes of exercise in older adults. Clin Interv Aging 2(1):3–16.
32. President's Council on Physical Fitness and Sports. June, 2001. Research Digest Series 3(13). http://fitness.gov/June2001Digest.pdf. Retrieved 1/10.
33. MacVicar, M. G., et al. 1989. Effects of aerobic interval training on cancer patients' functional capacity. Nurs Res 38(6):348–51.
34. Dimeo, F., et al. 1996. An aerobic exercise program for patients with haematological malignancies after bone marrow transplantation. Bone Marrow Transplant 18(6):1157–60.
35. Thune, I. et al. 1997. The influence of physical activity on lung cancer risk. Int J Cancer 70:57–62.
36. Thune, I. et al. 2001. Physical activity and cancer risk: Dose response and cancer, all sites and site specific. Med Sci Sports Exer 33:S530–S550.
37. Friedenreich, C. M., et al. 2002. Physical activity and cancer prevention: Etiologic evidence and biological mechanisms. J Nutr 132: 3456S–64S.
38. Mock, V. 2004. Evidence-Based Treatment for Cancer-Related Fatigue. J. Natl Cancer Inst Monogr 32:112–8.
39. National Cancer Institute. 2006. http://www.cancer.gov/cancertopics/pdq/supportivecare/fatigue/HealthProfessional/page6#Reference6.20. Retrieved 1/10.
40. Ohira, T. et al. 2006. Effects of weight training on quality of life in recent breast cancer survivors: The weight training for breast cancer survivors (WTBS) study. Cancer 106(9):2076–83.
41. De Backer, I. C., et al. 2009. Resistance training in cancer survivors: a systematic review. Int J Sports Med 30(10):703–12.
42. Schmitz, K. et al. 2002. Effects of a 9-month strength training intervention on insulin, insulin-like growth factor (IGF)-I, IGF-binding protein (IGFBP)-1, and IGFBP-3 in 30 50-year-old women. Cancer Epidem, Biom & Prev 11:1597.
43. U.S. Department of Health and Human Services. 2008. Physical Activity Guidelines for Americans. http://health.gov/paguidelines/pdf/paguide.pdf. Retrieved 1/10.
44. American College of Sports Medicine (ACSM). http://www.acsm.org. Retrieved 01/09.
45. http://www.laughteryoga.org. Retrieved 12/08.
46. Art of Living Foundation. http://www.artofliving.org. Retrieved 01/09.
47. Goldblatt, H. et al.. 1953. Induced malignancy in cells from rat myocardium subjected to intermittent anaerobiosis during long propagation in vitro, Journal of Experimental Medicine 97(4), 525.
48. On Otto Warburg, Director of the Max Planck Institute of Cell Physiology, Germany. http://en.wikipedia.org/wiki/Warburg_hypothesis. Retrieved 1/10.
49. Höckel, M. et al. 2001. Tumor Hypoxia: Definitions and Current Clinical, Biologic, and Molecular Aspects, Journal of the National Cancer Institute, 93(4):266–276.
50. Breathing: The Master Key to Self-Healing, Andew Weil M.D. Audiobook, 1st Edition. December 1999.
51. Dr. Weil's Self-Healing Newsletter. http://www.drweil.com/drw/u/ART00521/three-breathing-exercises.html.

52. Pal, G. K., et al. 2004. Effect of short-term practice of breathing exercises on autonomic functions in normal human volunteers. Indian J. Med Res 120(2):115–21.

53. Arambula, P., et al. 2001. The Physiological Correlates of Kundalini Yoga Meditation: A Study of a Yoga Master. Applied Psychophysiology and Biofeedback 26(2).

54. Ohnishi, S. & Ohnishi, T. 2006. The Nishino Breathing Method and ki-energy (life-energy): A challenge to traditional scientific thinking. Philadelphia Biomedical Research Institute, King of Prussia, PA and Department of Biochemistry and Biophysics, University of Pennsylvania School of Medicine, Philadelphia, PA eCAM 2006;3(2)191–200 doi:10.1093/ecam/nel004. http://ecam.oxfordjournals.org/cgi/content/full/3/2/191. Retrieved 1/10.

55. Tshuyoshi, S. et al. 2006. The Nishino Breathing Method and Ki-energy (Life energy). eCAM 3(2):191–200. http://www.nishinojuku.com/english/e_profile/e_pro_top.html. Retrieved 1/10.

56. Tanaka, Y. 2004. Beneficial effects of the Nishino breathing method on the microcirculatory response, the immune activity and the stress level. J Int Soc Life Inf Sci 22(2):450–454..

57. Kimura, H. et al. 2005. Beneficial effects of Nishino breathing method on immune activity and stress level. J of Alt and Comp Med 11(2): 285–291.

58. Selye, Hans, The Stress of Life (first published in 1956). 2nd Ed McGraw-Hill, 1978.

59. Writings of Richard S. Lazarus, possibly from Emotion and Adaptation, Oxford University Press, 1991.

60. Segerstrom, S. C. et al. 2004. Psychological Stress and the Human Immune System: A Meta-Analytic Study of 30 Years of Inquiry. Psychological Bulletin 130(4).

61. Antoni, M. et al. 2006. The influence of bio-behavioural factors on tumour biology: pathways and mechanisms. Nature Reviews Cancer 6:240–248.

62. American Psychological Association. http://www.apa.org/news/press/releases/2009/11/stress.aspx. Retrieved 1/10.

63. http://www.apa.org/pubinfo/anger.html. Retrieved 1/10.

64. Gouin, J. P., et al. 2008. The influence of anger expression on wound healing. Brain Behav Immun 22(5):699–708.

65. Gallacher, J. E., et al. 1999. Anger and incident heart disease in the Caerphilly Study. Psychosomatic Medicine 61:446–453.

66. Reilly, Patrick, M., Ph.D. and Shopshire, Michael S., Ph.D. 2002. Anger Management for Substance Abuse and Mental Health Clients. A Cognitive Behavioral Therapy Manual. U.S. Department of Health and Human Services Substance Abuse and Mental Health Services Administration Center for Substance Abuse Treatment.

67. Complementary and Alternative Medicine Index (CAM). University of Maryland Medical Center. http://http://www.umm.edu/altmed/articles/relaxation-techniques-000359.htm. Retrieved 1/10.

68. Autogenic Therapy, Dr. Johannes Schultz. British Autogenic Society. http://www.autogenic-therapy.org.uk. Retrieved 1/10.

69. Jacobson, Edmund. Progressive Relaxation, University of Chicago Press, Chicago, 1938.

70. Kwekkeboom, Kristine L. Ph.D. et al. 2008. Patients' perceptions of the effectiveness of guided imagery and progressive muscle relaxation interventions used for cancer pain. Complement Ther Clin Pract. 14(3):185–194.

71. NCCAM. National Center for Complementary and Alternative Medicine. http://nccam.nih.gov/health/meditation/overview.htm. Retrieved 1/10.

72. Coker, K. H. 1999. Meditation and prostate cancer: Integrating a mind/body intervention with traditional therapies. Semin Urol Oncol. 17:111–118.

73. Carlson, L. E., et al. 2003. Mindfulness-based stress reduction in relation to quality of life, mood, symptoms of stress, and immune parameters in breast and prostate cancer outpatients. Psychosom Med. 65:571–581.

74. Centers for Disease Conrol. Perceived insufficient rest or sleep among adults—United States, 2008. 2009. As reported in JAMA 302(23):2532–2539. MMWR. 2009;58:1175–1179. http://jama.ama-assn.org/cgi/content/full/302/23/2532. Retrieved 1/10.

75. Redwine, L., et al. 2000. Effects of sleep and sleep deprivation on interleukin-6,growth hormone, cortisol, and melatonin levels in humans. J Clinical Endocrin & Metab 85(10):3597–3603.

76. Toth, L. A., et al. 1993. Sleep as a prognostic indicator during infectious disease in rabbits. Proc Soc Exp Biol Med 203(2):179–92.

77. Palmblad, J. et al. 1979. Lymphocyte and granulocyte reactions during sleep deprivation. Psychosomatic Medicine 41(4):273–278.

78. Irwin, M., et al. 1994. Partial sleep deprivation reduces natural killer cell activity in humans. Psychosomatic Medicine 56:493–498.

79. Karni, A. et al. 1994. Dependence on REM sleep of overnight improvement of a perceptual skill. Science 265(5172):679–682.

80. Walker, M. P., et al. 2002. Cognitive flexibility across the sleep-wake cycle: REM-sleep enhancement of anagram problem solving. Brain Res Cogn Brain Res. 14(3):317–24.

81. Gottlieb, D. J., et al. 2005. Association of sleep time with diabetes mellitus and impaired glucose tolerance. Arch Intern Med. 165(8):863–7.

82. Wagner, U., et al. 2004. Sleep inspires insight. Nature 427:352–5.

83. Society of Clinical Psychology. http://www.psychology.sunysb.edu/eklonsky-/division12/treatments/insomnia_stimulus.html. Retrieved 1/10.

84. Sateia, M. J., et al. 2004. Insomnia. Lancet 3;364(9449):1959–73.

85. Smith A. 2002. Effects of caffeine on human behavior. Food Chem Toxicol 40(9):1243–55.

86. Reiter, A. M. 1994. Inhibitory effect of melatonin on cataract formation in newborn rats: Evidence for an antioxidative role of melatonin. J Pineal Res 17:94–100.

87. Agah, I. et al. 2009. Effect of melatonin on the antioxidant enzyme status in the liver of swiss albino laboratory mice in single circadian rhythm. Journal of Applied Biological Sciences 3(1):1–6.

88. Blask, D. E. & Hill, S. M. 1986. Effects of melatonin on cancer: studies on MCF-7 human breast cancer cells in culture. J Neural Transm Suppl. 21:433–449.

89. Basak, P. Y. et al. 2003. The effect of thermal injury and melatonin on incisional wound healing. Ulus Travma Acil Cerrahi Derg 9(2):96–101.

90. Petranka, J. et al. 1999. The oncostatic action of melatonin in an ovarian carcinoma cell line. Journal of Pineal Research 26(3):129–136.

91. Kanishi, Y. et al. 2000. Differential growth inhibitory effect of melatonin on two endometrial cancer cell lines. J of Pineal Research 28(4):227–233.

92. Hu, D. N. et al. 2000. Melatonin receptors in human uveal melanocytes and melanoma cells. J of Pineal Research 28(3):165–171.

93. Gilad, E. et al. 1999. Melatonin receptors in PC3 human prostate tumor cells. Journal of Pineal Research 26(4):211–220.

94. Anisimov, V. N. et al. 1997. Melatonin and colon carcinogenesis: I. Inhibitory effect of melatonin on development of intestinal tumors induced by 1, 2-dimethylhydrazine in rats. Carcinogenesis 18:1549–1553.

95. Carillo-Vico, A. et al. 2006. The modulatory role of melatonin on immune responsiveness. Curr Opin Investig Drugs 7(5):423–31.

96. Guerrero, J. M. et al. 2002. Melatonin-immune system relationships. Curr Top Med Chem 2(2):167–79.

97. FASEB, J. et al. 2004. Evidence of melatonin synthesis by human lymphocytes and its physiological significance: Possible role as intracrine, autocrine, and/or paracrine substance. 18(3):537–9.

98. Lissoni, P. et al. 1007. Treatment of cancer chemotherapy-induced toxicity with the pineal hormone melatonin. Support Care Cancer.5(2):126–9.

99. Castrillon, P. O. et al. 2000. Effect of melatonin treatment on 24-h variations in responses to mitogens and lymphocyte subset populations in rat submaxillary lymph nodes. J of Neuroendocrinology 12(8):758–765.

100. Cordain, L. et al. 2005. Origins and evolution of the Western diet: Health implications for the 21st Century. American Journal of Clin Nutr 81:341–54 9.

101. USDA Mypyramid. http://www.mypyramid.gov/index.html. Retrieved 08/10.

102. Harvard School of Public Health. http://www.hsph.harvard.edu/nutritionsource/what-should-you-eat/pyramid/. Retrieved 01/10.

103. Harvard Medical School. http://hms.harvard.edu/public/disease/nutrition/page2.html. Retrieved 01/10.

104. Colorado State University Extension. *http://www.ext.colostate.edu/pubs/foodnut09365.html.* Retrieved 08/10.

105. FDA U.S. Food and Drug Administration CFR-Code of Federal Regulations Title 21. http://www.accessdata.fda.gov/scripts/cdrh/cfdocs/cfcfr/CFRSearch.cfm?fr=101.22. Retrieved 01/10.

106. USHHS, Dietary Guidelines for Americans, 2010. http://www.health.gov/dietaryguidelines. Retrieved 08/10.

107. Andrews, K. S., et al. 2006. American Cancer Society Guidelines on Nutrition and Physical Activity for Cancer Prevention: Reducing the Risk of Cancer with Healthy Food Choices and Physical Activity. CA Cancer J Clin 56:254–281.

108. Lichtenstein, A. H., et al. 2006. Diet and Lifestyle Recommendations Revision 2006: A Scientific Statement From the American Heart Association Nutrition Committee. Circulation 114:82–96.

109. United States Department of Agriculture. http://fnic.nal.usda.gov/nal_display/index.php?info_center=4&tax_level=3&tax_subject=358&topic_id=1611&level3_id=5977&level4_id=0&level5_id=0&placement_default=0. Retrieved 01/10.

110. Harper, A. E. et al. 2003. Contributions of women scientists in the U.S. to the development of Recommended Dietary Allowances. J Nutr 133:3698–3702.

111. Dietary reference intakes for energy, carbohydrate, fiber, fat, fatty acids, cholesterol, protein, and amino acids (macronutrients). 2005. National Academy of Sciences. Institute of Medicine. Food and Nutrition Board. http://fnic.nal.usda.gov/nal_display/index.php?info_center=4&tax_level=4&tax_subject=256&topic_id=1342&level3_id=5141&level4_id=10588. Retrieved 01/10.

112. Simopoulos, A. P. et al. 2008. The importance of the omega-6/omega-3 fatty acid ratio in cardiovascular disease and other chronic diseases. Experimental Biology and Medicine 233:674–688.

113. Stoll, A. L. et al. 1999. Omega 3 fatty acids in bipolar disorder: A preliminary double-blind, placebo-controlled trial. Arch Gen Psychiatry. 56(5):407–12.

114. Rhodes, L. E. et al. 2003. Effect of eicosapentaenoic acid, an omega-3 polyunsaturated fatty acid, on UVR-related cancer risk in humans. An assessment of early genotoxic markers. Carcinogenesis 24(5):919–925.

115. Moison, R. M. et al. Dietary eicosapentaenoic acid prevents systemic immunosuppression in mice induced by UVB radiation. Radiat Res 156(1):36–44.

116. Okamoto M, Misunobu F, Ashida K, et al. 2000. Effects of dietary supplementation with n-3 fatty acids compared with n-6 fatty acids on bronchial asthma. Int Med 39(2):107–111.

117. USHHS, Dietary Guidelines for Americans, 2010. http://www.health.gov/dietaryguidelines. Retrieved 08/10.

118. Ulrich, et al., 2008. Vitamin and mineral supplement use among U.S. adults after cancer diagnosis; a systematic review. Journal of Clinical Oncology, 26(4):665–673.

119. Steinmetz K. A. et al. 1996. Vegetables, fruit, and cancer prevention: a review. J Am Diet Assoc 96(10):1027–1039.

120. Fontham, E. T. H. 1990. Protective dietary factors and lung cancer. Int J Epidemiol 19:S32–S42.

121. Block, G. et al. 1992. Fruit, vegetables, and cancer prevention: a review of the epidemiological evidence. Nutr Cancer 18(1):1–29.

122. van't Veer, P. et al. Fruits and vegetables in the prevention of cancer and cardiovascular disease. Public Health Nutrition 3:103–107.

123. World Cancer Research Fund, American Institute for Cancer Research. Food, nutrition, physical activity, and the prevention of cancer: A global perspective. Washington DC: AICR, 2007. http://www.dietandcancerreport.org/downloads/chapters/chapter_12.pdf. Retrieved 01/10.

124. Posner, G. 2002. Low-Calcemic Vitamin D analogs (deltanoids) for human cancer prevention. J Nutr 132:3802S–3S.

125. Chen, T. C. et al. 2003. Vitamin D and prostate cancer prevention and treatment. Trends Endocrinol Metab. 14(9):423–30.

126. Lappe, J. M. et al 2007. Vitamin D and calcium supplementation reduces cancer risk: results of a randomized trial. American J Clin Nutr 85(6):1586–1591.

127. Mehta, R. G. et al. 1997. Prevention of preneoplastic mammary lesion development by a novel vitamin D analogue, 1alpha-hydroxyvitamin D5. JNCI 89(3):212–218.

128. Mehta, R. G. et al. 2000. Differentiation of human breast carcinoma cells by a novel vitamin D analog: 1alpha-hydroxyvitamin D5. Int J Oncol 16(1):65–73.

129. Holt, P. R. et al. 1999. Dairy foods and prevention of colon cancer: Human studies. JACN 18(90005):379S–391S.

130. Gange, S. J. et al. 2000. Conceptually new deltanoids (vitamin D analogs) inhibit multistage skin tumorigenesis. Carcinogenesis 21(7):1341–1345.

131. Ainsleigh, H. G. et al. 1993. Beneficial effects of sun exposure on cancer mortality. Am J Prev Med 22(1):132–40.

132. Gorham, E. D. et al. 2007. Optimal vitamin D status for colorectal cancer prevention: A quantitative meta analysis. 32(3):210–6.

133. Lamprecht, S. A. et al. 2003. Chemoprevention of colon cancer by calcium, vitamin D and folate: Molecular mechanisms. Nat Rev Cancer 3(8):601–14.

134. Garland, C. et al. 1985. Dietary vitamin D and calcium and risk of colorectal cancer: A 19-year prospective study in men. Lancet 1:307–9.

135. Grant, W. B. et al. 2004. A critical review of studies on vitamin D in relation to colorectal cancer. Nutr Cancer 48(2):115–23.

136. Sieg, J. et al. 2006. Insufficient Vitamin D Supply as a Possible Co-factor in Colorectal Carcinogenesis. Anticancer Research 26(4A):2729–2733.

137. Jenab, M. et al. 2010. Association between pre-diagnostic circulating vitamin D concentration and risk of colorectal cancer in European populations: A nested case-control study. BMJ 340:b5500.

138. Lieberman, D. A. et al. 2003. Risk factors for advanced colonic neoplasia and hyperplastic polyps in asymptomatic individuals. J Am Med Assoc 290:2959–67.

139. Tangpricha, V. et al. 2001. 25-hydroxyvitamin D-1alpha-hydroxylase in normal and malignant colon tissue. Lancet. 26;357(9269):1673–4.

140. Deeb, K. K. et al. 2007. Vitamin D signalling pathways in cancer: potential for anticancer therapeutics. Nat Rev Cancer 7(9):684–700.

141. Ames, B. N. et al. 2983. Dietary carcinogens and anticarcinogens: Oxygen radicals and degenerative diseases. Science. 23;221(4617):1256–64.

142. Mergens, W. J. et al. 1978. Alpha-tocopherol: Uses in preventing nitrosamine formation. IARC Sci Publ. (19):199–212.

143. Meschino, James. 2007. Vitamin E Succinate: The Preferred Form of Vitamin E to combat breast, prostate and other cancers. Dynamic Chiropractic. http://biopharmasci.com/downloads/NanomegaESuccinate.pdf. Retrieved 01/10.

144. Carr, A. C. et al. 1999. Toward a new recommended dietary allowance for vitamin C based on antioxidant and health effects in humans. Am J Clin Nutr 69(6):1086–1107.

145. Kromhout, D. et al. 1987. Essential micronutrients in relation to carcinogenesis. Am J Clin Nutr 1987;45(5 Suppl):1361–1367.

146. Zhang, S. et al. 1999. Dietary carotenoids and vitamins A, C, and E and risk of breast cancer. J Natl Cancer Inst 91(6):547–556.144.

147. Michels, K. B. et al. 2001. Dietary antioxidant vitamins, retinol, and breast cancer incidence in a cohort of Swedish women. Int J Cancer 91(4):563–567.

148. Feiz, H. R. et al. 2002. Does vitamin C intake slow the progression of gastric cancer in Helicobacter pylori-infected populations? Nutr Rev 60(1):34–36.

149. Bender, David A. Nutritional biochemistry of the Vitamins, 2nd Edition, Cambridge University Press, 2003.

150. Liu, Z. et al. 2007. Mild Depletion of Dietary Folate Combined with Other B Vitamins Alters Multiple Components of the Wnt Pathway in Mouse Colon. J Nutr 137:2701–2708.

151. Schernhammer, E. et al. 2007. Plasma folate, vitamins B6, B12, and homocysteine and pancreatic cancer risk in four large cohorts. Cancer Research 67(11):5553.

152. Giovannucci, E. et al. 1998. Multivitamin use, folate, and colon cancer in women in the Nurses' Health Study. Annals of Internal Medicine 129(7):517–524.

153. Giovannucci, E. et al. 2004. Alcohol, one-carbon metabolism, and colorectal cancer: Recent insights from molecular studies. J Nutr 134:2475S–2481S.

154. National Cancer Institute. http://www.cancer.gov/drugdictionary/?CdrID=41719. Retrieved 01/10.

155. Chemocare.com, "Care during chemotherapy and beyond." http://www.chemocare.com/bio/folinic_acid. asp. Retrieved 01/10.

156. Keshava, C. et al. 1998. Inhibition of methotrexate-induced chromosomal damage by folinic acid in V79 cells. Mutat Res 397:221–8

157. Ganther, H. E., et al. 1999. Selenium metabolism, selenoproteins and mechanisms of cancer prevention: Complexities with thioredoxin reductase. Carcinogenesis 20(9):1657–1666.

158. Patterson, B. H. et al. 1997. Naturally occurring selenium compounds in cancer chemoprevention trials: A workshop summary. Cancer Epid Biom Prev 6(1): 63–69.

159. Fleet, J. C. et al. 1997. Dietary selenium repletion may reduce cancer incidence in people at high risk who live in areas with low soil selenium. Nutr Ruv 55(7):277–9.

160. Combs, G. F. et al. 2001. An analysis of cancer prevention by selenium. BioFactors 14; 153–9.

161. Clark, L. C. et al. 1996. Effects of selenium supplementation for cancer prevention in patients with carcinoma of the skin. A randomized controlled trial. Nutritional Prevention of Cancer Study Group. JAMA 276(24):1957–63.

162. Combs, G. F. Jr. et al. 1997. Reduction of cancer risk with an oral supplement of selenium. Biomed Environ Sci 10:227–34.

163. Fischer, J. L. et al. 2007. Chemotherapeutic selectivity conferred by selenium: a role for p53-dependent DNA repair Mol Cancer Ther 6;355.

164. Hongbo Hu, C. J. et al. Methylseleninic acid potentiates apoptosis induced by chemotherapeutic drugs in prostate cancer cells through enhancing caspase activation.2005. Proc Amer Assoc Cancer Res 46.

165. Nilsonne, G. et al. 2006. Selenite induces apoptosis in sarcomatoid malignant mesothelioma cells through oxidative stress. Free Radical Biol Med 41(6):874–885.

166. Vucelic, B. et al. 1994. Differences in serum selenium concentration in probands and patients with colorectal neoplasms in Zagreb, Croatia. Acta Med Austriaca 21(1):19–23.

167. Patterson, B. H. et al. 1997. Naturally occurring selenium compounds in cancer chemoprevention trials: a workshop summary. Cancer Epidemiol Biomarkers Prev 6(1):63–9.

168. Knekt, P. et al. 1998. Is low selenium status a risk factor for lung cancer? Am J Epidemiol 148:975–82.

169. Yamamura, K. Y. et al. 1990. Inhibitory effect of selenium on hamster pancreatic cancer induction by N'-nitrosobis(2-oxopropyl)amine. Int J Cancer 15;46(1):95–100.

170. McConnell, K. P. et al. 1980. The relationship of dietary selenium and breast cancer. J Surg Oncol 15(1):67–70.

171. Duffield-Lillico, A. J. et al. 2002. Baseline characteristics and the effect of selenium supplementation on cancer incidence in a randomized clinical trial: A summary report of the Nutritional Prevention of Cancer Trial. Cancer Epidemiol Biomarkers Prev 11(7):630–9.

172. Broome, C. S. et al. 2004. An increase in selenium intake improves immune function and poliovirus handling in adults with marginal selenium status. Amer J Clin Nutr 80(1):154–162.

173. Arthur, J. R. et al. 2003. Supplement: 11th International Symposium on Trace Elements in Man and Animals Selenium in the Immune System. J Nutr 133:1457S–1459S.

174. Wu, K. et al. 2002. Calcium intake and risk of colon cancer in women and men. J National Cancer Inst 94(6):437–446.

175. Park, Y. et al. 2009. Dairy food, calcium, and risk of cancer in the NIH-AARP Diet and Health Study. Archives of Int Med 169(4):391–401.

176. Larsson, S. C. et al. 2005. Magnesium intake in relation to risk of colorectal cancer in women. JAMA 5;293(1):86–9.

177. Folsom, A. R. et al. 2006. Magnesium intake and reduced risk of colon cancer in a prospective study of women. Am J Epidemiol 1;163(3):232–5.

178. van den Brandt, P. A. et al. 2007. Magnesium intake and colorectal cancer risk in the NetherlandsCohort Study. Netherlands British Journal of Cancer 96:510–513.

179. Saif, M. W. 2008. Management of hypomagnesemia in cancer patients receiving chemotherapy. Supportive Oncology 6(5); May/June.

180. Wang, A. et al. 1994. The inhibitory effect of magnesium hydroxide on the bile acid-induced cell proliferation of colon epithelium in rats with comparison to the action of calcium lactate. Carcinogenesis 15:2661–2663.

181. Hartwig, A. et al. 2001. Role of magnesium in genomic stability. Mutat Res 475:113–121.

182. Huerta, M. et al. 2005. Magnesium Deficiency Is Associated With Insulin Resistance in Obese Children. Diabetes Care 28(5):1175–1181.

183. Takaya, J. et al. 2004. Intracellular magnesium and insulin resistance. Magnes Res 17(2):126–36.

184. Paolisso, G. et al. 1992. Daily magnesium supplements improve glucose handling in elderly subjects. Am J Clin Nutr 55:1161–1167.

185. Rodriguez-Moran, M. et al. 2003. Oral magnesium supplementation improves insulin sensitivity and metabolic control in type 2 diabetic subjects: A randomized double-blind controlled trial. Diabetes Care 26:1147–1152.

186. Giovannucci, E. 1995. Insulin and colon cancer. Cancer Causes Control 6:164.

187. Schoen, R. E. 1999. Increased blood glucose and insulin, body size, and incident colorectal cancer. J Natl Cancer Inst 91:1147–1154.

188. Shankar, A. H. 1998. Zinc and immune function: The biological basis of altered resistance to infection. Am J Clin Nutr 68:447S–463S.

189. Abnet, C. et al. 2005. Zinc concentration in esophageal biopsy specimens measured by x-ray fluorescence and esophageal cancer risk. J Natl Cancer Inst 97(4):301–306.

190. Lin, Y. S. et al. 2009. Effects of zinc supplementation on the survival of patients who received concomitant chemotherapy and radiotherapy for advanced nasopharyngeal carcinoma: Follow-up of a double-blind randomized study with subgroup analysis. Laryngoscope 119(7):1348–52.

191. American Institute for Cancer Research. http://www.aicr.org. Retrieved 02/10.

192. National Cancer Institute. http://www.nci.org. Retrieved 04/10.

193. Centers for Disease Control and Prevention. http://www.fruitsandveggiesmatter.gov. Retrieved 04/10.

194. David Heber, What Color Is Your Diet?: The 7 Colors of Health, 1st Edition, William Morrow Publishers, 2001.

195. Rui, H. L. et al. 2004. Potential synergy of phytochemicals in cancer prevention: Mechanism of action. American Society for Nutritional Sciences 134:3479S–3485S.

196. Wu, A. H., et al. 1998. Soy intake and risk of breast cancer in Asians and Asian-Americans. American Journal of Clinical Nutrition 68(suppl);1437S–1443S.

197. Badger, T. M. et al. 2005. Soy Protein Isolate and Protection Against Cancer J Amer Coll Nutr 24(2)146S–149S.

198. Farina, A. et al. 2006. An improved synthesis of resveratrol. Nat Prod Res 20(3):247–52.

199. Jang, M. et al. 1997. Cancer chemopreventive activity of resveratrol, a natural product derived from grapes. Science 275(5297):218–20.

200. Athar, M. et al. 2007. Resveratrol: a review of preclinical studies for human cancer prevention. Toxicol Appl Pharmacol 224(3):274–83.

201. Garvin, S. et al. 2006. Resveratrol induces apoptosis and inhibits angiogenesis in human breast cancer xenografts in vivo. Cancer Lett 8;231(1):113–22.

202. Zhou, H. B. et al. 2003. Resveratrol induces apoptosis in human esophageal carcinoma cells. World J Gastroenterol 9(3):408–11.

203. Mateos-Aparicio, I. et al. 2008. Soybean, a promising health source. Nutr Hosp 23(4):305–31.

204. Chen, J. et al. 2002. Dietary flaxseed inhibits human breast cancer growth and metastasis and downregulates expression of insulin-like growth factor and epidermal growth factor receptor. Nutr Cancer 43(2):187–92.

205. Giovannucci, et al. 2002. A Prospective study of tomato products, lycopene, and prostate cancer risk. J National Cancer Institute 94(5):391–398.

206. Liu, R. H., et al. May 4, 2008. Potential Synergy of Phytochemicals in Cancer Prevention: Mechanism of Action. Department of Food Science, Cornell university. The Journal of Nutrition.

207. You, W. C., et al. 1989. Allium vegetables and reduced risk of stomach cancer. J National Cancer Institute 81(2):162–164.

208. Steinmetz, K., et al. 1994. Vegetables, fruit, and colon cancer in the Iowa Women's Health Study. Amer J of Epid 139(1):1–15.

209. Fleischauer, A. T. et al. 2001. Garlic and cancer: a critical review of the epidemiologic literature. J Nutr 131(3s):1032S–40S.

210. Hsing, A. W. et al. 2002. Allium vegetables and risk of prostate cancer: a population-based study. J Natl Cancer Inst 6;94(21):1648–51.

211. Galeone, C. et al. 2009. Allium vegetables intake and endometrial cancer risk. Public Health Nutr 12(9):1576–9.

212. Nakachi, K. et al. 1998. Influence of drinking green tea on breast cancer malignancy among Japanese patients. J Cancer Res 89:254–261.

213. World Health Organization. http://www.who.org. Retrieved 02/10.

214. Lilly, D. M. et al. 1965. Probiotics: Growth-promoting factors produced by microorganisms. Science 147(3659):747–748.

215. World Gastroenterology Organisation Practice Guideline. Probiotics and prebiotics. May, 2008. http://www.worldgastroenterology.org/assets/downloads/en/pdf/guidelines/19_probiotics_prebiotics.pdf. Retrieved 02/10.

216. Wollowski, I. et al. 2001. Protective role of probiotics and prebiotics in colon cancer. Amer J Clin Nutr 73(2):451S–455s.

217. van't Veer, P. et al. 1989. Consumption of fermented milk products and breast cancer: A Case-Control Study in the Netherlands. Cancer Research 49:4020–4023.

218. de Moreno de LeBlanc, A. et al. 2005. Effects of milk fermented by Lactobacillus helveticus R389 on a murine breast cancer model. Breast Cancer Research 7:R477–R486.

219. Naito, S. et al. 2007. Prevention of recurrence with epirubicin and Lactobacillus Casei After transurethral resection of bladder cancer J of Urology 179(2):485–490.

220. Nakamura, T. et al. 2002. Cloned cytosine deaminase gene expression of Bifidobacterium longum and application to enzyme/pro-drug therapy of hypoxic solid tumors. Biosci Biotechnol Biochem 66(11):2362–6.

221. Li, X. et al. 2003. Bifidobacterium adolescentis as a delivery system of endostatin for cancer gene therapy: Selective inhibitor of angiogenesis and hypoxic tumor growth. Cancer Gene Ther 10(2):105–11,

222. Broekaert, I. J. et al. 2006. Probiotics and chronic disease. J Clin Gastroenterol 40(3):270–4.

223. Nutrition Business Journal. http://www.nutritionbusinessjournal.com. Retrieved 01/10.

224. Organic Trade Association's 2009 Organic Industry Survey. http://www.ota.com/pics/documents/01a_OTAExecutiveSummary.pdf. Retrieved 02/10.

225. USDA. http://www.nal.usda.gov/afsic/pubs/ofp/ofp.shtml. Retrieved 02/10.

226. USDA Food Safety and Inspection Service (FSIS) http://www.fsis.usda.gov/. Retrieved 02/10.

227. Animal and Plant Health Inspection Service (APHIS). http://www.aphis.usda.gov. Retrieved 02/10.

228. Federal Trade Commission. http://www.ftc.gov. Retrieved 02/10.

229. Centers for Disease Control and Prevention http://www.cdc.gov. Retrieved 02/10.

230. Environmental Protection Agency. http://www.epa.gov. Retrieved 02/10.

231. Department of Commerce. http://www.commerce.gov. Retrieved 02/10.

232. Bureau of Alcohol, Tobacco and Firearms. http://www.atf.gov. Retrieved 02/10.

233. Dimitri, Carolyn and Oberholzer, Lydia. 2009. Marketing U.S. organic food: Recent trends from farms to consumers: A report from the economic research service economic information bulletin. #58 http://www.ers.usda.gov/publications/eib58/eib58.pdf. Retrieved 02/10.

234. USDA. http://www.ams.usda.gov/AMSv1.0/ams.fetchTemplateData.do?template=TemplateC&navID=PesticideDataProgram&rightNav1=PesticideDataProgram&topNav=&leftNav=ScienceandLaboratories&page=PesticideDataProgram&resultType. Retrieved 02/10.

235. United States Department of Agriculture Pesticide Data Program 2008. http://www.ams.usda.gov/AMSv1.0/getfile?dDocName=STELPRDC5081750. Retrieved 02/10.

236. Winter, C. K. et al. 2006. Organic Foods. J Food Science 71(9):117–124.

237. Daniels, J. et al. 1997. Pesticides and childhood cancers. Environmental Health Perspectives 105:1068–1077.

238. Jin Lee, W. et al. Cancer incidence among pesticide applicators exposed to chlorpyrifos in the Agricultural Health Study. 2004. J Natl Cancer Inst 96(23):1781–1789.

239. Xu, X., et al. 2010. Associations of serum concentrations of organochlorine pesticides with breast cancer and prostate cancer in U.S. adults. Env Health Persp 118(1).

240. Charlier, C. et al. 2003. Breast cancer and serum organochlorine residues. Occup Environ Med 60(5):348–51.

241. Kamel, F. et al. 2004. Association of pesticide exposure with neurological dysfunction and disease. Environ Health Perspec 112:950–958.

242. Longnecker, M. P. et al. 2001. Association between maternal serum concentration of the DDT metabolite DDE and preterm and small-for-gestational-age babies at birth. Lancet 358:110–14.

243. Silent Spring, Rachel Carson, Houghton Mifflin, 1962.

244. U.S. National Toxicology Program. http://www.ntp.niehs.nih.gov. Retrieved 02/10.

245. Environmental Protection Agency. http://www.epa.gov. Retrieved 02/10.

246. Rembialkowska, E. 2007. Quality of plant products from organic agriculture. J Sci of Food and Agric 87(15):2757–2762.

247. Wang, S. Y. et al. 2008. Fruit quality, antioxidant capacity, and flavonoid content of organically and conventionally grown blueberries. J Agric Food Chem 56(14):5788–5794.

248. Carbonaro, M. et al. 2002. Modulation of antioxidant compounds in organic vs. conventional fruit (peach, Prunus persica L., and pear, Pyrus communis L.) J Agric Food Chem 50:5458–5462.

249. Bergamo, P. et al. 2003. Fat-soluble vitamin contents and fatty acid composition in organic and conventional Italian dairy products. Food Chemistry 82(4):625–631.

250. Baxter, G. J. et al 2001. Salicylic acid in soups prepared from organically and non-organically grown vegetables. European Journal of Nutrition 40(6):289–292.

251. Kung, F. P., et al. 2009. Fatty acid composition of certified organic, conventional and omega-3 eggs. Food Chemistry 116(4):911–914.

252. Oregon State University Extension Service. http://extension.oregonstate.edu/fch/sites/default/files/documents/fcd_08-05eggsparticipantguide.pdf. "Eggs…They really are incredible." Participant handout January 2008. Retrieved 02/10.

253. David Wallinga, M.D. "Playing Chicken: Avoiding Arsenic in your Meat." Institute for Agriculture and Trade Policy Food and Health Program, April 2006. http://www.iatp.org/iatp/publications.cfm?accountID=421&refID=80529. Retrieved 02/10.

254. American Cancer Society Guidelines on Nutrition and Physical Activity for Cancer Prevention: Reducing the risk of cancer with healthy food choices and physical activity. http://www.cancer.org. http://caonline.amcancersoc.org/cgi/reprint/56/5/25. Retrieved 02/10.

255. Magee, P. et al. 1956. The production of malignant primary hepatic tumours in the rat by feeding dimethylnitrosamine. Br J Cancer 10(1):114–122.

256. Rocz Panstw Zakl Hig. 2006. A comparison of N-nitrosodimethylamine contents in selected meat products. 57(4):341–6.

257. Sandhu, M.S. et al. 2001. Systematic review of the prospective cohort studies on meat consumption and colorectal cancer risk: A metaanalytical approach. Cancer Epidemiol Biomarkers Prev 10:439–46.

258. Jakszyn, P. et al. 2006. Nitrosamine and related food intake and gastric and oesophageal cancer risk: A systematic review of the epidemiological evidence. World J Gastroenterol 12(27): 4296–4303.

259. Zucker, P. F. et al. 1988. Alterations in pancreatic islet function produced by carcinogenic nitrosamines in the Syrian hamster. Am J Patholology 133(3):573–577.

260. Zhang, C. M. et al. 2002. Diet and ovarian cancer risk: A case–control study in China. British Journal of Cancer (2002) 86, 712–717.

261. Morales, P. et al. 1998. Antimutagenic effect of fruit and vegetable aqueous extracts against N-nitrosamines evaluated by the Ames Test. J. Agric. Food Chem 46(12):5194–5200.

262. Erkekoglu, P. et al. 2010. Evaluation of the protective effect of ascorbic acid on nitrite- and nitrosamine-induced cytotoxicity and genotoxicity in human hepatoma line. Toxicology Mechanisms and Methods 20(2):45–52.

263. National Institutes of Health. http://ghr.nlm.nih.gov/glossary=freeradicals. Retrieved 02/10.

264. Dietary Reference Intakes: Proposed definition and plan for review of dietary antioxidants and related compounds. A report of the Standing Committee on the scientific Evaluation Dietary Reference Intakes and its Panel on Dietary Antioxidants and Related Compounds. Food and Nutrition Board, Institute of Medicine. http://www.nal.usda.gov/fnic/DRI//DRI_Dietary_Antioxidants_Review/antioxidants_full_report.pdf. (page 3) Retrieved 02/10.

265. Bowen, R. (Colorado State) 2003. http://www.vivo.colostate.edu/hbooks/pathphys/misc_topics/radicals.html. Retrieved 02/10.

266. Pon, Lisa A. and Schon, Eric A. Mitochondria, Volume 80, Second Edition (Methods in Cell Biology), Academic Press Publishing, 2007.

267. Halvorsen, B. L., et al. 2002. A systematic screening of total antioxidants in dietary plants. J Nutr 132:461–471.

268. Hu, J. et al. 2009. Dietary vitamin C, E, and carotenoid intake and risk of renal cell carcinoma. Cancer Causes Control 20(8):1451–1458.

269. Wong, G. Y. et al. 1997. Dose-ranging study of indole-3-carbinol for breast cancer prevention. J Cell Biochem Suppl 28–29:111–6.

270. Auvinen, M. et al. 1992. Ornithine decarboxylase activity is critical for cell transformation. Nature 360:355–358.

271. Mehta, K. et al. 1997. Antiproliferative effect of curcumin (diferuloylmethane) against human breast tumor cell lines. Anticancer Drugs 8(5):470–81.

272. Lamson, D. W. et al. 2000. Antioxidants and cancer, part 3: Quercetin. Altern Med Rev 5(3):196–208.

273. Hadley, C. W. et al. 2003. The consumption of processed tomato products enhances plasma lycopene concentrations in association with a reduced lipoprotein sensitivity to oxidative damage. Nutr 133:727–732.

274. Devaraj, S. et al. 3008. A dose-response study on the effects of purified lycopene supplementation on biomarkers of oxidative stress. J Am Coll Nutr 27(2):267–273.

275. Wintergerst. E. S. et al. 2006. Immune-enhancing role of vitamin C and zinc and effect on clinical conditions. Ann Nutr Metab 50(2):85–94.

276. Jacobs, E. J. et al. 2002. Vitamin C and vitamin E supplement use and bladder cancer mortality in a large cohort of us men and women. Am J Epidemiol 156:1002–1010.

277. Weitberg, A. B. et al. 1997. Effect of vitamin E and beta-carotene on DNA strand breakage induced by tobacco-specific nitrosamines and stimulated human phagocytes. J Exper & Clin Cancer Res 16(1):11–14.

278. Simbula, G. et al. 2007. Increased ROS generation and p53 activation in alpha-lipoic acid-induced apoptosis of hepatoma cells. Apoptosis 12(1):113–23.

279. Ma, Q. et al. 2007. L-arginine reduces cell proliferation and ornithine decarboxylase activity in patients with colorectal adenoma and adenocarcinoma. Clin Cancer Res 15;13(24):7407–12.

280. Saiko, P. et al. 2009. Avemar, a nontoxic fermented wheat germ extract, attenuates the growth of sensitive and 5-FdUrd/Ara-C cross-resistant H9 human lymphoma cells through induction of apoptosis. Oncol Rep 21(3):787–91.

281. Rhode, J. et al. 2007. Ginger inhibits cell growth and modulates angiogenic factors in ovarian cancer cells. BMC Complement Altern Med 20:7:44.

282. Ip, M. M. et al. 2003. Prevention of mammary cancer with conjugated linoleic acid: role of the stroma and the epithelium. J Mammary Gland Biol Neoplasia. 8(1):103–18.

283. Huang, D. et al. 2005. The Chemistry behind Antioxidant Capacity Assays. Journal of Agriculture and Food Chemisty. 53:1841–1856.

284. Cao, G. et al. 1998. Increases in human plasma antioxidant capacity after consumption of controlled diets high in fruit and vegetables 1–3. Am J Clin Nutr 68:1081–7.

285. Elevating Antioxidant Levels in Food through Organic Farming and Food Processing: An Organic Center State of Science Review. Charles M. Benbrook Ph.D. The Organic Center for Education and Promotion, 2005. http://www.organic-center.org/reportfiles/Antioxidant_SSR.pdf. Retrieved 02/10.

286. Ruch, R. et al. 1989. Prevention of cytotoxicity and inhibition of intercellular communication by antioxidant catechins isolated from Chinese green tea. Carcinogenesis 10:1003–1008.

287. Pillai, S. P. et al. 1999. J Environ Pathol Toxicol Oncol. Antimutagenic/antioxidant activity of green tea components and related compounds. 18(3):147–58.

288. Kurita, I. et al. 2010. Antihypertensive Effect of Benifuuki Tea Containing O-Methylated EGCG. J Agric Food Chem 58(3):1903–1908.

289. Yang, G. et al. 2007. Prospective cohort study of green tea consumption and colorectal cancer risk in women. Cancer Epidemiol Biomarkers Prev 16(6):1219–23.

290. Ui, A. et al. 2009. Green tea consumption and the risk of liver cancer in Japan: the Ohsaki Cohort study. Cancer Causes Control 20(10):1939–45.

291. Katiyar, S. et al. 2007. Green tea and skin cancer: photoimmunology, angiogenesis and DNA repair. J Nutr Biochem 18(5):287–96.

292. Can-Lan, S. et al. 2006. Green tea, black tea and breast cancer risk: a meta-analysis of epidemiological studies. Carcinogenesis 27(7):1310–5.

293. Yokoyama, S. et al. 2001. Inhibitory effect of epigallocatechin-gallate on brain tumor cell lines in vitro. Neuro Oncol 3(1):22–8.

294. Inoue, M. et al. 2009. Green tea consumption and gastric cancer in Japanese: a pooled analysis of six cohort studies. Gut 58(10):1323–32.

295. Friedman, M. 2007. Overview of antibacterial, antitoxin, antiviral, and antifungal activities of tea flavonoids and teas. Nutr Food Res 51:116–134.

296. Garbisa, S. et al. 2001. Tumor gelatinases and invasion inhibited by green tea flavanol epigallocatechin-3-gallate. Cancer 91:822–832.

297. Muto, S. et al. 2001. Inhibition by green tea catechins of metabolic activation of procarcinogens by human cytochrome P450. Mutat Res 479:197–206.

298. Kazi, A. et al. 2002. Inhibition of B.C.l-XL phosphorylation by tea polyphenols or epigallocatechin-3-gallate is associated with prostate cancer cell apoptosis. Molecular Pharmacology 62(4):765–771.

299. Smith, D. M. et al. 2001. Green tea polyphenol epigallocatechin inhibits DNA replication and consequently induces leukemia cell apoptosis. Int J Mol Med 7(6):645–52.

300. Cabrera, C. et al. 2006. Beneficial Effects of Green Tea—A review. J of the Amer College of Nutr 25(2):79–99.

301. Frei, B. et al. 2003. Antioxidant activity of tea polyphenols in vivo: evidence from animal studies. J Nutr 133(10):3275S–84S.

302. Stoner, G. et al. 2004. Polyphenols as cancer chemopreventive agents. J Cell Bioch 59(S22):169–180.

303. Leading Edge Antioxidants Research. Harold V. Panglossi, Editor. Nova Science Publishers, 2006.

304. Langley-Evans, S.C. et al. 2000. Antioxidant potential of green and black tea determined using the ferric reducing power (FRAP) assay. Int J Food Sci Nutr 51:181–188.

305. Benzie, I. F. et al. 1999. Consumption of green tea causes rapid increase in plasma antioxidant power in humans. Nutr Cancer 34:83–87.

306. Klaunig, J. et al. 1999. The effect of tea consumption on oxidative stress in smokers and nonsmokers. Proc Soc Exp Biol Med 220:249–254.

307. Maki, K. et al. 2009. Green tea catechin consumption enhances exercise-induced abdominal fat loss in overweight and obese adults. J Nutr 139(2):264–270.

308. Arab, L. et al. 2009. Green and black tea consumption and risk of stroke: A meta-analysis. Stroke 40:1786.

309. Venables, M. C. et al. 2008. Green tea extract ingestion, fat oxidation, and glucose tolerance in healthy humans. Am J Clin Nutr 87(3):778–84.

310. Mintel Market Research. http://www.mintel.com.

311. Freedonia Market Research. http://www.freedoniagroup.com.

312. Fahlberg, C. and Remsen, I. 1879. Ãœber die Oxydation des Orthotoluolsulfamids. Chemische Berichte 12:469–473.

313. Informational Hearing, "The Health Effects of Artificial Sweeteners," October 3, 2008. State Capitol, Room 126.

314. Reuber, M. D. et al. 1978. Carcinogenicity of saccharin. Environ Health Perspect 25:173–200.

315. Taylor, J. M. et al. 1980. Chronic toxicity and carcinogenicity to the urinary bladder of socium saccharin in the utero exposed rat. Toxicol Appl Pharmacol 54:57–75.

316. Squire, R. A. et al. 1985. Histopathological evaluation of rat urinary bladders from the IRDC two-generation bioassay of sodium saccharin. Food Chem Toxicol 23:491–497.

317. Soffritti, et al. 2006. First Experimental Demonstration of the Multipotential Carcinogenic Effects of Aspartame Administered in the Feed to Sprague-Dawley Rats. Environmental Health Perspectives 114(3).

318. Mead, N. N., 2006. Sour Finding on Popular Sweetener: Increased Cancer Incidence Associated with Low-Dose Aspartame Intake. Environ Health Perspect 114(3):A176.

319. Swithers, S. E. et al. 2008. A role for sweet taste: Calorie predictive relations in energy regulation by rats. Behavioral Neuroscience 122(1).

320. http://www.sucralose.com/About/Overview/Pages/Default.aspx. Retrieved 02/10.

321. Mercola, Joseph & Degen Pearsall, K. Sweet Deception: Why Splenda NutraSweet and the FDA May Be Hazardous to Your Health, Thomas Nelson Inc. Publishers, 2006.

322. Handbook of Food Analysis, Volume 2, Second Edition. Revised and Expanded Residues and other Food Component Analysis. Edited by Leo M. L. Nollet, Marcel Dekker, Inc., 2004.

323. Citizens for Health. The voice of the natural health consumer. http://www.citizens.org. Retrieved 02/10.

324. Dockets Management Branch, U.S. Food and Drug Administration. Citizens for Health (CFH) submits this petition pursuant to 21CFR10.30. April 3, 2006 James S. Turner, Esq. Chairman, Citizens for Health, c/o Swankin & Turner.

325. Panel on Dietary Reference Intakes for Electrolytes and Water, Standing Committee on the Scientific Evaluation of Dietary Reference Intakes. The National Academies Press, Washington, D. C., 2005.

326. EPA Office of Ground Water and Drinking Water (OGWDW), http://www.epa.gov/safewater/. Retrieved 01/09.

327. Stookey, J. D. et al, 1997. Letter to the Editor, Correspondence re: J. Shannon et. al, Relationship of food groups and water intake to colon cancer risk. Cancer Epidemiol, Biomarkers & Prev., 5:495–502. Cancer Epidemiol, Biomarkers & Prev 6:657–658.

328. Shannon, J. et al. 1996. Relationship of food groups and water intake to colon cancer risk. Cancer Epid Biom & Prev 5:495–502.

329. Michaud, D. S. et al. 1999. Fluid intake and the risk of bladder cancer in men. New Eng J Med 341:847–848.

330. Bitterman, W. A. et al. 1991.Environmental and nutritional factors significantly associated with cancer of the urinary tract in different ethnic groups. Urol Clin North Am 18:501–508.

331. Nweze Eunice Nnakwe, Community Nutrition Planning Health Promotion and Disease Prevention, Jones and Bartlett Publishers LLC, 2009.

332. Ivahnenko, T. et al. 2006. Sources and occurrence of chloroform and other trihalomethanes in drinking-water supply wells in the United States, 1986–2001: U.S. Geological Survey Scientific Investigations Report, 2006. 5015:13.

333. Cantor, K. P. et al. 1987. Bladder cancer, drinking water source, and tap water consumption: a case-control study. J Natl Cancer Inst 79(6):1269–79.

334. Environmental Protection Agency. http://www.epa.gov/safewater/ccl/index.html. Retrieved 02/10.

335. Rabin, R. et al. 2008. Public Health Then and Now. Amer J Public Health 98(9).

336. Thorton, J. 2002. Environmental impacts of polyvinyl chloride building materials. A Healthy Building Network Report. Washington, D. C. Retrieved 02/10.

337. Your Body's Many Cries For Water, Fereydoon Batmanghelidj, M.D., Global Health Solutions, Inc.; 3rd Ed. 2008.

CHAPTER 5: Mental Facets of Health

1. On Death and Dying, Elisabeth Kubler-Ross, Scribner, 1997.

2. http://www.authentichappiness.sas.upenn.edu/Default.aspx3. Retrieved 03/10.

3. Seligman, M. et al. 2004. A balanced psychology and a full life. Phil. Trans. R. Soc. London 359, 1379–1381.

4. Danner, D. D. et al. 2001. Positive emotions in early life and longevity: Findings from the Nun Study Journal of Personality and Social Psychology 80(5):804–813.

5. Segerstrom, S. C. et al. 1998. Optimism is associated with mood, coping, and immune change in response to stress. Journal of Personality and Social Psychology 74(6):1646–1655.

6. Shekelle, R. et al. 1981. Psychological depression and 17-year risk of death from cancer. Psychosomatic Medicine 43(2):117–125.

7. Irwin, M. et al. 2007. Depression and risk of cancer progression: An elusive link Michael R. Irwin *Journal of Clinical Oncology* 25(17):2343–2344.

8. Abbass, A. et al. 2002. The cost effectiveness of short-term dynamic psychotherapy. Journal of Pharmacoeconomics and Outcome Research 3:535–539.

9. Williams, S. et al. 2006. The effectiveness of treatment for depression/depressive symptoms in adults with cancer: a systematic review. Br J Cancer 13;94(3):372–90.

10. World Health Organization. http://www.who.org. Retrieved 03/10.

11. Report of the Surgeon General on Mental Health. http://www.surgeongeneral.gov/library/mentalhealth/pdfs/ExSummary-Final.pdf. Retrieved 01/09.

12. The Empowerment Partnership. (Neuro-liguistic Programming). http://www.nlp.com. Retrieved 01/09.

13. Montgomery, G. et al. 2007. A randomized clinical trial of a brief hypnosis intervention to control side effects in breast surgery patients. J Natl Cancer Inst 99(17):1304–12.

14. McRae, C. et al. 2004. Effects of perceived treatment on quality of life and medical outcomes in a double-blind placebo surgery trial. Arch Gen Psychiatry 61(4):412–20.

15. The Psychology of Winning, Denis Waitley, Berkley Press, 1986.

16. Brian Tracy's Website. http://www.briantracy.com. Retrieved 01/09.

17. Mischel, M. et al. 1989. Delay of gratification in children. Science 2(4):933–938.

18. Hom, H. L. Jr. et al. 1985. Low need achievers' performance. Personality & Social Psychology Bulletin 11(3):275–285.

19. The Mayo Clinic. http://www.mayoclinic.com/health/self-esteem/MH00129. Retrieved 03/10.

20. Imai, K. et al., 2001. Personality types, lifestyle, and sensitivity to mental stress in association with NK activity. Int'l J Hygiene & Env Health 204(1):67–73.

21. Falagas, M. et al. 2007. The effect of psychosocial factors on breast cancer outcome: A systematic review. Breast Cancer Research 9:R44.

22. Eysenck, H. et al. 1988. Personality, stress and cancer: Prediction and prophylaxis. Br I Med Psychol 61(Pt1):57–75.

23. Online Medical Dictionary. (http://www.online-medical-dictionary.org) Retrieved 03/10.

24. Mayo Clinic. 2009. Being assertive: Reduce stress and communicate better through assertiveness. http://http://www.mayoclinic.com/health/assertive/SR00042/NSECTIONGROUP=2. Retrieved 03/10.

25. Getting Well Again: A step-by-step, self-help guide to overcoming cancer. O. Carl Simonton, M.D., James Creighton, Ph.D. and Stephanie Matthews Simonton, Bantam Books, 1992.

26. Guided Imagery for Self-Healing, Martin Rossman, M.D. 2000. An H. J. Kramer Book, published in a joint venture with New World Library.

27. Eremin, O. et al. 2009. Immuno-modulatory effects of relaxation training and guided imagery in women with locally advanced breast cancer undergoing multimodality therapy: A randomised controlled trial. Breast. 18(1):17–25.

28. Fawzy, et al. 1990. A structured psychiatric intervention for cancer patients. I. Changer over time in methods of coping and affective disturbance. Arch Gen Psychiatry 47(8):720–5.

29. Benson, et al. 1988. Relaxation and imagery in the treatment of breast cancer. BMJ 297(6657):1169–72.

30. Guided Imagery Program at the Miller Family Heart & Vascular Institute at Cleveland Clinic http://my.clevelandclinic.org/heart/prevention/stress/guided_imagery.aspx. Retrieved 03/10.

31. Spiegel, D. et al. 1989. Effect of psychosocial treatment on survival of patients with metastatic breast cancer. Lancet 14(2):888–91.

32. Huth, M. M., et al. 2004. Imagery reduces children's post-operative pain. Pain 110(1–2):439–48.

33. Apóstolo, J. et al. 2009. The Effects of Guided Imagery on Comfort, Depression, Anxiety, and Stress of Psychiatric Inpatients with Depressive Disorders. Archives of Psychiatric Nursing 23(6):403–411.

34. National Cancer Institute, on the subject of depression. http://www.cancer.gov/cancertopics/pdq/supportivecare/depression/Patient/page2. Retrieved 03/10.

35. The Tibetan Book of Living and Dying, Sogyal Rinpoche, HarperCollins Publishers, Inc., New York, NY, 1992. Retrieved online at http://www.bibliotecapleyades.net/archivos_pdf/tibetanbook_livingdying.pdf, 03/10.

36. Meares, A. 1980. What can the cancer patient expect from intensive meditation? Aust Fam Physician 9(5):322–5.
37. Meares, Austin. 1977. Atavistic regression as a factor in the remission of cancer. Med J Aust 23;2(4):132–3.
38. Relief without Drugs: How You Can Overcome Tension, Anxiety and Pain. Ainslie Meares. Souvenir Press Ltd. 1994.
39. Austin, James. Zen and the Brain, MIT Press, 1999.
40. Borysenko, Joan. Minding the Body, Mending the Mind, Joan Borysenko, Bantam/Addison-Wesley Edition. 1987.
41. Benson, Herbert. The Relaxation Response, William Morrow and Company, 1975.
42. Benson, Herbert. Current Role Of Mind-Body Techniques In Wellness And Medical Care. http://www.integratedmeditation.com/docs/mind%20body%20in%20modern%20medicine.pdf. Retrieved 03/10.
43. Dusek, J. et al. 2008. Genomic counter-stress changes induced by the relaxation response. PLoS One 2;3(7):e2576.
44. Sharma, H. 2008. Gene expression profiling in practitioners of Sudarshan Kriya. J Psychosom Res. 64(2):213–8.
45. Lazar, S. W. et al. 2005. Meditation experience is associated with increased cortical thickness. Neuroreport 16(17):1893–1897.
46. Schneider, R. H. et al. 2005. Long-term Effects of Stress Reduction on Mortality in Persons >55 Years of Age With Systemic Hypertension. Am J Cardiol 95:1060–1064.
47. The Art of Spiritual Healing, Joel S. Goldsmith, HarperOne Publishers, 1992.
48. The Infinite Way, Joel S. Goldsmith, DeVorss Publications, 34th printing, 2006.
49. Spirituality: Living Our Connectedness, Margaret Burkhardt and Mary Gail Nagai-Jacobsen, Delmar Thomson Learning, Inc., 2002.
50. Berk, L. S. et al. 2001. Neuroendrocrine and stress hormone changes during mirthful laughter. Am J Med Sci 298(6):390–39.
51. Berk, L. S. et al. 2001. Modulation of neuroimmune parameters during the eustress of humor-associated mirthful laughter. Altern Ther Health Med 7(2):62–76).
52. A Life in Balance: Nourishing the Four Roots of True Happiness, Kathleen Hall, Amacom Publishing, 2006.
53. Huron, D. 2004. Auditory-Evoked Laughter: The Role of Expectation. Cognitive and Systematic Musicology Laboratory, School of Music & Center for Cognitive Science, Ohio State University. http://musiccog.ohio-state.edu/Huron/Talks/2004/Stanford/abstract.html. Retrieved 03/10.
54. Anatomy of an Illness as Perceived by the Patient: Reflections on Healing and Regeneration, Norman Cousins, W. W. Norton and Company, Inc, 1979.
55. Creating Humor: Life Studies of Comedy Writers, William F. Fry and Melanie Allen, Transaction Publishers, 1998.
56. The Cancer Treatment Centers of America (CTCA). http://www.cancercenter.com. Retrieved 03/10.
57. Nainis, N. et al. 2008. Approaches to Art Therapy for Cancer Inpatients: Research and Practice Considerations Journal of the Amer Art Ther Assoc 25(3):115–121.
58. Mandala: Luminous Symbols for Healing, 2nd Edition, Judith Cornell, 10th Anniversary Edition, Quest Books, 2006.
59. The Mandala Healing Kit, Using Sacred Symbols for Spiritual and Emotional Healin, Judith Cornell, Sounds True, Inc., 2006.
60. Burns, S. J. et al. 2001. A pilot study into the therapeutic effects of music therapy at a cancer help center. Altern Ther Health Med 7(1):48–56.
61. Cassileth, B. R. et al. 2003. Music therapy for mood disturbance during hospitalization for autologous stem cell transplantation: A randomized controlled trial. Cancer 98:2723–2729.
62. Bulfone, T. et al. 2009. Effectiveness of music therapy for anxiety reduction in women with breast cancer in chemotherapy treatment. Holist Nurs Pract 2009;23(4):238–42.
63. Barrera, M. E. et al. 2002. The effects of interactive music therapy on hospitalized children with cancer: A pilot study. Psychooncology 11:379–388.
64. Appendix to The Principia: Mathematical Principles of Natural Philosophy, Isaac Newton (circ. 1685). Published for the first time as an appendix to the 2nd (1713) edition of the Principia, the General Scholium reappeared in the 3rd (1726) edition with some amendments and additions. Retrieved 03/10.

65. Strawbridge, W. J. et al. 1997. Frequent attendance at religious services and mortality over 28 years. Am J Public Health 87(6):957–61.
66. Sephton, S. E. et al. 2001. Spiritual expression and immune status in women with metastatic breast cancer: an exploratory study. Breast J 7(5):345–53.
67. Thinking Outside The Box. http://www.sangraal.com/library/outside_the_box.htm. San Graal School of Sacred Geometry, Grassy Branch Loop, Sevierville, Tennessee. Retrieved 03/10.
68. A New Earth: Awakening To Your Life's Purpose, Eckhart Tolle, Penguin, 2005.
69. The Power of Intention, Wayne W. Dyer, Hay House; 1st Ed., 2005.

CHAPTER 6: Complementary and Alternative Medicines (CAM)

1. National Center for Complementary and Alternative Medicine. http://nccam.nih.gov/. Retrieved 03/10.
2. National Center for Complementary and Alternative Medicine. http://nccam.nih.gov/news/camstats/2007/camsurvey_fsl.htm#intro. Retrieved 03/10.
3. National Center for Complementary and Alternative Medicine. http://nccam.nih.gov/about/offices/od/directortestimony/0308.htm. Retrieved 03/10.
4. Ernst, E. 2000. The role of complementary and alternative medicine. BMJ 4; 321(7269): 1133–1135.
5. The Academic Consortium for Complementary and Alternative Health Care. http://www.accahc.org/. Retrieved 03/10.
6. 2002 National Health Interview Survey, National Center for Health Statistics (NCHS). http://nccam.nih.gov/health/acupuncture/introduction.htm. Retrieved 03/10.
7. Harris, R. E. et al. 2009. Traditional Chinese acupuncture and placebo (sham) acupuncture are differentiated by their effects on μ-opioid receptors (MORs). NeuroImage 47(3):1077–1085.
8. International Journal of Essential Oil Therapeutics. http://www.ijeot.com/. Retrieved 03/10.
9. National Center for Complementary and Alternative Medicine. http://nccam.nih.gov/health/ayurveda/introduction.htm. Retrieved 03/10.
10. National Center for Complementary and Alternative Medicine. http://nccam.nih.gov/health/chiropractic. Retrieved 03/10.
11. American Holistic Nurses Association. http://www.ahna.org/. Retrieved 03/10.
12. American Dietetic Association. http://www.eatright.org. Retrieved 03/10.
13. American Society for Nutrition. http://www.nutrition.org/. Retrieved 03/10.
14. British Nutrition Foundation. http://www.nutrition.org.uk/aboutbnf/values/who-we-are-what-we-do. Retrieved 03/10.
15. American Physical Therapy Association. http://www.apta.org. Retrieved from Bureau of Labor Statistics at http://www.bls.gov/oco/ocos080.htm. Retrieved 03/10.
16. Cassileth, B. R. et al. 2004. Massage therapy for symptom control: outcome study at a major cancer center. J Pain Symptom Manage 28(3):244–9.
17. Forchuk, C. et al. 2004. Postoperative arm massage: a support for women with lymph node dissection. Cancer Nurs 27(1):25–33.
18. Data compiled by the American Massage Therapy Association (AMTA), 2008. http://AMTAmassage.org/news/MTIndustryfactsheet.html.
19. Dr. Bernard Jensen's Guide to Better Bowel Care: A Complete Program for Tissue Cleansing Through Bowel Management ,Avery Trade; Revised edition, 1998.
20. Gut Wisdom:Understanding and Improving Your Intestinal Health, Alyce M. Sorokie, Career Press, Inc. 2008.
21. International Association for Colon Hydrotherapy (I-ACT). http://www.i-act.org/. Retrieved 12/08.
22. National Qigong Association. http://www.nqa.org . Retrieved 03/10.
23. National Center for Complementary and Alternative Medicine. http://nccam.nih.gov/. Retrieved 03/10.
24. The Herb Society. http://www.herbsociety.org. Retrieved 03/10.
25. Physicians Desk Reference (PDR), Thomson Healthcare, new editions yearly.
26. Physicians Desk Reference (PDR) for Herbal Medicine, 4th Edition. David Heber. Physicians Desk Reference, 2007.

27. Shah, S., et al. 2007. Evaluation of echinacea for the prevention and treatment of the common cold: A meta-analysis. Lancet 7(7):473–480.

28. Farnsworth, N. R. et al. 2001. The Value of Plants Used in Traditional Medicine for Drug Discovery. Environ Health Perspect 109(1):69–75.

29. National Institutes of Health. http://nccam.nih.gov/health/homeopathy/. Retrieved 03/10.

30. Association for Applied Psychophysiology and Biofeedback. http://www.AAPB.org. Retrieved 03/10.

31. Disease Control Priorities Project, June 2007. http://www.dcp2.org/file/5/DCPP-RiskFactors.pdf. Retrieved 03/10.

32. WHO Traditional Medicine Strategy 2002–2005. http://whqlibdoc.who.int/hq/2002/WHO_EDM_TRM_2002.1.pdf. Retrieved 03/10.

33. World Health Organization Fact Sheet: Traditional Medicine, No. 134. December 2008. http://www.who.int/mediacentre/factsheets/fs134/en/. Retrieved 03/10.

34. Disease Control Priorities Project. 2007. Complementary and Alternative Medicine may reduce risk of some diseases. http://www.dcp2.org/file/93/DCPP-CAM.pdf. Retrieved 03/10.

35. McLean T. W. et al. 2006. Complementary biochemical therapies in pediatric oncology. J Soc Integr Oncol 4(2):93–9.

36. Herman, P. et al. 2005. Is complementary and alternative medicine (CAM) cost-effective? A systematic review. BMC Complement Altern Med 5:11.

37. Spontaneous Healing: How to Discover and Embrace Your Body's Natural Ability, Andrew Weil, M.D. Random House Inc. 1995.

CHAPTER 7: Social Wellbeing

1. Author unknown, as quoted in The Heart Speaks: A Cardiologist Reveals the Secret Language of Healing, Mimi Guarneri, Touchstone, 2006.

2. National Association of Social Workers. http://www.naswdc.org/pressroom/features/general/profession.asp. Retrieved 04/10.

3. United States Department of Labor. http://www.bls.gov/oco/ocos060.htm. Retrieved 04/10.

4. National Cancer Institute. http://spores.nci.nih.gov/. Retrieved 04/10.

5. The American Cancer Society's National Cancer Information Center (NCIC) is a nationwide 1-800 help line. http://ww3.cancer.org/docroot/ESN/content/ESN_3_1X_ACS_National_Cancer_Information_Center.asp. Retrieved 09/10.

6. Association of Oncology Social Workers. http://www.aosw.org. Retrieved 04/10.

7. University of Michigan Comprehensive Cancer Center. Voices Art Gallery. http://www.cancer.med.umich.edu/support/voices_art_gallery.shtml. Retrieved 04/10.

8. Many Voices. "Words of Hope for People Recovering from Trauma & Dissociation, PTSD, DID, MPD, DSM-IV, multiple-personality." http://www.manyvoicespress.com. Retrieved 04/10.

9. Lutgendorf, S. K., et al. 2001. Quality of life and mood in women with gynecologic cancer: A one-year prospective study. Cancer 94(1):131–140.

10. Turner-Cobb, J. M. et al. 2000. Social support and salivary cortisol in women with metastatic breast cancer. Psychosom Med 62(3):337–45.

11. Kroenke, C. et al. 2006. Social networks, social support, and survival after breast cancer diagnosis. Journal of Clinical Oncology 24(7):1105–1111.

12. Psycho-Oncology, 2nd Edition, Jimmie C. Holland. Oxford University Press, 2010.

13. Shelby, R. et al. 2008. Optimism, social support and adjustment of African American women with breast cancer. Journal of Behavioral Medicine 31(5):433–444.

14. Wolf S. N. et al. 2005. Survivorship: An unmet need of the patient with cancer—implications of a survey of the Lance Armstrong Foundation. Journal of Clinical Oncology, ASCO Annual Meeting Proceedings. 23(16S):6032. As referenced at http://www.cancernetwork.com/survivorship/content/article/10165/1374232?verify=0. Retrieved 04/10.

15. Cancer Care for the Whole Patient: Meeting Psychosocial Health Needs, N. E. Adler and A. E. K. Page eds, National Academies Press, Washington, D.C., 2008. As referenced by http://www.cancernetwork.com/survivorship/content/article/10165/1374232?verify=0. Retrieved 04/10.

16. From Cancer Patient to Cancer Survivor: Lost in Transition, 2005. Committee on Cancer Survivorship: Improving Care and Quality of Life (Author), Institute of Medicine and National Research Council (Author), Maria Hewitt (Editor), Sheldon Greenfield (Editor), Ellen Stovall (Editor), National Academies Press; 1st edition.
17. American Cancer Society. http://www.acs.org. Retrieved 04/10.
18. National Cancer Institute. http://www.nci.org. Retrieved 04/10.
19. I Can Cope. Cancer support. http://www.cancer.org/docroot/ESN/content/ESN_3_1X_I_Can_Cope.asp?sitearea=SHR.
20. Oncochat. Cancer support. http://www.oncochat.org.
21. Cancer Support Community. Cancer Support. http://wpad.thewellnesscommunity.org/default.aspx. Retrieved 04/10.
22. Cancer Survivors Network. Cancer support. http://www.csn.cancer.org.
23. Gilda's Club. Cancer support. http://www.gildasclub.org.
24. American Brain Tumor Association. Cancer support. http://www.abta.org.
25. American Cancer Society, Man To Man Program. Cancer support. http://www.cancer.org/docroot/ESN/content/ESN_3_1X_Man_to_Man_36.asp.
26. American Cancer Society. http://www.lookgoodfeelbetter.org/general/facts.htm.
27. Reach to Recovery. http://www.cancer.org/docroot/ESN/content/ESN_3_1x_Reach_to_Recovery_5.asp
28. Colorectal Cancer Coalition. http//:fightcolorectalcancer.org.
29. Cancer Care Inc. http://www.cancercare.org.
30. Candlelighters Childhood Cancer Foundation. http://www.candlelighters.org.
31. Cancer Hope Network. http://www.cancerhopenetwork.org/.
32. Network of Strength http://www.networkofstrength.org/support/caring/husbands.php.
33. Susan G. Komen For The Cure. http://www.komen.org.
34. The Lance Armstrong Foundation. http://www.livestrong.org.
35. Lung Cancer Alliance http://www.lungcanceralliance.org/about/about.html.
36. The National Coalition for Cancer Survivorship. http://www.canceradvocacy.org/about.
37. Pink-Link. http://www.pink-link.org.
38. R. A. Bloch Cancer Foundation. http://www.blochcancer.org/about.
39. American Therapeutic Recreation Association. http://www.atra-tr.org.
40. United States Department of Labor. http://bls.gov/oco/ocos082.htm. Retrieved 04/10.
41. Centers for Disease Control and Prevention. http://www.cdc.gov/nccdphp/sgr/disab.htm. Retrieved 04/10.
42. United States Department of Labor. http://www.bls.gov/oco/ocos326.htm. Retrieved 04/10.
43. McIllmurray, M. B., et al. 2003. Psychosocial needs in cancer patients related to religious belief. Palliat Med 17(1):49–54.
44. Feher, S., et al. 1999. Coping with breast cancer in later life: the role of religious faith. Psychooncology 8(5):408–16.
45. Hobbies are Rich in Psychic Rewards, Eilene Zimmerman. New York Times. December 2, 2007. http://www.nytimes.com/2007/12/02/jobs/02career.html?_r=2&oref=slogin. Retrieved 04/10.
46. Creating Health: How to Wake up the Body's Intelligence, Deepak Chopra, Mariner Books, 1995.
47. Project Healing Waters Fly Fishing Inc. http://www.projecthealingwaters.org/.
48. Mediations and Devotions of the Late Cardinal Newman, 3rd Edition, Longmans, Green and Company, New York and London, 1903.
49. Anderson, W. P. et al. 1992. Pet ownership and risk factors for cardiovascular disease. Med J Aust 157(5):298–301.
50. Sandel, S. L., et al. 2005. Dance and movement program improves quality-of-life measures in breast cancer survivors. Cancer Nurs 28(4):301–9.

CHAPTER 8: Lifestyle

1. National Institutes of Health. http://www.nhlbisupport.com/bmi. Retrieved 04/10.
2. Toniolo, P. et al. 2000. Serum insulin-like growth factor-1 and breast cancer. Int. J. Cancer 88:828–832.
3. Hamelers, I. H. L. et al. 2003. Interactions between estrogen and insulin-like growth factor signaling pathways in human breast tumor cells. Endocrine-Related Cancer 10:331–345.
4. Stattin, P. et al. 2000. Plasma insulin-like growth factor-I, insulin-like growth factor-binding proteins, and prostate cancer risk: a prospective study. J Natl Cancer Inst 92(23):1910–7.
5. Giovannucci, E. et al. 2000. A prospective study of plasma insulin-like growth factor-1 and binding protein-3 and risk of colorectal neoplasia in women. Cancer Epidemiol Biomarkers Prev (4):345–9.
6. Brokaw, J. et al. 2007. IGF-I in epithelial ovarian cancer and its role in disease progression. Growth Factors 25(5):346–354.
7. Gable, K. L., et al. 2006. Diarylureas are small-molecule inhibitors of insulin-like growth factor I receptor signaling and breast cancer cell growth. Mol Cancer Ther 5(4):1079–86.
8. Michels, K. B. et al. 2004. Caloric Restriction and Incidence of Breast Cancer. JAMA. 2004;291:1226–1230.
9. Li, Y. et al. 2009. Glucose restriction can extend normal cell lifespan and impair precancerous cell growth through epigenetic control of hTERT and p16 expression. (Epub ahead of print.) FASEB Journal:DOI: 10.1096/fj.09–149328.
10. Morita, H. et al. 2005. Only two-week smoking cessation improves platelet aggregability and intraplatelet redox imbalance of long-term smokers. Journal of the American College of Cardiology 45(4):589–594.
11. National Cancer Institute. http://www.cancer.gov/cancertopics/smoking. Retrieved 12/09.
12. American Cancer Society. http://www.cancer.org/docroot/PED/content/PED_1_3X_Infectious_Agents_and_Cancer.asp.
13. National Cancer Institute. http://www.cancer.gov/cancertopics/factsheet/Risk/HPV. Retrieved 04/10.
14. Centers for Disease Control. http://www.cdc.gov/hepatitis. Retrieved 12/09.
15. Kassem, A. et al. 2008. Frequent detection of Merkel cell polyomavirus in human Merkel cell carcinomas and identification of a unique deletion in the VP1 gene. Cancer Res 68(13):5009–13.
16. Ornish, D. et al. 2005. Intensive lifestyle changes may affect the progression of prostate cancer. Journal of Urology 174(3):1065–1070.
17. Calafat, A. M., et al. 2007. Serum concentrations of 11 polyfluoroalkyl compounds in the U.S. population: Data from the National Health and Nutrition Examination Survey (NHANES) 1999–2000. Environ Sci Technol 41(7):2237–2242.
18. Environmental Protection Agency. http://www.epagov/oppt/pfoa. Retrieved 12/09.
19. Spinning Straw into Gold: Your Emotional Recovery from Breast Cancer, Ronnie Kaye, Lampost Press, Inc., 1991.

CHAPTER 9: Food for Thought (no references)

Addenum 1

Answer to "Thinking Outside The Box"

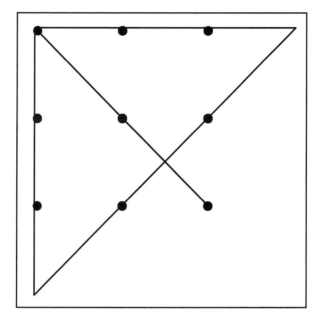

About the Author

Taking an active role in health and finding answers based on his own journey of having cancer has been important to Dr. Doug Levine since the age of 19. What he has learned is that it was not only the surgical, radiation, and chemotherapy treatments for Hodgkin's disease that he underwent, but the subsequent incorporation of significant lifestyle changes that have allowed him to experience the most dramatic and long-lasting results. Now over 30 years recovered, Dr. Levine continues to dedicate his life's work to increasing awareness relative to general health and cancer prevention.

Dr. Levine has a Bachelor's degree in Natural Science and Mathematics and a Master of Science in Nutrition. He has been a practicing chiropractor in Bergenfield, New Jersey for over 25 years. Dr. Levine is a guest speaker for the American Cancer Society and Cancer Care, where he provides groundbreaking presentations on cancer prevention and complementary medicine.

It is Dr. Levine's steadfast goal to educate and create public awareness about the importance of natural strategies—not only for lowering the risk of getting cancer, but for preventing it altogether. Please visit Dr. Levine's website for news and updates at *www.drdouglevine.com.*